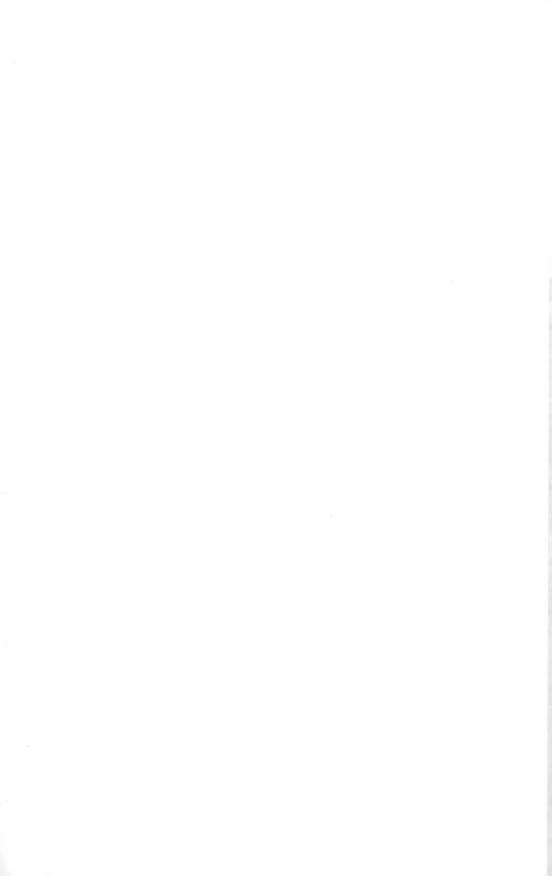

Global Health and International Community

Science Ethics and Society

GENERAL EDITORS: **Professors John Sulston and John Harris**
(respectively Chair and Director of the Institute for Science,
Ethics and Innovation (iSEI) at the University of Manchester)

In conjunction with the Institute for Science, Ethics and Innovation, this series examines the major issues surrounding the impact of science and technology and the ethical issues generated by new discoveries.

Books in the series highlight the interplay between science and society; new technological and scientific discoveries; how they impact on our understanding of ourselves and our place in society; and the responsibility of science to the wider world.

Themes covered in the series include:

- Global justice
- The scope, limits and future of humanity
- Public health
- Technological governance
- Intellectual property
- Chronic poverty
- Climate change
- Environment

The series will appeal to policy-makers, academic readers and students in diverse disciplines including sociology, international relations, law, bioethics, physical and life sciences and medicine.

Books already published in the series:
International Governance of Biotechnology Needs, Problems and Potential
Catherine Rhodes
ISBN 9781849660655 (Hardback)
ISBN 9781849660778 (Ebook)

Scientific Freedom
Edited by Simona Giordano, John Coggon and Marco Cappato
ISBN 9781849668996 (Hardback)
ISBN 9781849669016 (Ebook)

Families—Beyond the Nuclear Ideal
Edited by Daniela Cutas and Sarah Chan
9781780930107 (Hardback)
9781780930121 (Ebook)

Forthcoming:
Bioscience and the Good Life
Iain Brassington
ISBN 9781849663380 (Hardback)
ISBN 9781849663397 (Ebook)

Humans and Other Animals: Challenging the Boundaries of Humanity
Sarah Chan
ISBN 9781780932187 (Hardback)
ISBN 9781780932545 (Ebook)

Global Health and International Community

Ethical, Political and Regulatory Challenges

Edited by

John Coggon

Swati Gola

B L O O M S B U R Y

LONDON • NEW DELHI • NEW YORK • SYDNEY

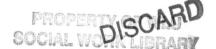

Bloomsbury Academic
An imprint of Bloomsbury Publishing Plc

50 Bedford Square
London
WC1B 3DP
UK

1385 Broadway
New York
NY 10018
USA

www.bloomsbury.com

Bloomsbury is a registered trademark of Bloomsbury Publishing Plc

First published 2013

British Library Cataloguing-in-Publication Data
A catalogue record for this book is available from the British Library.

ISBN: HB: 978-1-7809-3397-9
ePub: 978-1-7809-3559-1
ePDF: 978-1-7809-3558-4

Library of Congress Cataloging-in-Publication Data
A catalog record for this book is available from the Library of Congress.

Typeset by Newgen Knowledge Works (P) Ltd., Chennai, India
Printed and bound in Great Britain

For Margot Brazier, John Harris and Søren Holm:
My three mentors in Manchester

–JC

For parents and family for their unflinching support

–SG

Contents

Contributors

Richard Ashcroft is Professor of Bioethics at Queen Mary, University of London, where he teaches in the School of Law. He has worked in the medical schools of Queen Mary, Imperial College London and Bristol University, and in the philosophy department of Liverpool University. He trained in history and philosophy of science at Cambridge University. He has been Deputy Editor of the Journal of Medical Ethics, and is currently a member of the Tobacco Advisory Group of the Royal College of Physicians and of the Ethics of Research and Public Involvement Committee of the Medical Research Council. He is co-Director of the Centre for the Study of Incentives in Health, funded by the Wellcome Trust.

Solomon R. Benatar MBChB, DSc (Med) is Emeritus Professor of Medicine, Founding Director of the University of Cape Town's Bioethics Centre, and Professor in the Dalla Lana School of Public Health and Joint Centre for Bioethics, University of Toronto. Previously he was Professor of Medicine University of Cape Town and Chief Physician Groote Schuur Hospital (1980–2007), Vice-President, College of Medicine of South Africa (1989–95) and President of the International Association of Bioethics (2001–3). His academic interests and publications have included respiratory medicine, academic freedom, bioethics, human rights, health care systems, health economics and global health – on which topics he has published over 300 journal articles and book chapters. *Global Health and Global Health Ethics* (Editors Solomon Benatar and Gillian Brock) was published by Cambridge University Press in 2011. Some other recent publications include: Benatar S. R., Gill S. and Bakker I. C., 'Global health and the global economic crisis', *American Journal of Public Health* 2011; Nixon S. E. and Benatar S. R. A., 'Critical Public Health Ethics: Analysis of Canada's International Response to HIV', *Global Public Health* 2011; Benatar S. R., 'Global Leadership, Ethics and Global Health: The Search for New Paradigms', in Gill S. *The Global Crisis and the Crisis of Global Leadership,* CUP 2011; and Benatar S. R., Daar A. and Singer P. A., 'Global Health Ethics: The Rationale for Mutual Caring', *International Affairs,* 2003; 79: 107–38. Professor Benatar is an elected Foreign Associate Member of the US National Academy of Sciences' Institute of Medicine (1989); Honorary Fellow of the American College of Physicians (1993); Honorary Foreign Member of the American Academy of Arts and Sciences (1996); Fellow of the Royal Society of South Africa (1997); Fellow, Hastings Center (2004); Fellow, Faculty of Medicine, Imperial College London (2005).

John Coggon is Reader in Law in the School of Law, University of Southampton, United Kingdom. His research examines legal, moral and political theory, particularly in regard to human health and welfare. The main focus of his work is on public health broadly conceived, exploring questions concerning the source, scope and limits of the State's role in securing people's welfare, and the basis and extent of individual and social responsibility for doing so. He is also interested in global health; especially questions concerning the limits to transnational obligations for human welfare. He is the author of *What Makes Health Public?* (Cambridge: Cambridge University Press, 2012). With A. M. Viens and Anthony Kessel he is editor of *Criminal Law, Philosophy and Public Health Practice*, (Cambridge: Cambridge University Press, forthcoming) and with Simona Giordano and Marco Cappato, *Scientific Freedom*, (London: Bloomsbury Academic, 2012).

Malcolm Dando trained originally as a biologist (BSc and PhD at St Andrews). Since the early 1990s his research at Bradford University has focused on the problem of strengthening the Biological and Toxin Weapons Convention as concerns have increased about the advances in the life sciences potentially facilitating bioterrorism. His publications include co-editing *Deadly Cultures: Biological Weapons Since 1945*, Harvard University Press, 2006. Most recently he was part of the Royal Society Working Group that produced *Brain Waves Module 3: Neuroscience, Conflict, and Security*, 2012.

Thomas Gebauer is Executive Director of *medico international*, a Frankfurt-based social–medical relief and human rights organization. He received a diploma in psychology from the University of Frankfurt. Since 1979 he has been involved in advocacy and international campaigning on global health. In 1991 he co-founded the Nobel Peace Prize winning 'International Campaign to Ban Landmines'. He is member of the Steering Committee of the 'Joint Action and Learning Initiative' promoting the idea of a 'Framework Convention on Global Health'.

Swati Gola qualified as an advocate in India and did her first LLM in disabilities rights. She worked as a Policy Researcher with a Civil Society Organisation that worked for the empowerment of rural and tribal communities and for national laws and policies supportive of food and livelihood security. She then came to the United Kingdom and did her second LLM in International Trade Law and thereafter qualified to become a solicitor in England and Wales and practised in the area of criminal and prison law. She has now joined the University of Manchester as a Graduate Research Assistant and PhD Candidate. The focus of her research is to analyze and assess the impact of the international trade in hospital services on the right to health in developing countries. The research essentially looks into the right to health as a legal concept, that is as a fundamental right recognized, advocated and established under international law, as well as a social phenomenon, examining its importance in any given state, for economic, cultural and social growth, and identifying if and how the trade in health services impacts the exercise of the right to health in terms of accessibility, affordability and equity.

Lawrence O. Gostin is University Professor (Georgetown's highest academic rank) and Director of the O'Neill Institute for National and Global Health Law at Georgetown University Law Center. He also has academic appointments at the Johns Hopkins University, the University of Oxford, the University of Sydney and the University of the Witwatersrand, South Africa. The United Nations Secretary General endorsed his proposal for a Framework Convention on Global Health. He has two books by the University of California Press: *Public Health Law: Power, Duty, Restraint* (2nd edn, 2008) and *Public Health Law and Ethics: A Reader* (2nd edn, 2010). His book, *Global Health Law: International Law, Global Institutions, and World Health* will be published by Harvard University Press in 2013.

Rachel Hammonds JD is a researcher in the Public Health Department at the Institute of Tropical Medicine (Antwerp, Belgium) and a member of the Law and Development Research Group at the Law Faculty of the University of Antwerp. She studied law at the University of Ottawa and Edinburgh University and is a New York State licenced attorney. Her work focuses on the intersection of development policy, health and human rights.

Stephen R. Latham JD, PhD is Director of Yale University's Interdisciplinary Center for Bioethics. A graduate of Harvard College and Harvard Law School, Latham was a healthcare regulatory attorney prior to earning his doctorate from the UC Berkeley program in Jurisprudence and Social Policy. Latham served as Director of Ethics Standards at the American Medical Association before entering academia full time. He is a former graduate fellow of Harvard's Safra Center on Ethics and a former Research Fellow of the University of Edinburgh's Institute for Advanced Studies in the Humanities. He has served on Connecticut's Stem Cell Research Advisory Committee and on the board of the American Society for Bioethics and Humanities. His writings on health law, professionalism and bioethics have appeared in numerous peer-reviewed journals, law reviews and edited university-press books.

Lisbeth Witthøfft Nielsen, MA in Theology (cand.theol.) is a Research Associate at the Centre for Biomedical Ethics, Yong Loo Lin School of Medicine, National University of Singapore. In 2008 she finished a research project on the ethics of sustainability and the barriers to climate awareness. The project was carried out at the Centre for Ethics and Law and funded by the

Ministry of Climate and Energy, Copenhagen. Lisbeth's publications include the book Klimabevidsthedens barrierer, Tiderne skifter, 2009; and The Barriers to Climate Awareness – a Report on the Ethics of Sustainability, published by the Danish Ministry of Climate and Energy, 2009 (both with Peter Kemp). She was previously a project manager at the Centre for Ethics in Medicine, University of Bristol, United Kingdom (2006–7) on the project, ENHANCE, Enhancing Human Capacities: Ethics, Regulation and European Policy (2005–7), a European Commission funded project under the Sixth Framework Programme.

William Onzivu is a Lecturer in Law (tenured) at Bradford University Law School at the University of Bradford in the United Kingdom. He teaches environmental law, public law, international law, legal skills and law of contracts. He has prepared a Global Health Law module for the Law School's forthcoming LLM in Healthcare Law. He researches and writes in the areas of Global Health Law, Environmental Law and Regulation and Public International Law including their role in the promotion and protection of health. His recent published works include: '(Re) invigorating the World Health Organization's Governance of Health Rights: Repositing an evolving legal regime, its challenges and prospects,' *African Journal of Legal Studies* (2011) 4:3, 225–56; 'Health in Global Climate Change Law: The Long Road to an Effective Legal Regime Protecting Public Health and the Climate,' *Carbon and Climate Law Review*, (2010) 4, 364–82; and 'Eco-Patent Commons: Implications for Technology Transfer to Fight Climate Change in Developing Countries,' *Carbon and Climate Law Review*, (2010), 1, 13 (with Mark Van Hoorebek).

Gorik Ooms is a researcher in public health at the Institute of Tropical Medicine (Antwerp, Belgium), and adjunct professor of law at Georgetown University (Washington DC, United States). Trained as a lawyer with a special interest in human rights, Dr Ooms worked with Médecins Sans Frontières (Doctor without Borders) Belgium during many years, and as executive director from 2004 to 2008. He was appointed Global Justice Fellow at Yale University for the 2009–10 academic year. His work draws on human rights law, public health, philosophy and macroeconomics, but most importantly on the real-life struggle for essential social rights for all.

Sadie Regmi is studying for a degree in medicine at the University of Manchester. She is UK Coordinator of Universities Allied for Essential Medicines (UAEM), which aims to maximize global access to public health goods, and promote research into Neglected Tropical Diseases (NTDs). University students involved with UAEM from around the world are working to change the way universities commercialize drugs and other medical technologies. In 2011, Sadie co-founded the Manchester NTD Society, and has since been involved in research into NTDs. She works as a research assistant at the Institute for Science, Ethics and Innovation, where she has been involved in research on a variety of issues such as the ethics of interventions in sub-Saharan Africa, organ donation ethics, issues of ageism and equality and intellectual property rights and alternative ways of incentivizing innovation.

Catherine Rhodes is a Research Fellow in Science Ethics at the Institute for Science, Ethics and Innovation, University of Manchester. Bloomsbury Academic published her book *International Governance of Biotechnology: Need, Problems and Potential* in 2010. Catherine's research explores how science is governed internationally, and current projects focus on governance of genetic resources, the effects of increased patenting on academic research, and cooperation between international organizations on issues of common concern.

Doris Schroeder is Director of the Centre for Professional Ethics at the University of Central Lancashire, Preston, United Kingdom and Professorial Fellow at the Centre for Applied Philosophy and Public Ethics at the University of Melbourne, Australia. Her main areas of interest are global justice, human rights and health, benefit sharing and dignity. Her most recent book is a co-edited collection: 'Indigenous Peoples, Consent and Benefit Sharing— Learning Lessons from the San-Hoodia Case,' (2009) Springer, Berlin.

Keith Syrett is Professor of Public Health Law at Cardiff University, Wales, United Kingdom. His work focuses primarily upon the role for legal and regulatory mechanisms in addressing issues of public health, particularly in the context of climate change and access to scarce healthcare resources. He is the author of Law, Legitimacy and the Rationing of Health Care: a Contextual and Comparative Perspective (Cambridge: Cambridge University Press, 2007) and Foundations of Public Law: Principles and Problems of Power in the British Constitution (Basingstoke: Palgrave Macmillan, 2011). Professor Syrett is the founder of the Worldwide Universities Network Global Health Justice initiative (www.wun.ac.uk/research/ghjnetwork) and is Secretary of the British Association for Canadian Studies.

Peter West-Oram is an AHRC-funded PhD Candidate at the University of Birmingham. In 2011 he was awarded an AHRC-Kluge Center Fellowship to conduct research at the Library of Congress in Washington DC where he worked on issues relating to global justice and infectious disease. His doctoral research focuses on issues of health care, human rights and global justice, with an emphasis on duties to provide aid. He is currently working on a paper criticizing the commoditization of health care and essential medicines.

Heather Widdows is a well-known international researcher. In 2005 she was awarded a visiting fellowship at Harvard University, where she worked on issues of moral neo-colonialism. She has led a number of funded projects on issues of property in the body, reproductive rights, human tissue, war on terror and ownership and governance of the genome. Heather serves as a member of the UK Biobank Ethics and Governance Council and is also on the REF Philosophy Sub-Panel. Her recent publications include: *Global Ethics: An Introduction,* Durham: Acumen, 2011; *Global Social Justice*, Edited with Nicola Smith, Abingdon: Routledge, 2011; and *The Governance of Genetic Information: Who Decides?* Edited with Caroline Mullen, Cambridge: Cambridge University Press, 2009.

James Wilson is Lecturer in Philosophy and Health at University College, London. He has published widely in bioethics and in applied philosophy, specializing in public health ethics, the philosophy of intellectual property, resource allocation and research ethics. He is co-chair of the International Association of Bioethics' Philosophy and Bioethics Network. In 2011–12 Dr Wilson was seconded to the Royal Society, as co-lead of the Science as a Public Enterprise study. Open access versions of his papers are archived at http://discovery.ucl.ac.uk/view/people/JGSWI10.date.html.

Acknowledgements

We have produced this book following a meeting on 'Global Health, Global Goods, and International Community', hosted by the University of Manchester's Institute for Science, Ethics and Innovation (iSEI) in June 2011. We are very grateful for the support of iSEI and the Wellcome Strategic Programme on The Human Body, its Scope, Limits and Future. We would like too to thank Catherine Spanswick and Sam Walker for ensuring the conference, and the preparations for it, ran so smoothly. We are also grateful to iSEI for placing on its website podcasts of the conference papers, and the video and transcript of Lawrence Gostin's keynote lecture, which preceded the conference.[1] Along with this book, which is also available open access, we are delighted to see so many useful academic resources on Global Health made free to find at the touch of a button.

We are very pleased to thank all of the contributors to this volume for their chapters. The project is an ambitious one, and we have been lucky to draw together such a diverse authorship, combining people whose work proves impressively complementary. The span of chapters gives rise to a powerful conversation across and beyond academic disciplines. Earlier versions of most of the chapters were presented at the Manchester meeting. We thank their authors both for the care and attention given to preparing the chapters, and for making the Manchester meeting itself such a success. It was fantastic that these people came together and gave so generously of their time and energy. We would like individually to thank the authors of two further invited contributions. Richard Ashcroft was generous enough to produce a philosophical analysis of inequalities and health, whose importance we felt was foundational in a book such as this. And we are delighted that Lisbeth Nielsen allowed us to include her chapter on climate change and genetically modified organisms, which she originally presented at another iSEI conference, on 'Greening Humanity: Science, innovation, ethics and the green economy'.

The generosity of those who have contributed to this work serves as a mark of the importance of its subject matter. We are thankful to everyone who helped it to reach its completion, and hope that it will prove useful in developing understandings of how we should address some of the most complex questions that face humanity.

---

1 All available through: www.isei.manchester.ac.uk/research/conferences/globalhealth/.

Introduction:

Global Health and International Community

John Coggon and Swati Gola

Introduction

Global health arguably represents the most pressing issues facing humanity. Trends in international migration and transnational commerce render State boundaries increasingly porous. Human activity in one part of the world can lead to health impacts elsewhere. And animals, viruses and bacteria, as well as pandemics and environmental disasters, clearly do not recognize or respect political borders. Both in policy and the Academy, public health is rapidly growing as a source of specific and directed concern. It is widely accepted that a global perspective is needed if we are to understand fully the nature of threats to health and how best to respond to them. And such a perspective simultaneously draws into question matters of justice, fairness and equity. While theories of morality tend to appeal to concepts of universality, global politics presents a gross imbalance in freedoms, rights, capabilities, duties and entitlements.

University curricula, researchers, pressure groups and policy bodies are therefore now assuming a keen focus on questions in public and global health, and seeking to identify and address a broad range of problems. With this book, we aim to provide a foundational text accessible to readers from across disciplines, and from outside of the university system, concerned with these issues. The book contains essays by internationally leading experts. Its balanced combination of critical analysis and practically focused policy pieces will make it, we hope, a valuable and enduring resource for researchers, students, activists and policy-makers across the globe. The multi-disciplinarity of the contributors, covering areas such as ethics, human rights, international relations, law, philosophy and politics, is underwritten by many of the contributors' practical experience in national and international policy. The book thereby adds positively to a literature that is of central and growing importance. This introductory chapter allows us to provide an outline of the book's contents, and to explain the structure that we have adopted.

The book's structure

We have separated the book's chapters into three parts. Broadly, these reflect three distinctive ways of coming to debates on global health: first, we have chapters exploring 'big picture' philosophical questions; second, questions relating to specific moral and regulatory problems in global health; and third, large-scale regulatory responses to global health governance. The divisions necessarily involve a level of artificiality, and readers might, of course, read the chapters in an alternative order. Nevertheless, we hope to have given the work a logical progression. While the chapters were each written independently of one another, we do see a flow throughout the work. We outline here how and why we have structured the book as we have.

Part One – framing global ethics and international justice

Part One addresses philosophical concerns and questions about how, as a matter of ethics or justice, we should approach and frame an analysis of global health. Given the stark self-evidence (to many minds) of current global injustices, some might question what role at all a moral theorist has in a work on global health: are the moral problems, it might be asked, not just obvious? While we have some sympathy with this view, we think it misses various crucial questions whose import spreads far beyond debates that might take place in the 'ivory tower'. Nevertheless, we agree that it is important to question properly what value moral theorizing lends to debates in global health. As such, the five chapters in Part One explore various theoretical challenges. Understanding both the role and limits of theory is crucial to making sound use of principled arguments. Without coherent principles on which to base moral imperatives, we lack the understanding needed to support coherent claims about how we and our governments should perceive our responsibilities and then choose to act. While on the face of things protagonists in global health might appeal to apparent widespread agreement about global injustices, it is not far below the surface that radical differences present themselves. Furthermore, we cannot ignore that there are nuanced philosophical arguments that (more or less) support the global *status quo*,[1] and their practical strength is reinforced by contemporary international political practices. Therefore, those who seek large-scale change – policy-makers, activists and students alike – must be able to speak to and refute the arguments that they would reject, and present a persuasive position in favour of reform.

---

1 Most notably, John Rawls, *The Law of Peoples* (Cambridge, MA: Harvard University Press, 2001).

Consequently, we begin Part One with two chapters that challenge the idea that 'global health ethics' or 'global health justice' present straightforwardly compelling ideals. Neither chapter is given to undermining the agendas or ends of global health activism, but each gives reason to consider carefully the moral basis – the *reasons* – for wanting to advocate for change. In other words, each asks us to be sure about what our fundamental concern is: is it *health*, is it at base something else, or is it health *among other things*. Furthermore, Chapter 1, by Stephen Latham, questions the very value of theory in debates on global health justice; he presents and examines problems for *any* theory of global health justice. Latham's arguments provide a constructive but challenging position. If we argue that health is what motivates our concerns in justice, might that not undermine rather than reinforce what we really mean by moral respect? For example, when arguing about women's reproductive autonomy, should this not be something that is directly due morally, rather than something we value because it is good for women's health? And does a similar point not stand in relation to arguments in favour of education, peace, job opportunities and so on? Arguments based on 'health justice' seem to ask us to value these things not in themselves, but because – and insofar as – they are good for health. Latham also urges us to recognize the complex nature of the world itself, and the resultant limits to theories' explanatory value. He notes the importance of being clear about whom the theory would address, of accounting for a theory's demandingness and of dealing with conflicts of value. Furthermore, he asks, in the context of practical debates on global health, what value should be given to a theory of global (health) justice. Is it really concerns for justice that motivate actors in global health, or would it be wiser to appeal to potentially more motivating reasons, such as prudence?

Chapter 1, then, presents an important and complex challenge to moral theorists working in global health, and to those who appeal to theory. In Chapter 2, Richard Ashcroft further adds to the challenge by interrogating the question of global health inequalities. It is common in arguments concerning global health to find appeals to health inequalities, both internationally and within nation States. While these seem of themselves to present an injustice, Ashcroft asks whether it is health inequalities themselves that are fundamental to concerns about global injustice, or whether they are rather indicators of the actual injustices that (should) concern us. Ashcroft unpacks several distinct lines of argument. These include the problems of being clear about what we mean when discussing 'health' or saying that someone's health is bad, and on deciding how we define the groups that we will compare with one another. He argues that when comparing in justice two groups, we will be building an analysis on *status inequality* rather than *health inequality*. At the root of an injustice that we would seek to remediate, he suggests, is an unmet need rather than simply a health inequality. Injustices give rise to claims for corrective action in the form of redistribution of resources, and health is not something that can be redistributed in the relevant sense. We help someone who is in ill health because of a basic need; not because someone else is healthy at the cost of that person's health. In short, Ashcroft's argument is that resolving the conceptual difficulties implicated in claims about health inequalities requires a great deal of prior normative analysis about matters such as what we are measuring when we say we are measuring health, what we are comparing and which groups we are comparing. He agrees that health inequalities signal injustice and need, but his paper presents a strong argument that the *moral* concern is not ultimately with health inequalities themselves.

It is with Chapters 1 and 2 in mind, therefore, that we label Part One 'Framing Global Ethics and International Justice', rather than make explicit mention of health. Both chapters seem to suggest that those who are concerned about using moral theory should perhaps make their focal concern global justice, rather than global *health* justice. Against the backdrop that these chapters provide, it is instructive to read the remaining three chapters of Part One. Chapter 3, by Heather Widdows and Peter West-Oram, provides a positive argument for why (bio)ethics must be considered as a global endeavour. Although their practical focus is on health, their claims could clearly have a wider application, rather than be reduced to a theory of global health justice in the sense criticized by Latham or Ashcroft. In essence, their argument is that as medical and scientific problems are global, and as medical and scientific practices are global, ignoring their global nature will lead to injustice. These points allow that many questions will also be local rather than global. Likewise, their argument is about ethics; they are not advancing a case for global homogenization or standardization of health *policies*. Rather, the ethics of the framework within which health policies are developed must account for their global reach. Having made the case for (bio)ethics being global, Widdows and West-Oram finally note three characteristics that they find across arguments in global ethics: the frame is global, the approach is multidisciplinary, and it combines theory and practice. Rather than reduce ethics either to individuals' obligations or the justice of institutions, they argue that both of these must be addressed.

Solomon Benatar's approach, in Chapter 4, reinforces Widdows' and West-Oram's argument by demonstrating the three characteristics that they describe: a global frame; a concern for multidisciplinarity; and a concern for combining theory and practice. Benatar's chapter presents stark facts both about inter- and intranational inequalities in health. He then usefully considers various ways in which the term 'global health' is used before arguing in favour of his preferred definition. For Benatar, global health should be thought of like public health, when the latter is seen as a mission aimed at eradicating or lessening disease.[2] Following a short history of public health efforts, Benatar

---

2 See the parallels with the influential definition of public health in C.-E. A. Winslow, 'The Untilled Fields of Public Health', (1920) *Science* 51:1306, 23–33, 30.

places the late 1970s as a turning point at which neo-liberal economics took hold, to the advantage of a global minority and to the detriment of the global majority. The minority's 'distorted values', such as hyper-individualism, short-termism and restricted concepts of rights are the root, Benatar argues, of unjust global disparities. He goes on, therefore, to consider how the position might be ameliorated. To do so, he provides 11 'moral lenses' through which to view international obligations to improve health globally: historical, social justice, self-interest and security, ecological, human rights, needs, solidarity, finite resources, moral global economy, international professional standards, and global crises. Benatar's message is strong and urgent: the *status quo* is unjust and unsustainable, addressing the problem is a matter for scholars from across disciplines.

Chapter 5, the final chapter in Part One, is by Gorik Ooms and Rachel Hammonds. Ooms and Hammonds note that to say that global inequalities are inequities requires a theory of global justice. They also recognize that there are principled arguments that hold that the nation State is special and thus gives rise to special obligations that do not obtain internationally. They note too that such a position can be argued to reflect practical reality. Their chapter, however, aims to weaken the claims for finding that ethical obligations end with national boundaries. They do so by taking to task the influential work of John Rawls who, as noted above, purports to defend a means of limiting the more demanding obligations in justice to bounded political communities, rather than allow them a global scope. In questioning the coherence of Rawls' theory in this regard, Ooms and Hammonds draw from the claims that Rawls makes in relation to justice within a single State.[3] The demands of justice can limit what individuals should be free to do, and the same should hold, they argue, internationally. Furthermore, in their conception global justice is not simply about the rights and duties held between States, but at base is about individuals' rights and duties, held across national boundaries. Beyond even questions of principle, Ooms and Hammonds argue convincingly about people's global connectedness; that it is implausible to claim that the world's population comprises different people living in completely separate, isolated and self-contained systems of cooperation. Rather, there are many layers of cooperation. While they accept that political reality means that complete global justice is out of reach, there is scope for increased justice as global cooperation intensifies. Included in their argument here is the case for a global social justice scheme. With a firm basis in concerns for global justice, and with due account given to practical and political reality, this proposal presents a fascinating practical note on which to end Part One.

---

3   See John Rawls, *A Theory of Justice. Revised Edition* (Cambridge, MA: The Belknap Press of the Harvard University Press, 1999).

Part Two – practical challenges in global health governance

In Part Two, the book's focus moves to various specific problems that feature large in debates on global health. We do not aim, or pretend, to provide anything nearing an exhaustive span of problems in global health, or of scholarly approaches to responding to them. Nevertheless, the points of focus are representative of the scale and nature of the problems in global health, and both in themselves and by implication point to the sorts of considerations that need to be raised in seeking to address them. The chapters present perspectives from a broad range of approaches: law, philosophy and ethics, economics and regulation, international governance and international security. The problems studied are diverse, though overlaps also emerge between the chapters, which cover: climate change; sustainability policies based on the use of genetically modified organisms; access to essential medicines; access to antibiotics and 'ownership' of their effectiveness; international governance of biotechnologies; and controlling threats to global health in the form of bioterrorism and State offensive biological weapons programmes. In combination, the chapters demonstrate the breadth of ground and range of analyses relevant to global health.

Keith Syrett, in Chapter 6, examines the potential utility of human rights adjudication – specifically that based on the human right to health – in response to climate change. Climate change, as Syrett notes, has clear implications for populations globally, and furthermore will affect disproportionately people who are already relatively disadvantaged. While, he argues, climate change may bar the *realization* of human rights, including the right to health, for adjudication the important question is whether there has been a *breach* of these rights in a strict, legal sense. Reflecting on the work of the Office of the High Commissioner for Human Rights (OHCHR) on this question, Syrett notes several potential problems: attributing responsibility, causation, and the presence or immediacy of a rights violation. Furthermore, he notes the complexities of establishing who could litigate, problems of legal standing and questions of whether the right to health is justiciable. Even in the face of these problems, Syrett suggests that we should not give up on securing accountability through judicial or quasi-judicial mechanisms. Instead, he develops an argument in favour of a wider concept of accountability than that taken by the OHCHR, drawing from contemporary analyses of judicial approaches to socioeconomic rights, with particular reference to those protected under South Africa's constitution. Courts' decisions on this view, noting that they are given wide publicity, serve as a 'catalyst for further public dialogue'. In this sense, the judicial process may be viewed as part of a wider system of accountability and deliberative democracy, meaning that even when litigants fail in their legal case, the case itself potentially advances their cause. As such, we move beyond adjudication being seen as a zero-sum game, to a productive and ongoing democratic discourse. Syrett's view is certainly not that such an approach would form the only strategy for effecting political change, but he is clear that it serves well as a means of supplementing such efforts.

Chapter 7, by Lisbeth Nielsen, also begins with reference to the effects of climate change and the challenges it raises. Nielsen's focus is on possible scientific responses to food shortages and sustainability, through the development and use of genetically modified organisms. Her analysis leads to a focus both on ethics and regulation. Again, her argument is advanced as part of a wider possible response to a practical problem. Her position is framed against a context, particularly within the European Union, of scepticism about genetic modification. Nielsen argues that the ethics of sustainability can be seen as being based on three responsibilities to compensate. First, there is corrective justice, which requires actors to compensate for harms that they have caused, and to correct negative trends through mitigation practices. Second, there is a shared responsibility to avoid further harm to vulnerable populations, which Nielsen characterizes as being comparable to the Rawlsian 'difference principle'. Finally, there is the responsibility to protect nature, a term that she argues should be taken to include the atmosphere. In order to overcome scepticism of genetically modified organisms, Nielsen addresses ethical concerns about 'the unnatural', noting among other things that these are driven by context, and that overall, given the fact of anthropogenic climate change, we may ultimately need anyway to alter the natural to save the natural. Her chapter goes on to provide a detailed account of the matters that those contemplating introducing genetically modified organisms should bring into an all things considered evaluation. It is clear too that public support is needed, both through funding and coordination of practices. While the institution of measures will be made locally, Nielsen insists that a global outlook is needed.

Sadie Regmi's focus in Chapter 8 is on another problem that is at the fore in many debates within global health: the question of access to essential medicines. As Regmi notes, millions of people die avoidably every year from diseases for which treatments exist but which, to those people, are unaffordable. Regmi describes the regulatory regime surrounding intellectual property, which is the main cause of the high price of medicines: rather than production costs, the prices are largely due to monopoly rights. Unaffordability of medicines itself logically affects those with fewer resources, compounding global inequities. But a further effect, given economic incentives, is that the global burden of disease is not reflected in research spending priorities, which are driven to respond to the problems of the world's richest people, thus further heightening inequalities. Against the justice-based concerns for global health to which this situation gives rise, Regmi's chapter evaluates intellectual property regimes, with a view to understanding whether global health outcomes are optimized within the current system. Regmi argues that we can find two presumptions underpinning justifications for current intellectual property regulation: first, it incentivizes innovation; and second, the effects on innovation outweigh any public health concerns that would speak against protecting monopoly rights. There is, she suggests, reason to doubt these premises. And given the failure of the current system to meet the healthcare needs of so many people in low- and middle-income countries, she explores possible alternatives. First she considers public–private partnerships. Then she looks at the idea of a health impact fund, as famously advocated by Thomas Pogge.[4] Although Regmi favours this approach, she acknowledges that as richer countries would be the greater contributors, politics may get in the way of it overcoming all equity-based concerns. Finally, she considers arguments for the development of a Medical Research and Development Treaty. Her overall conclusion is clear: a rethink is needed on how we protect intellectual property rights, whose drawbacks within the current system are too great to make the system defensible.

In Chapter 9, James Wilson's focus is also on access to treatments. However, the subject of his chapter is narrower than that of Regmi's. Wilson's essay considers the problem of antibiotic resistance. The discovery of antibiotics has revolutionized medicine. However, as any particular antibiotic becomes ineffective, there are especial questions of justice that give reason to doubt the appropriateness of the current intellectual property regime. Wilson notes three principal, complementary strategies that may be employed to control antibiotic resistance: first, limit their use by ensuring they are prescribed only where they will be effective; second, consider opportunity costs when prescribing, so even if their potential efficacy is not in doubt, accept that overall not prescribing may be more sensible in a given case; and third, replace the available antibiotics as they lose their effectiveness. Wilson notes that at present replacement happens more slowly than expiration of existing antibiotics. As such, he frames a convincing argument that we should conceive of an antibiotic's effectiveness as a limited resource, such as oil or coal. The time-limited nature of their effectiveness distinguishes antibiotics, and thus gives us reason to doubt whether they are subject to the general arguments that we find made in favour of granting a patent. The public interest arguments that would support granting time-limited monopolies to innovators, in order to incentivize innovation, make sense, Wilson argues, because then a public benefit is secured. In the case of effective treatment by antibiotics, however, this is not true because effectiveness will not be ongoing. He therefore contends that there cannot be a moral entitlement to 'own' antibiotic effectiveness. Rather, such effectiveness 'remains the common property of humanity', and should be subject to public controls.

Catherine Rhodes, in Chapter 10, looks more widely at the potential for biotechnologies to fulfil global health needs. Her analysis is framed through consideration of international governance, examining what could be done in the ideal to maximize benefits, manage risks, minimize harms and promote

---

4   See www.yale.edu/macmillan/igh/.

capacity building. She looks then at shortcomings in the current approach to international governance of biotechnologies. Finally, her chapter provides an argument for what could be done given the wider realities of the international system. Rhodes notes two distinct complicating matters. First, a significant upshot of advances in biotechnological innovation is the entrenchment of global inequalities. Second, health regulation is substantially intertwined with other areas of regulation. In echo of Widdows' and West-Oram's chapter, Rhodes points out that the global nature of biotechnology is born of its impact on inequalities, and in the way one country's policy may have effects beyond its borders (thinking, for example, about the possible effects of a country allowing xenotransplantation). States are interdependent, and there are clear areas where international cooperation is needed. In regard to biotechnology, Rhodes lists the following areas wherein international interdependence is high: arms control, development, drugs control, environmental protection, health, social impacts of genetics, and trade. In the governance of biotechnology, there are three strands of regulation that are of particular relevance: disease control, laboratory biosafety and biosecurity, and food safety. Having evaluated both areas where we can find signs of progress and key obstacles to progress, Rhodes considers the problem that States tend to assess national interest in economic terms, with a view on short-term gain rather than long-term welfare improvements.

The final chapter of Part Two, Chapter 11, by Malcolm Dando, examines an area of key importance in global health, albeit one that often receives less attention than it arguably should do. Dando divides threats to global health into three: those coming from natural disease; those coming from accidental disease; and those coming from deliberately caused disease by use of biological and chemical agents. While there are many discussions of public health measures to respond to the first type of threat, and of biosafety measures in regard to the second, Dando works to draw attention to the third. Knowledge and understanding of risks of deliberately caused disease, be it by bioterrorism or a State's biological weapons programme, are of key importance in global health. Dando therefore draws attention to international prohibitions found in the Biological and Toxin Weapons Convention (BTWC) and the Chemical Weapons Convention. His concern in the chapter is that properly to implement the BTWC, it is necessary to ensure that life scientists have a good awareness of the Convention's norms. Without this, they will not be able to assure due oversight to overcome the problem of misuses of technologies, or even to know what activities contravene the Convention. Dando presents strong evidence that internationally the scientific community is greatly under-informed on these matters, and in the main that life-scientists do not consider themselves as creating a significant risk of their work contributing to a biological or chemical weapons programme. Dando outlines how he and his colleagues have responded to this gap in education for life scientists, and reflects on the problem and the development of their response to it. The programme they have designed, of which he presents an overview in the chapter, is not intended to prevent scientific advances or limit scientific freedom, but rather is to guard against misuse of science, preventing only exceptionally dangerous research and publication.

Part Three – political and regulatory responses in global health

With a view to bringing us almost 'full circle', Part Three again focuses on 'big picture' challenges, this time in the development of large-scale political and regulatory responses to global health problems. The final four chapters of the book contain analyses of particular problems, and are also heavily influenced by concerns from ethical theory. We collect them separately, however, because they also offer broader-ranging practical approaches than those considered in Part Two. The scales of the problems they seek to address demonstrate clearly the ambition required for a practical exercise in global health. Nevertheless, by articulating how global governance for health can work, they offer good reason to think that the challenges of global health are not *over*-ambitious and that they should be taken seriously. A research agenda has been set, and Chapters 12–15 suggest practical means of responding to it.

Chapter 12, by Doris Schroeder, bridges well Parts Two and Three. Schroeder's chapter focuses on what must be the most famous and politically effective single measure in global health: the human right to health. The work that theorists and activists ask this right to do is quite staggering, and we can only imagine that its presence in academic and public debates will increase over the coming decades. As already seen in Syrett's chapter, the potential of the right expands well beyond questions of its justiciability, or its successful use in litigation. Nevertheless, by purporting to articulate grounded, enforceable rights, the right to health is neither reducible to an abstract moral requirement, nor to a political slogan. Thus, while Schroeder gives her chapter practical focus by using the case study of access to life-saving medicines, her analysis is of much broader relevance. The chapter explores the important question of whose obligation is triggered by the right to health, considering its potential implications for governments, rich individuals, non-governmental organisations (NGOs) and pharmaceutical companies. With regard to governments, the argument seems straightforward: where they have signed up to the right to health, they have assumed definite duties under the right to health. Affluent, private individuals are in a different position. They are able to ameliorate the positions of people who are worse off than them. Furthermore, many distinct philosophical theories can support claims about strong duties to help others.

Nevertheless, Schroeder argues, these duties are not necessarily to protect those things that would be guarded by the right to health; *that* specific right is not only not enforceable in a legal sense, but also one that is harder to ground even in a moral sense (Schroeder makes the point by reference to Kant's idea of 'imperfect duties'). Still, she notes, moral arguments can be made against affluent individuals, as they have been by Pogge. Moving to NGOs, Schroeder is clear that their obligations are voluntarily assumed and charity-based. Thus, while they assume a role in addressing matters that would fall under the right to health, they do not do so as a matter of obligation in the relevant sense. Schroeder argues that pharmaceutical companies, however, are arguably subject to obligations under the right to health. Her argument is based on how such companies benefit, in a unique way, from the intellectual property regime, in goods that are necessary to benefit basic human needs.

Thomas Gebauer begins Chapter 13 by stressing that global health is not just about controlling pandemics or making structural or managerial improvements; it is a call to reconceive responsibility for health in a globalized world. Drawing from the World Health Organisation (WHO)'s famous aspiration of 'Health for All', Gebauer works towards an analysis of global health responsibilities, considering both ethical and practical concerns. The problem with achieving the ideal of health for all is not, he suggests, insufficient money; it is rather the need for better redistribution of existing wealth. This, of course, means a need too for a change in political will and public pressure. In echo of Benatar's chapter, Gebauer laments the neo-liberal promise of a regime that would benefit everyone; under neo-liberalism, inequalities have grown. In bringing a practical focus to his arguments, Gebauer emphasizes two big problems in global health: theses on the social determinants of health; and questions concerning the provision of universal healthcare. He acknowledges the importance of the former, but focuses the practical aspects of his arguments on the latter. His position can be summarized by noting his agreement with the observation that poverty fuels ill-health, and ill-health poverty. Given this, Gebauer argues, healthcare cannot sensibly be linked to individual purchasing power. He therefore frames an argument around five requirements: the need to challenge neoliberal ideology; health governance reform; the need to reduce out of pocket payments for healthcare; the need to create pooled funds; and the need to build the system on the principle of solidarity. Whether the healthcare system is financed through general taxation or a social health insurance scheme, Gebauer insists that solidarity is key. Arguing along lines advocated by Ooms and Hammonds, Gebauer pushes for a global system for redistributing wealth. He draws a normative basis for doing so from the Universal Declaration on Human Rights, and practical inspiration from the longstanding cooperation found in the equalization payment mechanism in the Universal Postal Union. He argues that a treaty, such as that advocated for in Lawrence Gostin's chapter, is needed to assure an International Fund for Health. His arguments would thus reframe global health commitments to ones based in entitlement rather than charity.

In Chapter 14, William Onzivu demonstrates the scale of the challenge of global governance for health. Globalization has altered the spread of health threats, both through infectious and non-infectious diseases. And at the same time, the complexity of global health governance, which involves a vast array of actors including States, international organizations, and other non-state actors, presents a huge challenge in terms of shaping governance. In the face of this situation, Onzivu's argument is that 'adaptive governance' offers a good solution. He outlines the nature of adaptive governance, describing how it originates from complexity theory. Its strength comes in its being adaptable, flexible and responsive. To demonstrate how, Onzivu focuses on and explores five features of adaptive governance: continuous learning; policy making as experimentation; avoiding irreversible harm, monitoring and feedback; and pluralism and process. He then considers the role of adaptive governance within the context of WHO law. The need for flexibility demonstrated by the WHO's constitution, and the complexity of its governance, reinforce Onzivu's arguments for adaptive governance. As well as describing the array of different actors implicated in global health governance, he applies his arguments in the context of the WHO Framework Convention on Tobacco Control, and the International Health Regulations. He ends the chapter by addressing the benefits and problems of adaptive governance. Positively, it facilitates policy experimentation, promotes global health co-regulation and promotes implementation of WHO law and policy. However, there are concerns about its potential to undermine WHO law's binding nature, about regulatory capture and about robbing global health law of its 'public' character. For Onzivu, these problems are not compelling, and he advocates for the use of an adaptive governance framework.

The book's closing chapter, by Lawrence Gostin, details the project of developing a Framework Convention on Global Health. In Gostin's own summary, 'My proposal for a Framework Convention in a nutshell is to establish fair terms of international cooperation, with agreed-upon mutually binding obligations to create enduring health system capacities, meet basic survival needs and reduce unconscionable inequalities in global health.' The chapter is a valuable resource for scholars and activists alike, considering both our reasons for wanting to develop such a Convention, and the principles that it would enshrine. Gostin is clear that when international assistance is conceived as 'aid' we undermine the strong arguments that health is a shared responsibility internationally; as such, he characterizes global governance for health as a 'partnership', based on common goals. As a matter of justice, he argues, we can found obligations to protect health globally. In his framing, this is best explained by reference to a theory of human functioning, with health as a foundational human capacity. He also notes that States might be persuaded of the importance of global health by reference to national interests. However, he argues, recognizing health inequalities as a problem does not of itself tell us where we find the duties to respond to the problem. In Gostin's assessment, globally we need to act just as nation States (should) do to protect the health of their own citizens. That is, in addressing major determinants of ill health, by providing, for example, sanitation and sewerage, clean air and water and healthcare, the international community could meet its responsibilities to ameliorate global health. In working toward this, law has an important role to play to galvanize responsibilities and offer much-needed coordination. Gostin sees it best provided through a Framework Convention on Global Health, drawing inspiration from international environmental treaties that are also founded on the idea of shared responsibility, shared resources and the need for international cooperation. He outlines the proposed Convention's principles, and highlights its strengths, which would be ethical, practical and political. Gostin recognizes that problems will remain that the Convention could not overcome, given, for example, entrenched economic interests of powerful global actors. He also notes the risks of adopting a strategy of developing such a Convention, but argues that all things considered it is worth pursuing. His closing message is to remind us of the cost of failing to agree on fair terms of cooperation between States in relation to the enormous problems of global health.

Global health: Intellectual and practical challenges

The chapters collected in this volume add to the growing literature on the vast but important range of matters implicated in a study of global health, from theoretical and political concerns, through practical questions, to matters of law and governance.[5] It is common in texts on these issues, as has been the case in this introduction, to find multiple references to 'challenges'. Global

---

5   Our hope is that the volume complements and sits well alongside other works in this growing area, including: Wolfgang Hein and Lars Kohlmorgen (eds), *Globalisation, Global Health Governance and National Health Politics in Developing Countries – An Exploration into the Dynamics of Interfaces* (Hamburg: DÜI, 2003); Sudhir Anand, Fabienne Peter, Amartya Sen (eds), *Public Health, Ethics, and Equity* (Oxford: Oxford University Press, 2004); Belinda Bennett and George F. Tomossy (eds), *Globalization and Health: Challenges for Health Law and Bioethics* (Springer, 2006); Andrew F. Cooper, John J. Kirton, and Ted Schrecker (eds), *Governing Global Health: Challenge, Response, Innovation* (Ashgate, 2007); Michael Boylan (ed), International Public Health Policy and Ethics (Springer, 2008); Robert Beaglehole and Ruth Bonita (eds), Global Public Health – A New Era (2nd edn) (Oxford: Oxford University Press, 2009); Michael J. Selgelid and Thomas Pogge, *Health Rights* (Ashgate, 2010); Richard Parker and Marni Sommer (eds), *Routledge Handbook in Global Public Health* (New York: Routledge, 2011); Michael Boylan (ed), *The Morality and Global Justice Reader* (Westview Press, 2011); Solomon Benatar and Gillian Brock (eds), *Global Health and Global Health Ethics* (Cambridge: Cambridge University Press, 2011).

health does indeed present enormous challenges. Many projects are given to responding to them, and we are pleased to point interested readers to some of the impressive single-authored book-length treatments of questions in global health from ethics, philosophy and governance perspectives.[6] The challenges of global health – both intellectual and practical – are enormous, but we should draw inspiration from the contributors to this book. The subject demands attention and true communication between scholars, activists, citizens and policy-makers. The urgency of the questions raised cannot be overstated, and their resolution requires a substantive, informed, respectful discourse.

6   While not at all comprehensive, we would here single out: David Fidler, *International Law and Public Health* (Ardsley, NY: Transnational Publishers, 2000); Peter Singer, *One World: The Ethics of Globalization* (New Haven, CT: Yale University Press, 2004); Norman Daniels, *Just Health: Meeting Health Needs Fairly* (Cambridge: Cambridge University Press, 2008); Thomas Pogge, *World Poverty and Human Rights – Second Edition* (Cambridge: Polity, 2008); Amartya Sen, *The Idea of Justice* (London: Penguin, 2009); Thomas Pogge, *Politics as Usual* (Cambridge: Polity, 2010); Michael Boylan, *Morality and Global Justice: Justifications and Applications* (Westview Press, 2011); Heather Widdows, *Global Ethics: An Introduction* (Acumen Publishing, 2011); Jonathan Wolff, *The Human Right to Health* (New York, NY: W. W. Norton & Company, 2012); Lawrence O. Gostin, *Global Health Law: International Law, Global Institutions, and World Health* (Cambridge, MA: Harvard University Press, forthcoming).

PART ONE

Framing Global Ethics and International Justice

1

On Some Difficulties for Any Theory of Global Health Justice

Stephen R. Latham

[Moral philosophy] has received more over-general and
over-simplified systematization, while inviting it less, than virtually
any other part of philosophy.

Bernard Williams[1]

In theory, theory and practice are the same, but in practice, they're not

Yogi Berra

Introduction

In this chapter, I shall raise a number of different objections to the enterprise
of creating any theory of global health justice. Some of these objections are
simply applications to the global health justice arena of familiar objections to
ethical theory-making in general, some are specific to the problems of theory-
making about global health in particular. Different theories of global health
justice can deal, to some extent, with some of the objections; but none, I think,
can overcome them all.

Of course, one can't get very far with a critique of ethical theory without
offering some definition of what it is that one is critiquing. Not every abstract
discussion of matters ethical counts as the creation of an ethical theory, after
all, and a large amount of such abstract discussion is tremendously useful.
I mean here only to raise objections to a certain ambitious form of theorizing
about global health justice: the form in which the theory, minimally, purports
to explain most of our well-considered views about health justice by means
of some fairly simple machinery which, when applied to new cases, can guide
our judgements about justice and the steps we should take to establish it. I take
theories of justice to be a particular variety of ethical theory. I take my view of
'ambitious' theory to be fairly straightforward, and to apply not only to rationalist
and universalist ethical theories such as Utilitarianism and Kantianism, but also to

1 Bernard A. O. Williams, *Morality: An Introduction to Ethics* (Cambridge: Cambridge
University Press, 1972), xx.

coherentist and historicist theories such as one might arrive at by way of a process of reflective equilibrium. Any plausible theory of justice will explain most of our well-considered views on the subject; if it did not, it would not be a plausible theory. Its explanation will come by means of some fairly simple machinery (a social contract mechanism, a utility calculation, a specification of a few basic and coherent principles). Complex and comprehensive descriptions of moral life such as one might encounter in a novel or a work of social history are therefore not theories. And finally, an ambitious ethical theory of the sort I am here challenging claims that its machinery can be used to guide our judgements and conduct in new or difficult cases. (I mean here to be following Bernard Williams's view of ethical theory as 'a philosophical structure which, together with some degree of empirical fact, will yield a decision procedure for moral reasoning'.[2])

There is another preliminary matter to straighten out: it is important to understand that the claim that an ethical theory or a theory of justice cannot usefully capture or guide decisions about the demands of global health justice is not a denial that such demands exist. Certainly some anti-theorists in ethics have been anti-realists in meta-ethics,[3] but the two positions needn't always come as a package. Scepticism about the functioning of ethical theory is completely compatible with a wide range of meta-ethical commitments, from realism to historicist relativism, about global health justice itself. It is completely consistent, for example, to claim that justice demands that we improve the health of children in Sierra Leone, while also claiming that no theory of global health justice can adequately capture our understanding of the requirements of global justice. The sceptical claim is simply that a theory of global health justice cannot get us all the way to an understanding of what justice actually requires, or all the way to concrete on-the-ground prescriptions for interventions; it will always need to be augmented by historical and situational considerations which the theory fails to marshal or organize. This position, I think, is not particularly novel. We can agree on what needs to be done without reference to a theory of justice that prescribes exactly what we've agreed to. And that is because no theory of justice can be as sensitive to historical and situational variables as we can. A theory of justice can, at best, set some outer limits to our judgements about what justice requires in particular circumstances.

Theory

There is good reason to be sceptical about the enterprise of ethics theory-making. Ethical theory can of course be illuminating, bringing to our attention various

---

2   Bernard A. O. Williams, *Moral Luck* (Cambridge, MA: Harvard University Press, 1981), ix–x.
3   See Stanley G. Clarke and Evan Simpson, 'Introduction: The Primacy of Moral Practice', in Stanley G. Clarke and Evan Simpson (eds), *Anti-Theory in Ethics and Moral Conservatism* (Albany: State University of New York, 1989), 12ff.

important considerations that inform our ethical judgements, and the contests among rival ethical theories are especially valuable insofar as they pinpoint tensions and contradictions among those various considerations. But there are many reasons to think that no normative ethical theory can either fully explain our settled ethical judgements or guide our responses to new ethical questions.

Scepticism about the enterprise of ethical theory-making can arise with regard to any of the parts of the definition of ethical theory that I've offered. Consider, first, the fact that nearly every ethical theory is constructed with (explicit or implicit) reference to our moral intuitions. An ethical theory, to be plausible, must confirm and underwrite at least an important percentage of our core ethical beliefs. But intuitions cannot simply be permitted to play the same role for moral theory creation as observations do in the creation of scientific theory.[4] To the extent they are permitted to do so, then any ethical theory created on that basis risks being a mere formalization of our prejudices.

Second, consider the idea that ethical theory purports to capture and motivate the full variety of our ethical judgements using only a few relatively simple concepts and variables: a single telos, a small set of coherent principles, a single imagined procedure, a short list of basic human capabilities. That a small number of variables or principles should capture the universe of our ethical judgements is, on its face, quite unlikely, if we consider for a moment the complex historical and social roots of such ethics-laden phenomena as our notions of property ownership, of family structure, of social status, or of sexual ethics. All of these notions are both subjects of, and considerations within, day-to-day ethical judgements. Why *would* we expect a small number of concepts to bring order to this all-too-human mix?[5] To the extent that ethical theory illuminates ethical judgement, it does so precisely by simplifying. This simplification shows the power of certain kinds of considerations. In fact, it is not too much to say that abstraction from real ethical cases and judgements is in the very nature of any theory of ethics, for it is precisely abstraction that permits any theory to apply across multiple and diverse circumstances, and to assist us in reasoning about novel cases. But it may be that the required abstraction actually comes at the cost of irrelevance, or impotence, with regard to particular cases; that is, the very simplification that seems to makes ethical theory attractive and useful actually strips away all of the historical and social complexity which in fact informs many of our core ethical beliefs and judgements. Thus the language of ethical theory is often characterized by the use of highly abstract concepts such as justice, right, good and duty, and seldom employs more complex and situationally variable ideas such as indebtedness, regret, loyalty, admiration,

---

4   This point is made by Cheryl N. Noble in 'Normative Ethical Theories', in Clarke and
    Simpson (eds), *Anti-Theory in Ethics* 58ff.
5   See ibid., 50ff.

humiliation, or cowardice. A novel or a social history is not a theory of ethics – but it may well be that ethical problems and decisions are better characterized in novels and social histories than in theories.

Consider, for example, the ethical question whether someone is justified in feeling affronted at another person's behaviour. Various well-known ethical theories will clearly concentrate on different aspects of the problem: the consequences of the behaviour in question, and of the affronted response to it; the virtues of the two people involved; the principles underwriting their actions. But it matters, in answering the question, whether our social pair is interacting in Tokugawa Japan, in Victorian England, or in contemporary Manhattan. Any reasonable account of 'justified affront' will have historical and cultural content that none of the theories can provide. It matters, also, what sort of personal history and mutual understanding our two characters share. A theory can attempt to import that detailed historical and personal content, under the rubric of 'consequences', for example – but this just means that much of the work in generating an ethical decision is done by ethical knowledge and understanding acquired, so to speak, from outside the theory. Of course, every reasonable ethical theory can generate answers to *some* ethical questions (else they'd be poor candidates for the title of 'reasonable ethical theory'). The questions it can best answer will be those where our judgement is dominantly driven by the kinds of considerations that the theory, by its selective simplification of moral judgement, highlights. But no ethical theory can capture all of the detailed nuances of real ethical decision-making. At best, it can call our attention usefully to one, or some, of the most important considerations guiding our final judgements.

The problem of abstraction and simplification in ethical theory raises the question whether ethical theory really can be action-guiding. But that question can also be raised in another way. Some philosophers have alleged that ethical theorizing simply does no necessary work: most people through most of history have successfully made ethical judgements without reference to ethical theory, and people who justify their judgements by reference to theory today may well be engaged in mere post hoc justification of their intuitions. There is also a related question whether knowledge of ethical theory is an effective motivator, let alone the most effective motivator, for ethical action.

These brief comments are little more than a swift summary of well-known arguments against ethical theorizing. I turn now to some considerations that bear more particularly on the question of theorizing about global health justice.

Health

The subject-matter of any theory of global health justice will necessarily be 'health'. This raises some notorious problems of definition for the aspiring theorist: health has been defined narrowly as the absence of disease, and famously broadly (by the World Health Organization) as a complete state of physical, mental and social well-being. It has been seen by some theorists as a fundamentally normative concept, and by others as a purely descriptive one. It can be defined according to strict objective criteria, or subjectively according to the preferences and feelings of the patient or population in question. The choice of one (or some combination of) these definitions will of course have profound consequences for the shape of a theory of health justice.[6]

These well-known definitional problems apart, however, it remains that 'health', however defined, will be some state (broad or narrow, subjective or objective, normative or descriptive) of human beings. It cannot therefore be distributed among persons, and this makes it a difficult subject for any theory of justice. A theory of health justice will of course be concerned with health inequalities (those caused by, or indicative of, injustice), and will address itself to distributing something or other to rectify those inequalities. But what should the theory aim at distributing? It may appear simplest for the theorist to concentrate on distribution of and access to medical treatments. The have the virtue, at least, of being fairly easily quantifiable and of having an obvious connection to health. But that connection, though obvious, is not terribly deep. Improved access to medical treatment is far from synonymous with improved health. Particularly in the developing world (with which theories of global health justice are primarily concerned), health status is determined not primarily by access to medical interventions, but by non-medical health determinants such as access to clean water and nutritious food, access to education, peace, absence of social oppression, opportunity to work, control over reproductive choices and so on.[7] Given this fact, even a theory of global health justice that uses a narrow and objectively determined definition of 'health' will find itself becoming a theory of the just distribution of everything. Such a broad range of social phenomena has implications for health that a 'theory of health justice' will have considerable difficulty defining its own limits.

An interesting consequence of this difficulty is a problem that we might term 'the problem of misplaced concern'. It flows directly from the effort to create a theory of justice related specifically to health (as opposed to creating a theory of justice which in some way takes account of health). The theorist of global health justice will observe, for example, that women who lack reproductive autonomy

---

6   For a fuller discussion of these various definitional approaches and their consequences for theories of health justice, see John Coggon, *What Makes Health Public?* (Cambridge: Cambridge University Press, 2012), 11–23.

7   Jennifer Prah Ruger specifically declines, in her elaboration of Sen's health-capability theory, to take account of the social determinants of health. Jennifer Prah Ruger, *Health and Social Justice* (Oxford: Oxford University Press, 2010), 98–103. Another Sen-inspired health-capability theorist, Sridhar Venkatapuram, takes her to task for this narrow approach, Sridhar Venkatapuram, *Health Justice* (Cambridge: Polity, 2011), 153–4.

are at considerable health risk from unwanted and ill-timed pregnancy. Health justice, then, will seem to require women's reproductive autonomy. But it requires reproductive autonomy for what immediately seems to be the wrong reason, or not the core reason; it requires reproductive autonomy for the sake of the woman's health, rather than on the more compelling ground that reproductive autonomy is what women, as persons, deserve. Similar difficulties will arise in connection with concerns for education, peace, job opportunities and so on: the global health theorist's concern for them will be based in health, because she is a health theorist, and that kind of concern for those important items will ring hollow.

Global

A theory of global health justice must necessarily include the whole globe in its concerns, and the globe is a large and complicated place. Any theory that can cover the whole globe will have to be fairly thin, and given that thinness will hover high above the troposphere. Its prescriptive reach will not extend all the way down to the ground.

A theory of justice in global health may purport to tell us to whom better health is owed, but it cannot tell us much about how that health is to be delivered without running into messy facts about governance, politics, law and logistics. 'Ought' implies 'can'; a theory of global health that directs us to do things that are in fact impossible on the ground is for that reason a poor theory. (This is not to say that a theory can't aim at helping us imagine and lobby for better institutions and strategies that would make some previously impossible tasks possible.) Where the rubber meets the road, and we contemplate delivering actual vaccines or water or building materials or money to those in need, theory will have to yield to the insights of politics, law, management and logistics. It is insights from those disciplines that will tell us which interventions are possible, how much those interventions will cost and how successful they are apt to be at improving human health. The practical disciplines will therefore determine how our priorities are set, and where scarce resources are to be deployed.

A number of important theorists of global health justice have recognized this point explicitly. Amartya Sen has drawn attention to the problem; practical problems are one reason why his view of justice remains 'incompletely theorized', and why the relative weights of different capabilities are to be determined differently in different cases.[8] Norman Daniels admits that the principles of justice as fairness are 'too general and indeterminate to resolve many reasonable disputes about how to allocate resources fairly', and relies

8   Amartya Sen, *The Idea of Justice* (Cambridge, MA: Belknap/Harvard University Press, 2009).

instead on procedural principles of reasonableness and public accountability to guide concrete choices.[9]

Justice

Justice, let us agree, requires that people be given their due: a platitude, and one that leaves undone most of the work of specifying what it is that justice demands. But even the platitude is enough to raise for us the question: is there good reason to think that people all around the globe are due the same things, and that the demands of justice fall uniformly upon people around the globe?

Suppose, for example, that we follow Thomas Pogge in believing that much of world poverty (and the poor health that is closely associated with it) results not from bad luck, but from the deliberate and damaging policies of developed countries.[10] Protectionist US agricultural price supports, for example, prevent developing countries from being able to export their agricultural products at decent prices and therefore keep farmers in those countries poor. Developed-world lending institutions prevent poorer countries from borrowing in useful and productive ways, and developed-world manufacturers dump their shoddy products into developing-world markets, and their industrial waste into developing-world landfills. These allegations are used by Pogge to ground a duty of rich countries to help poorer countries not in distributive justice, but in retributive justice – or, to put it another way, to ground the claims of the world's poor not in positive rights ('you must help us') but in negative rights ('you must stop hurting us'). The point is not just to eliminate an unfair inequality, but to eliminate an unfair inequality for which many of the wealthiest countries are directly culpable.

But these claims of Pogge's, as compelling as they are, nonetheless imply that the demands of justice do not fall uniformly on wealthy countries around the globe. The culpability of wealthy countries for the world's poverty is not perfectly general or uniform; it is grounded in particular countries' histories as colonial powers, as hosts to particular multinational firms, as sponsors of particularly damaging institutions and exponents of particular damaging policies. The United States, for example, is undoubtedly more to blame for the poverty of certain Central American states than is Kuwait – or, for that matter, Denmark. Kuwait and Denmark are both wealthy, but their wealth has not been established with policies that undermine the ability of Central American states to compete in world agricultural markets. Kuwait was not

---

9   Norman Daniels, *Just Health: Meeting Health Needs Fairly* (Cambridge: Cambridge University Press, 2008), 117.

10 Thomas Pogge, *World Poverty and Human Rights: Cosmopolitan Responsibilities and Reforms*, 2nd edn (Cambridge: Polity, 2008).

the home of the National Fruit company, did not support farming economies based on monoculture, and does not now have agricultural price supports that diminish central American countries' ability to export food. Similarly, there may be some poor countries – Kazakhstan, for example – whose poverty has comparatively little to do with US policy, and much more to do with the ruinous economic and environmental policies of the former Soviet Union. To the extent that health justice is bound up with retributive justice, in other words, it is a mistake to expect it to have some uniformly 'global' character. This is because injustice, both past and continuing, has its roots in complex stories about history, economics, geography and religion.

Particular details about the historical relationships among wealthy and poor countries may also have consequences for the best means of redressing injustice. Some poor countries enjoy special historical or geographical relationships with certain wealthier countries: former colonies, for example. Certain African countries have sent their elites to be educated in France, others in Spain. South and Central American elites have commonly been educated in the United States, and commonly also have relations there. These kinds of connections relate not only to past injustices, but also to the efficiency with which some countries are capable of addressing others' problems. On some theory of global health justice, the United Kingdom (perhaps as a nation, or perhaps as a convenient representative of all its individually obligated citizens) owes health-related assistance both to India and to Senegal. For a thousand different reasons, it will likely be more effective at delivering that assistance to India.

Most theories of global health justice are grounded not in past and continuing injustice, but in various assertions about what human beings as such need or deserve. The 'capabilities approach' associated with Amartya Sen and Martha Nussbaum bases claims of justice on certain core capabilities necessary for free human flourishing;[11] Daniels specifies basic health needs necessary to achieve the fair equality of opportunity that characterizes a just (Rawlsian) society;[12] Powers and Faden argue for six dimensions of human well-being (one of which is health).[13] Any such approach, when applied not to a single society but to the global community, raises what might be termed a 'problem of address'. To whom are the demands of global justice – the demands of each needy human being – addressed? The countries of those in great need often lack the means or the political motivation to respond to the demands of justice. And above the level of the nation-state, there is a remarkable dearth of global institutions

---

11   See Sen, *The Idea of Justice*; and Martha Craven Nussbaum, *Frontiers of Justice: Disability, Nationality, Species Membership* (Cambridge, MA: Harvard University Press, 2007); Martha Craven Nussbaum, *Women and Human Development: The Capabilities Approach* (Cambridge: Cambridge University Press, 2001).

12   Daniels, *Just Health*.

13   Madison Powers and Ruth Faden, *Social Justice: The Moral Foundations of Public Health and Health Policy* (Oxford: Oxford University Press, 2006).

capable of carrying out the work of global health justice, however that might be described. In fact, most of the work currently being done to eliminate health inequalities is being done by wealthy countries, by foundations and by alliances of these. Many of those efforts are focused on particular diseases (AIDS, malaria) or particular interventions (fistula surgery, say, or childhood vaccination). It is difficult to see how most of these already-working institutions can be cast even as partial vindicators of the demands of any comprehensive theory of global health justice. Setting aside the question whether the diseases they target and the interventions they champion are precisely those that a theory of global health justice would prioritize, these institutions operate for the most part under the banner not of justice but of charity. Institutions of global health justice should be of the sort to which victims of injustice can address not requests, but demands. This near-absence of global-justice institutions poses a serious '"ought" implies "can"' problem for the framing of a theory of global health justice. It seems fruitless to prescribe actions which no one is well-situated to carry out, or to describe rights for which no one bears correlative duties – and equally fruitless, though not valueless, to imagine new global institutions which are quite unlikely to be created anytime soon.

Uniquely among global-health theorists, Peter Singer entirely avoids this problem of address. He is explicit that the demands of justice fall on each of us, individually.[14] We may attempt to meet them, in part, by lobbying for better global institutions or greater governmental interventions in global health, but the obligations are ours. Each of us is obligated to help the world's poor, using our own resources; it is wrong for us to permit human suffering to continue if we could alleviate it at a lesser cost (in terms of suffering) to ourselves.

This leads us, however, directly to another difficulty for theories of global health justice: the problem of 'demandingness'.[15] The problem has been most discussed in connection with utilitarian theory, though it is of broader applicability. The problem (using the familiar utilitarian example) runs this way: utilitarianism is the view that actions are good just insofar as they have the consequence of creating social utility (conceived variously as the net of pleasure and pain, welfare, preference satisfaction, etc.). It therefore demands that, as between any two actions, an agent should perform the one which will create the greatest net utility among the persons affected. The upshot of this is that a good utilitarian should always be doing the one action available to her which will produce the largest amount of utility. And what this means is that, taken seriously, the theory takes over her life, treating her as a machine for generating social utility, and leaving her no space to choose actions on

14 These arguments of Singer's were first, and forcefully, made in Peter Singer, 'Famine, Affluence and Morality', *Philosophy and Public Affairs*, 1972, 1: 229–43.

15 This problem has its classic articulation in Bernard Williams's essay in J. J. C. Smart and Bernard A. O. Williams, *Utilitarianism: For and against* (Cambridge: Cambridge University Press, 1973).

non-utilitarian grounds (e.g. because of their special meaning for her, or because of some non-moral preference of hers). Utilitarianism is therefore too demanding, not in the sense common to many moral views that its standards are too high for ordinary, erring mortals consistently to live up to, but in the sense that those standards leave the utilitarian agent no life of her own.

Peter Singer sees this issue and simply embraces it. He sees no reason to reject the idea that morality requires us to give of our resources to the poor until we spend ourselves all the way down to their level. This extreme view of course raises all kinds of issues internal to utilitarian analysis – notably questions about interpersonal comparisons of utility and lingering questions about our ability to judge the real utility effects of our intended interventions across the globe. It also raises important questions about utilitarian theory itself – for example, its discomfiting demand that we transfer our resources not to those most desperately in need, but to those whose lives the resources are most apt to improve. But our present concern is with demandingness. If, as Singer claims, justice demands that each of us devote our personal energy and productive capacity to the improvement of the lives of everyone less well-off than ourselves, this leaves very little for our lives to be about. Neither we nor those we assist, for example, are justified in devoting any of our resources to art or amusement while there exists a single person whose utility we could improve by more than the utility cost to us of bringing about the improvement. In any world with seriously scarce resources, the utilitarian moral life seems to consist entirely in our keeping one another (barely) alive.

The demandingness problem is conveniently illustrated by, but is certainly not limited to, utilitarian theory. So stark are global health inequalities that if any significant portion of them is properly conceived of as unjust, then the requirements of any general theory of global health justice that addresses its demands to individuals will threaten to consume the lives of the better off among us in something like this way. Again, this is not simply a question of the demands of global health justice hijacking all available social resources (though this is a problem, too); it is instead a deeper question of those demands, if taken seriously, requiring so much of our time and resources as to leave us no ability to lead our own lives. An analogous problem occurs for theories of global health justice addressing themselves to governments. What state could justify any investment in arts or education or medical research or highway construction if justice demands that it attend, first, to infant mortality and infectious disease in the poorest parts of the world? Is it not wrong for the United Kingdom to spend resources on medical research, or on historical research, given the dire levels of global health need?

These concerns with demandingness are easily caricatured either as selfishness or as hyperbole. An earnest concern with demandingness, the demanding theorist can jeer, is just convenient cover for the fact that we'd rather buy a new iPad than send money to help children in Africa. And how many of us, after all, are in any real danger of reducing ourselves to poverty to meet others' health needs? Not even Peter Singer actually does that. Our wealthy governments are giving next to nothing in aid to the world's poor, and show no sign of failing to give priority to the needs of their own comparatively well-off citizens.

But the demandingness objection should not, I think, be so easily dismissed. Either a theory means what it says or it does not. If the consequences of a theory, were that theory to be fully realized, would be offensive to our deepest views about the meaning, point and best uses of a human life; or would threaten our core notions of the legitimate function of government; then the theory should not be able to excuse itself via claims that it is not, in fact, apt to be fully realized.

Next we must consider the vexed problem of conflict of values. Such conflicts will occur both within any theory of global health justice (Which diseases is it more important to eradicate? Should we allocate more funds to saving infant's lives, or to improving the quality of adult's lives?) and between the demands of health justice and other moral concerns (Should we allocate more resources to medical interventions or to lawyer training? Will we gain more utility by paying for healthcare for the poor, or by developing technologies to control climate change?). Theories that attempt to achieve health justice by addressing social determinants of health may find the former conflicts more vexing than the latter, because most any competing candidates for resource allocation (governance, education, security, physical infrastructure, trade) will have positive payoffs for health. But this leaves them, once more, with the problem of misplaced concern – supporting better education, for example, for the sake of its health payoffs rather than out of concern for the minds of those educated.

There will also be conflicts between the demands of health justice and other non-moral concerns. How important is health justice compared to other things that are important without being morally important? Should every country stop funding military bands and expensive non-combat dress uniforms in order to allocate those funds to health justice? Neither the ability to play the national anthem at ceremonial events, nor the appearance of crisp military whites, is morally important. They're just important.

The problem, in sum, is that no theory of global health justice can determine its own weight. This is a problem for any topic-specific ethical theory. A theory of medical ethics can articulate the demands of medical ethics, but cannot adjudicate conflicts between those demands and the demands of public economy. A theory of legal ethics cannot adjudicate conflicts between itself and democratic theory. The problem, which may seem trivial, is in fact serious. It means that no theory of global health ethics can ever do anything more than weigh in on an allocation problem from its own point of view. The answer to the question, 'What, all things considered, is to be done?' will always be determined from outside the theory, in the world where it competes with other theories, and struggles with other priorities both moral and non-moral.

Finally there is the purely prudential question, alluded to earlier, of the motivational power of any theory of global health justice. The fact that most of the world's existing global health institutions are structured as 'charitable', rather than cast as vindicating claims of justice, may be a mistake – but if it is, it is a mistake that speaks volumes about what motivates nations and people to help strangers. We are used, normally, to thinking that the claims of justice are stronger than the claims to charity, but there is no reason to expect this always to be true, and in global health it seems simply to be the fact that charitable motivations – along with the selfish desires for borders secure from disease and from uncontrolled immigration – are more motivating than the claims of global justice. What necessary role, then, does a theory of global health justice play in actually helping to meet the demands of justice?

The positive uses of ambitious theory

I have thus far argued that any theory of global health justice will stumble on definitional problems with health and on the problem of what to distribute in order to attain health justice, and ultimately founder on the 'problem of misplaced concern'; that no theory of global health justice will be able to supply practical, ground-level prescriptions, but will instead have to cede territory to the practical disciplines of politics, law and logistics; that no theory of global health justice will take adequate account of the historical and local character of claims in retributive justice; that the lack of institutions available to vindicate the actual demands of global health justice will act to render theories of global health justice irrelevant; that theories of global health justice will face a problem of demandingness; that they will never be able to resolve problems of conflicting values; and that they are, as a prudential matter, poor motivators to action compared to charity and security.

Of course, as J. L. Austin is said to have remarked, 'There's the part where you say it, and the part where you take it back'. None of my comments are meant to imply that the enterprise of ambitious theorizing about global health justice is not at all worthwhile. The implication is only that such theorizing cannot succeed on its own terms: it cannot fully explain or describe our convictions about what justice requires, or reliably guide us to correct judgements in novel cases. What it can do, though, is clarify our thinking in a large number of helpful ways: by highlighting, in a simplified and approachable way (as Singer's and Pogge's analyses have) specific considerations that ought to inform or challenge our settled beliefs about health justice; by offering (as the capabilities approach has done) powerful critiques of, or methods of evaluating, real-life global health interventions; by proposing potentially useful future institutions for the betterment of human health; and so on.

It might be worthwhile, in closing, to consider an analogy between the field of global health justice and the better-established field of clinical ethics.[16] It is surely the case that ambitious moral theorists have helped bioethicists think through their ethical convictions in a number of important ways. Bioethics would surely be worse off without the contributions of such ethical theorists as Frances Kamm, Jeff McMahon, and, yes, Peter Singer.

But it is also worth recalling in this connection that practical, clinical ethics has long had a generally anti-theoretical cast, and that there have been both prudential and philosophical reasons for this. Clinical ethicists have avoided theory-talk mostly as a matter of prudence. Where a bedside decision needs to be made, discussions about background theoretical commitments are beside the point, and could create distracting disagreement unnecessarily. Moreover, reference to ethical theory could mark the ethicist as 'flighty' and out of touch with the realities of the clinic. Ethicists on public commissions and policy-making bodies have avoided discussion of theoretical commitments for similar reasons.

The two major 'methods' in clinical ethics – the Beauchamp and Childress 'principles' method[17] and the so-called Four-Box method – are each explicitly anti-theoretical. The 'Four-Box' method, originating in Jonsen, Siegler and Winslade's book *Clinical Ethics*,[18] is essentially a method for focusing the discussion of cases in all of their concrete detail. It is designed to facilitate and guide a casuistic process of case analysis, so that new cases can properly be assimilated to previously considered paradigm cases. Discussion of each new case is focused around four topics (medical indications, patient preferences, quality of life and contextual features), each of which is further specified and broken down into sub-topics. No claim is made about the origins of these topics in any ethical theory; instead, the idea is to make every case discussion both uniform and thorough, so that areas of commonality with settled paradigm cases can easily be identified. Later versions of the approach note that discussion of each of the topics will be guided by consideration of ethical principles, and that analogies between new cases and paradigm cases will be drawn on the basis of principles; but again, no particular claims are made about the origins of principles in ethical theory.

Beauchamp and Childress have changed their view of the relationship of their 'principles' approach to ethical theory over time. Early editions of their classic

---

16 I am indebted, in this section, to John Arras's extensive and illuminating discussion of the relationship of theory to bioethics in his 'Theory and Bioethics', *Stanford Encyclopedia of Bioethics*, Edward N. Zalta (ed.), available at http://plato.stanford.edu/archives/sum2010/entries/theory-bioethics/.

17 See Tom L. Beauchamp and James F. Childress, *Principles of Biomedical Ethics*, 6th edn (Oxford: Oxford University Press, 2009).

18 Albert R. Jonsen, Mark Seigler and William J. Winslade, *Clinical Ethics: A Practical Approach to Ethical Decisions in Clinical Medicine*, 7th edn (New York: McGraw Hill Medical, 2010).

Principles of Biomedical Ethics claimed that the 'mid-level' principles they use to frame discussion of bioethics cases could be generated by any number of ethical theories. Both Mill and Kant believed in the importance of permitting people to make their own choices, for example, and both were concerned to limit harm done by agents to others. Certainly both were committed to distributional justice. Their conflicting theoretical grounds for supporting these mid-level ethical principles could therefore safely be ignored, and the discussion of concrete cases begun without reference to them. In more recent editions of the same book, though, the story has changed. 'Mid-level principles', instead of having their origin 'top down' from any number of higher-order ethical theories, are imagined as having their origins 'bottom up', as generalizations from ground-level judgements about concrete cases.

These two main methods of clinical ethics have therefore drifted together over time. In one, concrete case discussion is treated as the core method, but ethical principles have an acknowledged role to play in framing case discussion and comparing cases. In the other, the core method involves application of ethical principles to new cases, but those principles are acknowledged as having had their origin in concrete case discussion. Both methods are well-established as practical and useful. In the United States, for example, thousands of hospitals have clinical ethics consultation services which make use of one or another of these methods, and dozens of legal cases have featured the testimony of clinical ethics experts versed in both. Neither method evokes, in its application, any connection to any full-blown ethical theory. Both rely on context-heavy intuition and judgement, especially when principles conflict, or when relevant paradigms seem inconsistent. Both methods are consistent with a broad range of meta-ethical commitments, as well as commitments to professional, religious and common secular moral views. Both have proven practically useful, and neither implies any scepticism about the reality of the ethical conclusions they facilitate.

It may be that what global health justice needs now is not better theory, but more attention to method.

2

Ethics and Global Health Inequalities*

Richard Ashcroft

Introduction

Life expectancy varies widely between countries. So too do the incidences of the principal causes of mortality and morbidity. There is no question but that avoidable mortality and morbidity is of moral concern. Exactly what form that concern should take, and what actions and policies it should mandate is of central importance in epidemiology, public health, health policy and development policy. My argument in this chapter is that we can, and should, acknowledge all of this, but nevertheless be sceptical about whether *health inequalities* should be a matter of moral concern. To give an example: suppose in country A a patient who is HIV positive can expect to live 25 years after diagnosis, whereas in country B a patient who is HIV positive can expect to live only two years after diagnosis. Suppose that the reason for the difference is that in country A antiretroviral treatment is cheaply and generally available, whereas in country B it is neither. There are two different ways of responding to this difference which I wish to distinguish morally: we might say that we have an obligation to aid someone in need where there is an avoidable cause of premature mortality, here, the lack of access to treatment. Or we might say that we have an obligation to reduce the inequality between country A and country B. My general view, which I develop here, is that it is *not* the inequality which motivates us to act to assist patients in country B. Rather it is the unmet need. Comparison of country A and B provides us a *signal* of the extent of that need. But it is not the signal we care about; it is the unmet need itself.

Broadly speaking, writers in global ethics (including global health ethics) can be divided into two groups: those who are concerned with global injustice, and those who are concerned with global welfare.[1] The argument sketched so far suggests that I am more in the latter camp than in the former. However,

---

* A version of this chapter was presented at the Current Legal Issues Colloquium on law and global health, held at University College London, 5–6 July 2012.

1 Representative of the justice school is the work of Thomas Pogge, in particular *World Poverty and Human Rights* (Oxford: Blackwell, 2007) (2nd edn). Representative of the welfare school is the work of Peter Singer, for instance *The Life You Can Save: Acting Now to End World Poverty* (London: Picador, 2009).

as the chapter develops, we will see that a concern with injustice is perfectly appropriate in the case of health. It is just that a focus on health inequality is not the best way to frame that concern with injustice.

Comparison problems

If we want to talk about health inequalities at all, of course, we need to compare. In other words, we need to be able to define a relation 'healthier than' over a set of individuals or relata. We need the proposition 'A is healthier than B' to mean something. This is quite tricky. I have a cold, but am basically fit; you don't have a cold but do have a calf-strain; she is physically well but is depressed; he has asympomatic HIV infection. Just as comparing individuals in this simple way is difficult, we have even more trouble when we have to take age into account. At 85 I am less healthy than I was at 25, but that is to be expected. On the other hand, in terms of comparative life expectancy, I might be healthier than someone who cannot expect to live beyond 50 years of age in another country, and indeed than my own birth cohort if the life expectancy of that cohort was 75 years of age. Defining our relation 'healthier than' over the set of individuals is fraught with ambiguity and it is hard to see how we can derive any reasonably general, reasonably robust way of comparing any two individuals in a population in terms of their general health. Those measures of health which do seem to support comparison relationships, like QALYs (Quality Adjusted Life Years) or DALYs (Disability Adjusted Life Years) work best either where the comparison is defined over a rather narrow class of individuals and to measure the impact of some intervention, or where we are comparing large groups treated as aggregates. An example of the former is the comparison we might make over the set of individuals with early stage breast cancer, to see whether one drug is superior to another in terms of promoting five-year survival post treatment. An example of the latter is comparing expectancies of healthy years of life in two different countries using DALYs, as in Murray and Lopez's study of the Global Burden of Disease. In this study, comparison is made between different countries' performance in respect of carefully chosen indicators of health: in other words it is a multidimensional comparison, rather than a simple 'healthier than' relation. The problems of measuring, computing and comparing or evaluating QALYs and DALYs are well known, and have been central to conceptual debates on justice in healthcare rationing for a generation.[2]

2 See for a comprehensive overview of the conceptual issues and a wealth of data, Christopher J. L. Murray and Alan D. Lopez (eds) *Global Health Statistics* (Cambridge, MA: Harvard University Press, 1996).

In other words, there is nothing simple about comparing health states, or health expectations, between individuals. What we want to say about inequalities in health very much depends on why we want to know, what we are able to measure and what moral importance we attach to that measure. Suppose we can sort out the conceptual problems with the measures of health and the kinds of comparison we want to make with our measures of health. We also have to decide which groups we want to compare. Some intergroup comparisons make sense and are probably important – comparisons between men's and women's health, for instance. Some intergroup comparisons make sense but are probably unimportant – comparisons between redheads' health and blondes' health, for instance. And some intergroup comparisons may be meaningless and/or unimportant – comparisons between the health of people born on Saturdays with the health of people born on Sundays, for instance.

The issue I am concerned with here is this: if we think that health inequalities between groups matter morally, then we have to be very careful both about the measure we use and about the groups over which we make the comparison. Since the selection of both groups and measure involve judgements of importance, we need to be very careful that we are not begging the question about why health inequalities matter. It is one thing to say that women live longer than men and that's wrong *because* it's an inequality, and quite another to say that it's wrong because it's an *inequality between men and women*. In the latter claim we are importing a concern about the relationships between men and women which is prior to a concern about this particular numerical inequality between men and women. The concern with justice precedes the concern with inequality, and it's arguably that concern with gender injustice which grants the inequality between men and women according to the measure of interest some importance. If so, the importance we attach to the inequality measure is as a *signal* of that injustice.

Put another way, consider interventions to do something about gender injustice. We could choose to motivate such interventions by pointing to health inequalities between men and women, and seek to identify interventions which aim to reduce such inequalities. Or we could take such inequalities as signals of underlying causes which apply unjustly, and intervene to modify those. For instance, women and men vary categorically in their exposure to perinatal health problems attendant on pregnancy and giving birth. That is not in itself a signal of injustice. On the other hand, we might conclude on the basis of some other comparison that women's perinatal health does not attract sufficient investment or research or good quality healthcare. But insofar as we are making a male/female comparison here, it will be the economic or status inequality which drives our analysis, rather than the health inequality, and it will be the avoidable mortality and morbidity (welfare concerns) which may be more important than health justice concerns per se.

Connectedness and circumstances

It is not enough to ground a concern with health inequality on the choice of a robust and meaningful measure and a meaningful class of groups over which to use the measure. Suppose we compare the health of HIV positive women in Brazil with the health of HIV positive women in South Africa. Very likely there are differences, which are meaningful, between these groups on several meaningful and robust measures of health. Some of these differences will be quite informative, and might guide policy or choice of interventions – call this learning from experience. But it is most unlikely that we would conclude that there is something unfair about these inequalities unless we can say something further to warrant that judgement of unfairness. We might say that there is something unfair in the inequality if in some way the difference is *caused* by the relationship between these two groups of women, or, perhaps, between some contexts in which these groups are embedded. Suppose women who are HIV positive in Brazil do better than women who are HIV positive in South Africa, and suppose that is due to something problematic about trade relations between the two countries, or their respective position vis-a-vis third party or international trade relations. Then we might have reason to say that the inequality between the two groups of women has a basis in an injustice between the two countries, or between the two countries and the international system. However, in such a case once again we have shown that the health inequality signals some other, more fundamental injustice, in this case in political economy. In other words, for an inequality in health to be unjust in and of itself we need to show a causal relationship between the relata in the comparison, which has a direct impact on health: they need to be connected, and somehow a relationship of responsibility must exist between the two groups, in what David Hume called the 'circumstances of justice'.[3] Of course, difference between the two groups may lack this feature. It may still matter as a signal that something is wrong in, say, South Africa. But once again, we are treating the inequality as a signal rather than a wrong in itself.

Health inequality and resource inequality

Part of the appeal of the concept of health inequality, I suspect, is that a rather slippery analogy is made with resource inequality. On the one hand, we might want to say that the unfairness of differential distribution of health is like the unfairness of (some) differential distribution of resources.

---

3   See Brian Barry, *Theories of Justice* (Berkeley, CA: University of California Press, 1989), chapter 4 for a lucid exposition of the theory.

Individuals who think about health with a Rawlsian turn of mind find it difficult to imagine how fairness on the Rawlsian model could permit a wide variation in distribution of health states.[4] Behind the veil of ignorance, no one would choose such an outcome, the thought goes. On the other hand, you might think that health inequalities are *worse* than resource inequalities, for a variety of reasons. Ill health is not chosen, it is far less under the control of the individual (luck plays a greater part, perhaps), and so even if you are prepared to tolerate some resource inequalities, unjust health inequalities should be even more motivating to action than unjust resource inequalities. This line of reasoning goes some way to explaining why many people who are concerned with local or global injustice choose, as a matter of political practice, to focus on health inequalities. Intuitively it seems more wrong that poor people are more prone to ill health or early death than rich people, than the fact that they are poor or rich. Wealth, one might think, has to do with effort, talent, imagination, risk-taking … but illness is sheer misfortune. How can it be right that the poor are more exposed to sheer misfortune? Of course, some kinds of misfortunes are preventable, or can be managed with prudence, and it is true that the wish to buy security and protection from misfortune is a powerful motivator to find ways out of poverty. Nevertheless, at some basic level it just seems wrong that health misfortunes should cluster along with poverty, poor housing, low access to education and unemployment or low paid, long hours of work. The interaction between these factors is also rather obvious: if one is ill a lot, one cannot work very much; conversely, if one works very long hours, or is unable to find regular work, one may be more liable to fall ill. It is rather important that needs do not simply cluster as a mere empirical fact, but that there are discoverable causal relationships which show how and why they cluster.

In terms of making sense of health inequalities, however, as objects of moral concern, there is a difficulty. Health is not a resource, since it is not transferrable: I cannot give, and you cannot take, some of my health, in the way that I can transfer money, property, or even social status.[5] Thus many of the usual ways of responding to resource inequality (redistributive taxation, resource transfers and welfare payments, for example) do not apply in the health context. It

---

4   Of course, the difficulty of interpreting health and disability within Rawls's own theory is well known, and modern successors to Rawls, in particular Norman Daniels, have wrestled with the problem with greater or lesser success. My point here is simply that if you think health is *like* a resource, then you could try to think about health inequalities in the way Rawlsians think about resource inequalities. Norman Daniels, *Just Health: Meeting Health Needs Fairly* (Cambridge: Cambridge University Press, 2007) is the most important and best Rawlsian approach to health, and my brief characterization of a 'Rawlsian' approach here is not intended in any way to capture the sophistication or insight of that book.
5   Of course, you can damage my health by infecting me with something nasty. This is not the point. No one would argue that the cause of health justice, or health welfare, is advanced by levelling some people's health down by making them more ill.

may be more promising to think in terms of 'luck egalitarianism'.[6] According to luck egalitarians, what matters is not equality of resources, but equality of fortune. Ex ante, we should all start out in life with similar chances and opportunities; and, as Segall puts it, 'it is unjust for individuals to be worse off than others due to outcomes that it would have been unreasonable to expect them to avoid'.[7] There are many problems with this definition as a proposal about injustice as such – it neglects all the concerns I have sketched above about the meaningfulness of certain kinds of comparison as the way to think about differences which are unjust. But it does give us a clue as to what might be wrong with health inequality. Health inequality is wrong where it maps outcomes 'that it would be unreasonable to expect agents to avoid'. This seems right. The unfairness of differential outcomes derives, in part, from the ways in which some kinds of poor health are unavoidable, and thus cause differences in income or social status or human rights protection which fall on some but not on others, for reasons they cannot control. And in part, it comes from the way in which the *avoidability* of some kinds of poor health is controlled by still other differences (in economic or social status, or human rights protection, or employment conditions, or educational opportunities) which again may be outside the agent's control or prudent foresight.

The promise of luck egalitarianism for those who want to take health inequalities as morally important in their own right is precisely the link between health and luck. On the theory that inequalities are wrong where person A is worse off than person B for reasons it would be unreasonable to expect person A to avoid, as is the case with health inequalities much of the time, person A's ill health is not just unlucky, it is unjust. Injustice requires some kind of corrective action. But consider what we are saying here. We are not saying that there is an unjust distribution of health between A and B. B owes nothing to A in view of A's ill health being somehow to the advantage of B. B might owe something to A out of a duty of beneficence, as a welfarist would certainly agree. So the thesis that A's ill health is unjust seems to collapse into the claim, accepted at the outset of this chapter, that A's need should motivate us to aid A. And the argument from justice has added nothing. So what could we say that would make an argument from this health inequality to claims of injustice useful?

One of the common responses to A's ill health relative to B is to deny, with more or less force, that A's ill health relative to B should prompt or even require B to aid A in some way. We could say that B has no *obligation* to aid A, although of course if B does so it will, other things being equal, be praiseworthy. As my focus in this chapter is not on welfarist arguments about duties to aid, but on injustice, I will not explore this idea, but simply note that it is a commonly

---

6 The important recent book by Shlomi Segall, *Health, Luck and Justice* (Princeton, NJ: Princeton University Press, 2010) explores this proposal in detail.

7 Ibid., 13.

held intuition. If you acknowledge the fact of the health inequality, and you go further and accept that A is in need and you agree that this is regrettable, but do not agree that you are under any obligation to do something about it, what can I say? I can say that it is *unfair* that A is worse off than B. This claim is meant to add something to my motivation to aid A, tipping it into action and a recognition of an obligation to help. If the claim of injustice is meant to be more than a forceful rhetorical restatement of your claim that I do really have an obligation on welfarist grounds, then it will need to explain something about the relationship between us and A.[8]

Health inequalities and 'structural violence'

The idea that a significant proportion of health inequality can be explained by *structural* factors is the strongest and most important element of the theory of health inequality. Robust and detailed work has been done since the 1970s exploring the ways in which social structure can explain the ways in which mortality and morbidity, across a whole range of measures from life expectancy to disease incidences to biochemical markers of stress, is patterned within and between societies. Although some of this patterning can be explained by reference to genetic or cultural factors, a large proportion of the variation in health in a society can be explained by 'material' factors including access to services, employment opportunities, health and safety at work, the ways social hierarchies function in the economic sphere and beyond and so on.[9] In a telling phrase, the public health physician and humanitarian Paul Farmer has labeled the health consequences of poverty, discrimination and oppression 'structural violence'. The idea is that the consequences for the health of the worst off are indistinguishable from the consequences of individualized physical violence; but that they are brought about by the ways the social structure operates to perpetuate and intensify patterns of social and economic inequality rather than, or in addition to, specific acts of violence or oppression by identifiable individuals. The language of structural violence is particularly apposite in the

8 I am not going to explore here the idea that we might have a prima facie obligation to aid A, in need, but that this is *blocked* either because A is ill or less healthy due to A's own conduct or imprudence (the responsibility for health issue) or because someone else – perhaps some institution, in the global health case A's own government perhaps, is better placed or under a stronger obligation to help. These are important issues, but are generic problems in theories of justice. We could substitute 'wealth' for 'health' in these arguments without too much strain, and their form would be broadly the same. My focus here is on the moral status of health inequalities per se, so I leave these generic issues to one side.

9 For instance, see Richard Wilkinson and Kate Pickett, *The Spirit Level: Why Equality Is Better for Everyone* (London: Penguin, 2010); Michael Marmot and Richard Wilkinson, *Social Determinants of Health* (Oxford: Oxford University Press, 2005); and the classic Margaret Whitehead, Peter Townsend, Nicholas Davidson, *Inequalities in Health: The Black Report and The Health Divide* (London: Penguin, 1992) (2nd edn).

countries where Farmer works, notably Haiti and Rwanda, but he claims that it is a mistake to think of structural violence as being exceptional and localized. Rather he sees it as a global phenomenon, which varies in its form from place to place, but whose underlying causes are quite general.[10]

What the structural violence argument does is construct a powerful empirical and causal argument to show both how structural causes operate to bring about differences in health across populations locally, nationally and internationally and how the connectedness requirement we discussed above applies. Hence, we can conclude that considerations of justice do apply internationally, indeed globally, and we can also conclude that differences in health do fit into any sensible account of global justice. However, what the structural violence argument does not do is show that health inequalities are fundamental in a theory of global justice, nor that they are our primary object of concern. There is perhaps a rhetorical trick here: Farmer and other public health experts on health inequality know that for most people there is something intuitively outrageous about variations in health and illness which are associated with poverty and oppression.[11] This is how they grab our attention. But having grabbed our attention, they then show how actually it is the injustice – violence – of global political economy which should really attract our anger and our efforts. In this they adopt a broadly similar tactic to non-governmental organizations which motivate us to donate to causes which will generally improve development and fairness by badging them as focusing primarily on child poverty. It is much easier to attract the interest of the ordinary well-meaning person by flagging up child poverty, which seems cruel and unfair, than 'general' poverty, which 'is always with us'.

Conceptually, then, the structural violence argument does show that arguments from justice have a place in our thinking about health inequalities. But I do not think they show that health inequalities are unjust in themselves, or that our obligations of justice require us to reduce *health inequalities* as such. They show something else, just as important, but different. They show that where someone is relatively unhealthy we have both the ordinary obligations of beneficence toward someone in need *and* the obligations of justice which arise from our position of relative advantage in a structurally unjust context, a context which we can show we do truly share with the apparently remote Other. So, returning to my theme throughout this chapter, we see health inequalities as a *signal* of injustice, rather than as something inherently unjust.

---

10   See Paul Farmer, *Pathologies of Power: Health, Human Rights and the New War on the Poor* (Berkeley, CA: University of California Press, 2004) (2nd edn) for a general overview of his argument.

11   It is not *just* a rhetorical trick, of course. It is clear that Farmer and others believe sincerely in the importance of health inequalities. And besides, as doctors and public health physicians they naturally focus on the health and medical dimension as what they are trained to understand and research.

Capabilities and health

Have I been too quick? Consider the following argument. My argument so far has been to show that health inequalities are not appropriate objects of moral concern. They are useful signals of more fundamental problems – including inequalities – which are appropriate objects of moral concern, either because they support obligations of beneficence or because they support well-grounded concerns of justice or both. I argued that health needs do support obligations of beneficence, but that health differences do not; and I argued that health differences may signal obligations of justice which relate to the structural causes of health differences. There is a difficulty with this argument. It seems implicitly to assume that health, and health inequalities, arise from some set of causes which are more fundamental. This is puzzling, since surely health is an operating cause in social structure, not simply an epiphenomenon of that structure. Even if we agree that the pattern in society of incidence of heart disease has a significant socioeconomic or gender component, for instance, we should not forget that it is a physical illness, and that social causes are mediated through biological ones. And more obviously still, for some disorders and disabilities the socioeconomic component will be less significant than in others. Indeed, for many disorders and disabilities the incidence may not be socially patterned to any great extent; instead the *consequences* of those disorders and disabilities are where the social patterning is most apparent, and in these cases we would want to say that it is the health difference which causes the social difference, and not the other way around.

I can accept all of this without abandoning my overall thesis. Suppose we identify a class of causes of ill health which are not socially patterned in their incidence, but which give rise to social patterning of disadvantage. If so, the justice argument for correcting health inequalities *still* does not apply. There is nothing *unfair* about the incidence of these illnesses and disabilities (except perhaps in a cosmic sense – but we are not concerned with cosmic justice here, just the ordinary human kind). The need/beneficence argument certainly does. The injustice arising from the emergent disadvantage brought about by the interaction of the disorder or disability and socioeconomic structure once again directs our attention to justice-based obligations to help remedy the causes and consequences of the disorder or disability. And so the argument that some health conditions are primary operating causes of disadvantage is true, but it does not establish the sui generis importance of health inequalities. Rather, it reinforces the importance of structural inequality as the basis of obligations of justice.[12]

---

12   On disadvantage, see Jonathan Wolff and Avner de Shalit, *Disadvantage* (Oxford: Oxford University Press, 2007).

I believe this makes my approach, surprisingly perhaps, consistent both with the luck egalitarian approach favoured by Segall and with the capabilities approach recently developed in the global health context by Sridhar Venkatapuram. Building on the work of Nussbaum, Sen and others in elaborating 'capability theory' as a normative theory for justice and social choice, Venkatapuram develops a book-length argument for making a 'capability to be healthy' central to any account of global health justice. Capability theory was developed initially as a technical approach for dealing with the limitations of welfare-based utilitarianisms and models of rational choice in economic theory. It focuses on a set of basic human 'capabilities' to live and flourish, to which everyone is entitled as the conditions of a minimally decent life. Venkatapuram develops a detailed account of both a 'capability to be healthy' and a concept of health *as* capability. The former places health alongside other capabilities, such as the capability for life, emotional relationships, or affiliation with others.[13] The latter takes health as a global 'meta-capability' which gives a measure or index of one's overall flourishing in light of the functioning of one's basic capabilities. So far as health as capability is concerned, we could think of this as a more structured kind of welfare concept, and a debate about inequalities in that would be far more general than the debate we are considering here about health in the more common-or-garden sense. So I take it that debates about health inequality, if they are to use the capabilities framework, will more likely focus on the 'capability to be healthy'. If so, I claim that the focus on inequalities which this approach would motivate is not one on inequalities in health, but one on inequalities in 'capability to be healthy'. And that capability is in turn a construct out of a range of social, economic, structural and institutional factors. So even if you are attracted to the idea of capability theory as a way of saying what is special about health – and it has much to recommend it – it won't tell you what is special about health inequalities. Rather it will give you further reasons to want to attend to the human causes of health inequalities.

Conclusion

In this chapter, I have argued that health inequalities are important signals of injustice and need, but that they are not directly objects of moral concern themselves. I showed that there are significant conceptual difficulties in grasping health inequalities without making a series of prior, normatively loaded decisions

---

13   Sridhar Venkatapuram, *Health Justice*, (Cambridge: Polity, 2011). For capabilities, more generally, see Amartya Sen, *The Idea of Justice*, (London: Penguin, 2010); Martha Nussbaum, *Creating Capabilities: The Human Development Approach* (Cambridge, MA: Harvard University Press, 2011).

about what to measure, what to compare and which groups are of concern. I argued that this imports the set of moral concerns into the measure of health inequalities, rather than 'finding it there'. I argued further that if we distinguish between obligations of beneficence and obligations of justice then our concern with health inequalities can collapse into ordinary concerns with the health needs of others which do not rest on claims about the unfairness of differential need. In so far as we are concerned with justice, however, this requires us to consider the necessary conditions of connectedness and mutual responsibility. These turn out to be well-described and well-understood within the literature on inequalities in health, but the twist is that they are described primarily in terms of socioeconomic structure and its impact on individual welfare – the structural violence theory. As a result, whether we are Rawlsians, luck egalitarians, capability theorists our primary focus ends up being on the injustice inherent in socioeconomic arrangements rather than on inequality in health per se. And this remains so even when we allow for the fact that some kinds of ill-health involve a greater sheerly biological element than others. From the point of view of ethics, which is concerned with human responsibility and human action, it should not be very surprising that our fundamental proper concern is with the fairness or otherwise of our socioeconomic arrangements.[14]

---

14 For a very different route to a similar conclusion, consider the literature on the 'human right to health', in particular Jonathan Wolff, *The Human Right to Health* (New York: W. W. Norton, 2012).

3

Why Bioethics *Must* Be Global

Heather Widdows and Peter West-Oram

Introduction

This chapter considers what type of bioethics is necessary to address contemporary issues in global health. It explores what kind of ethics, or bioethics, is needed to adequately address such concerns, and argues that because the most pressing ethical dilemmas are global, a global framework must be adopted. Moreover, it argues that to adopt a local model of ethics (whether one community, one nation state or one area of jurisdiction) will fail to illuminate key issues of injustice and thus will ultimately fail as an ethical framework. In short, the global nature of current health issues requires that ethics is global. This argument is a practical one, and one which should be uncontroversial given the clear need for this response. Thus this chapter goes on to explore why, if the need for a global ethical approach is so clearly required by the global nature of health concerns, there is still a debate about whether ethics can or should be global. Thus the chapter looks briefly at the arguments against a global approach to ethics and goes on to suggest a global model of ethics which addresses at least some of these concerns.

In order to make this argument the chapter begins by outlining why only a global bioethics or ethics is appropriate. It will argue that global bioethics is necessary for both practical and ethical reasons. As a matter of practicality a global approach to bioethics is necessary as health issues are essentially global; and ethically, not to recognize the global implications of health issues is to endorse the significant injustice which occurs in the arena of global health. Given this the chapter will then go on to consider why, given the overwhelming reasons for adopting a global ethical framework, that the debate about whether ethics should be local or global is still ongoing. The chapter will finish with a brief overview of the global ethics model and will suggest that it might address some of the concerns of those who are wary of global approaches.

Global ethics and bioethics

Global ethics is an emerging and growing area – which from some perspectives includes bioethics as one subsidiary aspect necessary for effective global ethics. Others do not see global ethics as a separate field, but rather regard bioethics as the overarching discipline; one which occasionally has to address global issues as and when they are relevant to the bioethical concern they are working on. From this perspective global ethics is seen in one of two ways; either, not as an area in itself or, as essentially a sub-section of bioethics; on this view global ethics is only relevant to, or only intersects with, bioethical issues when these issues cross into the international sphere. This chapter argues that the latter is not a defensible view – and that it is no longer possible to endorse a predominantly local ethics – as bioethics tends to be – or only to be concerned with global ethics now and again when international issues arise.

The prevalence of 'local bioethics' is shown in a paper by Engelhardt, which actually argues *against* the possibility of a global bioethical framework.[1] In this paper Engelhardt endorses a specific 'American' view of bioethical norms and expectations and states that bioethics cannot be global for both economic and cultural reasons. According to Engelhardt existing (American) norms and expectations are incompatible with other cultural perspectives,[2] and therefore global bioethics is impossible. Importantly however, while he attempts to argue against global bioethics, Engelhardt actually provides an inadvertent suggestion of why it is necessary. Engelhardt's view is that the 'American' framework is incompatible with other perspectives and practices,[3] this may well be true. However, what this shows us is merely that one particular form of American, local, bioethics is inappropriate for application to the global stage, and not that all global ethical frameworks are inappropriate.

On the contrary, global frameworks are needed if contemporary ethical issues are to be addressed and this is true in bioethics no less than in other areas of ethics. This claim about global frameworks needs some justification and explanation. It is not a blanket claim – that every possible issue must be considered globally – it may well be that there are some areas where to adopt a predominantly local framework might be appropriate, for instance, if the issue is contained in a particular jurisdiction or a smaller group. This is not to say that there may be no global implications of local decisions, but rather to recognize that there are areas where local ethics is appropriate within a broader global framework (and that to demand consideration of ethical issues from a global perspective in these areas would be detrimental).

Think, for instance, of resource allocation within the NHS. While such decisions should not ignore possible global consequences (for instance, that to ban organ and egg sale in the United Kingdom might lead to more medical tourism)[4] it is appropriate that the dominant ethical framework for

---

1   Tristram H. Engelhardt, 'Critical Care: Why There Is No Global Bioethics', *Journal of Medicine and Philosophy*, 1998, 23: 643–51.
2   Ibid., 643–4, 650.
3   Ibid., 644.
4   Heather Widdows, 'Localized Past, Globalized Future: Towards an Effective Bioethical Framework Using Examples From Population Genetics and Medical Tourism', *Bioethics*,

some limited decisions is national. Accordingly the claim is not that all ethics should be global, or that there is no place whatsoever for local ethics – clearly there is. Rather the claim is that there are some areas where ethics must be global and that not to have global ethics in these areas is either to ignore the reality of practice, and thus to promote ineffective ethical frameworks which ignore key injustices. Or, and worse, it is to deliberately promote local ethics as sufficient, knowing that in fact it is not and that it only considers the rights and interests of some, in order to deliberately advantage one group over another, and thus to permit injustice. For example, Gillian Brock argues that by actively recruiting health-care workers from poor countries, wealthy countries are actively depriving the most vulnerable people around the world of adequate health care.[5] In this case, the local focus of the ethical concerns taken into consideration by wealthy countries means that those poor countries who can afford to train health-care workers are actually subsidizing the health-care costs of the wealthy.[6] This seems to be a clear case of injustice, and one which is fostered by a failure to approach the issue with a global perspective.[7]

For a local approach to be justified it must ensure that it is not ignoring pertinent information and thus endorsing or allowing injustice. Therefore, even 'narrow focus' ethics must consider those beyond the defined limit of the 'in-group' to justify a local approach – it must show that the local approach is not unjust or harmful for those beyond and outside the 'local' (however that is defined); thus to some extent a global ethical framework is necessary. Of course, when it comes to working out practice and policy, in some instances the local may dominate. However, as this chapter shows the areas in which an overtly global framework will be required are increasing and it may be that there are fewer and fewer areas where the global consequences of policy and practice are so small that a local framework can be dominant.

There are many possible contenders for global ethical frameworks; including human rights,[8] basic welfare standards,[9] cosmopolitan duties of

2011, 25: 84, 87; As has been noted elsewhere, restrictions on certain technologies in one country do not mean that wealthy persons who wish to make use of that technology will not travel to other, more permissive countries, to gain a benefit from available medical services. This is discussed in more detail later in the chapter.

5   Gillian Brock, *Global Justice: A Cosmopolitan Account* (Oxford: Oxford University Press, 2009), 198–203.

6   Ibid., 201–2.

7   Brock suggests several methods for addressing this injustice, including refusing to employ health-care workers from poor countries until they have worked for a set period of time in the country which trained them, or requiring wealthy countries to pay large subsidies of one kind or another to poor countries from which they recruit health-care workers (Brock, *Global Justice*, 201–3).

8   The United Nations General Assembly, *The Universal Declaration of Human Rights* (Paris, France: The United Nations, 1948), www.un.org/millennium/declaration/ares552e.pdf.

9   Henry Shue, *Basic Rights: Subsistence, Affluence and U.S. Foreign Policy* (Princeton, NJ: Princeton University Press, 1980).

justice,[10] international laws, standards and guidelines, capability approaches,[11] benefit sharing and trust models[12] and development goals and milestones like the Millennium Development Goals.[13] This chapter is not arguing for any one of these models, but rather suggests that some form of global scope or frame is necessary when it comes to addressing core global issues. In fact, these disparate approaches can often be used together and in complementary ways to promote effective policies which lead to more just outcomes. In this way they can all be seen as 'tools' in the 'ethical toolbox'.[14] Increasingly, this view is gaining recognition with perception of the need for global approaches becoming standard. Perhaps the most obvious examples are debates about national security and climate change,[15] where to suggest a national or local response which fails to take into account global issues is clearly ineffective. This chapter will argue that it is just as ineffective to adopt local approaches to health issues as it is to issues of security and climate change; this will be shown using examples from healthcare and medical and scientific research and practice.

The global requirement

In the climate change and security debates global ethics is regarded as necessary for three key reasons: first, global problems need global solutions; second, if

10 Simon Caney, 'Cosmopolitan Justice and Equalizing Opportunities', *Metaphilosophy*, 2001, 32: 113–34; Simon Caney, *Justice Beyond Borders: A Global Political Theory* (Oxford: Oxford University Press, 2005); Brock, *Global Justice*.

11 Martha Nussbaum, 'Capabilities as Fundamental Entitlements: Sen and Social Justice', *Feminist Economics*, 2003, 9: 35–59; Martha Nussbaum, 'Creating Capabilities: The Human Development Approach and Its Implementation', *Hyparia*, 2009, 24: 211–15; Amartya Sen, 'Development as Capabilities Expansion', *The Journal of Development Planning*, 1989, 19: 41–58.

12 Bartha Maria Knoppers, Ruth Chadwick, Hiraku Takebe, Michael Kirby, Kare Berg, Ren-Zong Qiu, et al., *HUGO Ethics Committee, Statement on Benefit Sharing* (Vancouver: Human Genome Organisation, 2000), www.hugo-international.org/img/benefit_sharing_2000.pdf; Bartha Maria Knoppers, Ruth F. Chadwick, Ishwar C. Verma, Kare Berg, Jose Maria Cantu, Abdallah Daar, et al., *HUGO Ethics Committee: Statement on Human Genomic Databases* (Singapore: Human Genome Organisation, 2002), www.hugo-international.org/img/genomic_2002.pdf; World Health Organization, *The Ethical, Legal and Social Implications of Pharmacogenomics in Developing Countries: Report of an International Group of Experts* (Geneva, Switzerland: World Health Organization, 2007), http://whqlibdoc.who.int/publications/2007/9789241595469_eng.pdf.

13 United Nations General Assembly, *United Nations Millennium Declaration* (The United Nations, 2000), www.un.org/millennium/declaration/ares552e.pdf.

14 Heather Widdows, *Global Ethics: An Introduction* (Durham: Acumen Press, 2011), 2.

15 Henry Shue, 'Ethics, the Environment and the Changing International Order', *International Affairs (Royal Institute of International Affairs*, 1995, 71: 459; Stephen M. Gardiner, 'Ethics and Global Climate Change', *Ethics*, 2004, 114: 555–6.

practice is global then non-global forms of ethics and governance are ineffective; and third, that to ignore the interconnections that exist between locations and jurisdictions leads to injustice (usually manifested in the exploitation of the weaker by the stronger or the poorer by the richer). These three conditions will form the basis for the subsequent argument for why health is global and thus why bioethics must also be global. The rationale behind these three reasons can be seen clearly if we take the environmental crisis – for some *the* overarching contemporary global ethical dilemma – as an example.[16]

First, the environmental crisis is clearly a global problem in need of a global solution. It makes little sense to construct a less than global ethical community when considering how to address global threats such as climate change – our 'shared ecological destiny'[17] means that we must have a global approach to the problems of climate change. Second, because climate change is a global problem, non-global ethics and governance will be ineffective. No nation or region can address climate change alone. Only a shared response, where everyone takes the actions necessary, will be effective. Climate change is no respecter of national borders and the behaviour of one nation or region impacts on others. For example, the risks of climate change to atoll countries are severe. Already vulnerable due to poverty, lack of resources and relative isolation, citizens of atoll countries are among those most at risk of climate-change-induced harm.[18] Atoll countries are frequently poor[19] and lack the resources which may enable them to adapt to climate change. Further, with a mean height above sea-level of around 2 m,[20] any rise in sea-level poses significant risk of harm. The sources of these emissions also suggest possible injustice; Caney notes that the United States of America and the European Union contributed 60 per cent of 'energy-related carbon emissions' between 1850 and 2000.[21] It is the wealthiest

16   Roderick comments that 'there can be no bigger dispute than over the future of our planet' (Peter E. Roderick, 'Foreword', in William C. G. Burns and Hari M. Osofsky (eds), *Adjudicating Climate Change* (Cambridge, UK; New York, NY: Cambridge University Press, 2009) vii–viii), when he discusses the importance of addressing the effects and causes of Climate Change. Similarly, McMichael states that the 'most serious potential consequence of global environmental change is the erosion of Earth's life-support systems' (Anthony J. McMichael, *Planetary Overload: Global Environmental Change and the Health of the Human Species* (Cambridge: Cambridge University Press, 1993), xiii). This human effect on our environment he argues is likely to have a devastating impact on the health prospects of all people, particularly the poor and vulnerable (Ibid., 66).

17   McMichael, *Planetary Overload*, 318.

18   Jon Barnett and Neil Adger, 'Climate Dangers and Atoll Countries', *Climatic Change*, 2003, 61: 321–2.

19   Barnett and Adger note that three of the five countries comprised entirely of low-lying atolls, Kiribati, the Maldives and Tuvalu, are on the UN's least developed countries list (Barnett & Adger, 'Climate Dangers', 322).

20   Barnett and Adger, 'Climate Dangers', 322.

21   Simon Caney, 'Justice and the Distribution of Greenhouse Gas Emissions', in Heather Widdows and Nicola J. Smith (eds), *Global Social Justice* (London and New York: Routledge, 2011), 59.

countries that have produced the majority of the climate change problem, yet it is the poorest that face the greatest risk because of it.[22]

Third, to ignore the interconnections between between locations and jurisdictions is often to ignore the unethical effects of the actions of one group on the lives of others. In climate change this is particularly clear as to do nothing is effectively to make the plight of the poorest worse – thus to actually cause harm as climate change compounds other already existing injustices such as vast wealth disparities that exist between the wealthy and the global poor.[23] We find a similar issue when considering how climate change should be addressed. Henry Shue notes that the wealthy countries, which emitted the vast majority of greenhouse gases, are now attempting to impose emission limits on poorer countries in order to reduce the speed of climate change. They are in effect demanding that other countries, which were disadvantaged by the actions of wealthy nations, pay the price of dealing with the problem.[24] Wealthy, industrialized nations created the problem of climate change, reaped the benefits of their industrialization and are now creating 'an expanding inequality'[25] through their demand for concessions from the poor.

Importantly, those who are already living a subsistence existence have no spare resources with which to cushion themselves from the effects of severe weather events caused by climate change, such as drought or flood.[26] In the event of a large increase in sea-level for example, which could be caused by the melting of the Greenland ice sheet, 'the rights to life, health, and subsistence of inhabitants of small island states and all those who live or work on the coast' would be 'devastated'.[27] Nor do the global poor have the means to attain increasingly scarce natural resources, such as water and productive land; as weather patterns change and land that was once fertile becomes uninhabitable the total resources available diminish, further endangering the most vulnerable. As well as exacerbating economic injustice, other forms of injustice also increase – in an environmentally unstable context accessing basic health and security becomes more difficult.[28] As natural resources – of fertile land, energy, water and food – become increasingly scarce the likelihood that there will be conflict to secure them increases. Such conflict need not be violent to have

---

22 See also McMichael for a brief outline of the potential impact of climate change on Bangladesh ('rising seas, cyclones, storms and flooding'), a country with roughly 2 per cent of the world's population but responsible for only 0.1 per cent of global greenhouse gas emissions (McMichael *Planetary Overload*, 319).

23 McMichael, *Planetary Overload*, 319.

24 Henry Shue, 'Global Environment and International Inequality', *International Affairs*, 1999, 75: 531–45.

25 Ibid., 533.

26 McMichael, *Planetary Overload*, 319; Barnett and Adger, 'Climate Dangers', 322.

27 Simon Caney, 'Climate Change and the Future: Discounting for Time, Wealth, and Risk', *Journal of Social Philosophy*, 2009, 40: 178.

28 Ibid., 178.

violent effects; as Barnett and Adger note, as sea-level rises,[29] and vulnerable countries have to adapt to smaller national boundaries or to displacement, the sovereignty atoll countries have over their exclusive economic zones (EEZ) may be jeopardized.[30] The loss of sovereignty, and hence economic authority, over a state's EEZ may have disastrous economic effects for such already vulnerable people. Thus an ethical focus which ignores effects beyond the local actually results in harm to others, thus meeting the third criterion.

In this example of environmental ethics the global requirement is shown. The environmental crisis requires a global ethical response for ethics to be effective. This chapter argues that if healthcare and research also fit these criteria then bioethics too should be global. Our aim in the next section is to show that the following three criteria or conditions are clearly met: that medical and scientific problems are global, that medical and scientific practice and research is global and that ignoring the global nature of such practices leads to injustice.

Healthcare and research and the global criteria

This section shows that in a parallel way as environmental ethics, healthcare and medical and scientific research and practice fit the three criteria required for a global ethic to be necessary. This has been done using five arguments and examples to show how the three conditions set out above with reference to environmental ethics, are met in the health debate.

First, and uncontroversially, many bioethical laws, norms and guidelines are already global. Thus some ideals, norms and standards, as well as some practices, are global. An obvious example is the Declaration of Helsinki, which is referred to globally and used as an international benchmark for regulating research.[31] Other examples of international governance are WHO definitions and guidelines. For example, the WHO defines health as 'a state of complete physical, mental and social well-being and not merely the absence of disease or infirmity'.[32] In addition, global health aspirations are expressed in the right to Health, part of article 25 of the Universal Declaration of Human Rights

---

29 As will almost certainly happen even in the unlikely event that all countries meet their Kyoto protocol commitments and greenhouse gas emissions cease by 2020 (Barnett & Adger, 'Climate Dangers', 323).

30 Barnett and Adger, 'Climate Dangers', 327.

31 World Medical Association General Assembly, *WMA Declaration of Helsinki – Ethical Principles for Medical Research Involving Human Subjects* (1964), www.wma.net/en/30publications/10policies/b3/index.html.pdf?print-media-type&footer-right=[page]/[toPage].

32 World Health Organization, *Preamble to the Constitution of the World Health Organization as adopted by the International Health Conference, New York, 19 June – 22 July 1946* (2006), 1: www.who.int/governance/eb/who_constitution_en.pdf.

which specifies the right to an adequate standard of living.[33] In such global governance practices the second and third conditions, as set out above, are met – current practice is global (condition two); and when global standards are not met (or are inadequately met), for instance when the declaration of Helsinki ignored, injustice occurs (condition three).

Second, medical research is global. The pharmaceutical companies who fund and engage in research are multinational corporations; the funding and practice of research takes place in multi-site settings;[34] and the resulting products, drugs and services of research are utilized and marketed globally. The AIDS pandemic and the (hugely unequal) distribution of treatment demonstrate both the global nature of health issues and the existence of world markets in health care.[35] In fact, so ingrained is the global nature of medical and scientific research, it is almost impossible to imagine what it would mean to reverse this and have 'local' research only: where drugs are developed and tested in one bounded locality, by scientists trained only within that locality from medical knowledge developed there. To deny the global community and produce bounded research communities seems so farfetched that the reality of current global practice is forcibly shown. This is true for all research. All research is global, from the testing of drugs and interventions for efficacy and safety to research on populations, such as biobank research.[36]

Biobanks and population genetics generally emphasize the global nature of research.[37] This is for a number of reasons, some of which are scientific, for instance biobanks, with their focus on population research are more effective if they are larger and contain more data;[38] however, there are also more idealistic reasons. For example, the human genome is rhetorically spoken about, for instance by HUGO, as the 'common heritage of humanity'[39] and in some sense it is regarded as belonging to all. This communal vision is clearly rhetorical

33   United Nations, *The Universal Declaration of Human Rights*, Article 25.
34   Jeremy Howells, 'The Internationalization of R & D and the Development of Global Research Networks', *Regional Studies: The Journal of the Regional Studies Association*, 1990, 24: 496–7; For example, the pharmaceutical company Glaxo (now GlaxoSmithKline) went from having two, UK-based, research centres employing 750 researchers in 1968, to having four primary international research centres and four secondary international centres by 1988 (Howells, 'The Internationalization of R & D', 501).
35   John H. Barton, 'TRIPS and the Global Pharmaceutical Market,' *Health Affairs*, 2004, 23: 146; World Health Organization, *Global Report: UNAIDS Report on the Global AIDS Epidemic 2010* (Geneva, Switzerland: World Health Organization, 2010), 20–1, 23, www.unaids.org/globalreport/documents/20101123_GlobalReport_full_en.pdf.
36   Biobank UK, *UK Biobank: Protocol for a Large-Scale Prospective Epidemiological Resource* (Stockport, UK: Biobank UK, 2007), 3, www.ukbiobank.ac.uk/docs/UKBProtocolfinal.pdf.
37   M. Asslaber and K. Zatloukal, 'Biobanks: Transnational, European and Global Networks', *Briefings in Functional Genomics & Proteomics*, 2007, 6: 197–200.
38   Ibid., 197.
39   Knoppers, Chadwick, Verma, Berg, Cantu, Daar, et al., *HUGO Ethics Committee: Statement on Human Genomic Databases*, 1.

in some cases; for instance, it is hard to sustain when genetic sequences and 'junk DNA' are routinely patented and thus kept private rather than shared. But in some areas of genetic research the communal and connective conception is overtly manifest, to return to the example of biobanking the tendency is to grow larger and connect: to construct ever larger biobanks, to link smaller biobanks to larger ones and to share between biobanks.[40] Research then is a practical manifestation of the global nature of research which meets condition two – to be ethical, local frameworks alone are not sufficient.

Third, intellectual property regimes are global, which profoundly affects not only research but also global health. The nature of intellectual property laws and norms dramatically impacts on both the sorts of diseases researched and the way in which research is carried out. For instance, consider controversies regarding the global market in drugs and the limits imposed by TRIPS on the manufacture and export of generic drugs.[41] The global nature of the market in drugs, and the effects of the TRIPS regime, dramatically limits what is available. For example, Trouiller et al. found that of the 1393 new drugs developed between 1975 and 1999, only 16 were for tropical diseases or tuberculosis.[42] The reason for this is clear, because the people that these diseases predominantly affect are poor, there is little incentive for pharmaceutical companies to invest in researching drugs for these people; the poor cannot afford to pay for drugs[43] they desperately need, and so the drugs do not get made.[44] The TRIPS regime has also created problems even for middle-income countries (and the poor in wealthy countries) as it has drastically reduced the freedom of producers of generic medicines, such as the Indian pharmaceutical industry, to produce generic versions of new drugs.[45] The TRIPS regime has thus closed off one of

40 Asslaber and Zatloukal, 'Biobanks: Transnational, European and Global Networks', 193–201; Biobank UK, *UK Biobank: Protocol for a Large-Scale Prospective Epidemiological Resource*, 16; Heather Widdows and Sean Cordell, 'The Ethics of Biobanking: Key Issues and Controversies', *Health Care Analysis*, 2011, 19: 215.

41 Barton, 'TRIPS and the Global Pharmaceutical Market', 149–50; Tim Hubbard and James Love, 'A New Trade Framework for Global Healthcare R&D', *PLoS Biology*, 2004, 2: 147; Aidan Hollis and Thomas Pogge, *The Health Impact Fund: Making New Medicines Accessible for All* (New Haven, Connecticut: Incentives for Global Health, 2008), 3, www.yale.edu/macmillan/igh/hif_book.pdf; Amitava Banerjee, Aidan Hollis and Thomas Pogge, 'The Health Impact Fund: Incentives for Improving Access to Medicines', *The Lancet*, 2010, 375: 166.

42 Patrice Trouiller, Peiro Olliaro, Els Torreele, James Orbinski, Richard Laing, and Nathan Ford, 'Drug Development for Neglected Diseases: A Deficient Market and a Public-Health Policy Failure', *The Lancet*, 2002, 359: 2188.

43 As William Ryan notes 'the facts are plain: their health is bad. The cause is plain: health costs money, and they don't have money' (*Blaming the Victim: Revised, Updated Edition* (New York: Pantheon Books, 1971), 170).

44 Alimuddin Zumla (in 'Drugs for Neglected Diseases', *The Lancet: Infectious Diseases*, 2002, 2: 393) (among others) has also noted that only 10 per cent of all research funding for new drugs is spent on the diseases which account for 90per cent of the global burden of disease. See also Hollis & Pogge, *The Health Impact Fund*, 5 and Thomas Pogge, *World Poverty and Human Rights Second Edition* (Cambridge: Polity Press, 2008), 236.

45 Barton, 'TRIPS and the Global Pharmaceutical Market', 147–9.

the only sources of cheap essential medicines that the poor could access.[46] This again speaks to all three conditions; the problem of lack of access to affordable and effective drugs is global (condition 1); the legislation is currently global (condition 2); and currently injustices result from not taking global conditions into account (condition 3).

Fourth, medical and reproductive tourism is globalized. The medical tourist moves from one legislative area to another in order to obtain treatment or procedures that are not available (or are less easily available) in their own country. Medical tourism includes travelling to Switzerland for physician-assisted suicide;[47] travelling to countries with public health services to access free or cheap treatment;[48] travelling for cheaper cosmetic surgery (sometimes combined with holidays in the sun: the 'cut and beach');[49] and travelling to relatively poor counties to purchase organs from live 'donors'.[50] It also includes 'reproductive tourism'.[51] Reproductive tourism is very similar to medical tourism for the purchase of transplantable organs, with the difference that what are bought and sold are human eggs or sperm.[52] Not only is medical tourism by definition international, as it only happens because one travels between nations, but also, as evidenced in the organ and gamete markets, it is certainly global: shown well in the recent films like 'Google Baby'[53] – where eggs are bought on-line from US donors, gestated in Indian wombs, for Israeli recipients – and 'Made in India'[54] which documents the practice of surrogacy warehousing.[55] Again all three conditions are met – and the third ethical condition very starkly.

Fifth – and glaringly obvious – is the global nature of health threats. The interconnectedness of populations means that health threats, such as pandemics, are always global. Think of the trajectory of AIDS, which as Farmer puts it,

46   Ibid., 150.
47   BBC News Online, 'Dignitas: Swiss Suicide Helpers', *BBC News: Health* (2009), http://news. bbc.co.uk/2/hi/4643196.stm.
48   John Connell, 'Medical Tourism: Sea, Sun, Sand and . . . Surgery', *Tourism Management*, 2006, 27: 1096–7.
49   While not specializing in cosmetic surgery, Thailand, for example, has been a destination for those seeking sex change operations since the 1970s (Connell, 'Medical Tourism', 1095).
50   Nancy Scheper-Hughes, 'A Beastly Trade in "Parts": The Organ Market is Dehumanizing the World's Poor', *Los Angeles Times*, 29 July 2003, B.15; Nancy Scheper-Hughes, 'Keeping an Eye on the Global Traffic in Human Organs', *The Lancet*, 2003, 361: 1645–8.
51   Antony Barnett and Helena Smith, 'Cruel Cost of the Human Egg Trade', *Observer*, 29 April 2006, 6.
52   Guido Pennings, 'Reproductive Tourism as Moral Pluralism in Motion', *Journal of Medical Ethics*, 28 (2002), 337.
53   Z. Brand Frank, *Google Baby* (Brandcom Productions and HBO Documentary Films, 2009).
54   R. Haimowitz and V. Sinha, *Made in India* (Women Make Movies, 2010).
55   For a discussion of some of the (many) ethical concerns surrounding egg sale or donation, see (Heather Widdows, 'Border Disputes across Bodies: Exploitation in Trafficking for Prostitution and Egg Sale for Stem Cell Research', *International Journal of Feminist Approaches to Bioethics*, 2009, 2: 10–16).

has 'brought connections, not discontinuities, into relief'[56] – AIDS is certainly a global threat (although the resulting burdens fall differently depending on the resources of different countries). Other more recent threats – such as Severe Acute Respiratory Syndrome (SARS)[57] or Swine Flu (H1N1)[58] also demonstrate the increasingly global nature of infectious disease, arguably facilitated by the greater prevalence of cheap international travel.[59] No longer can such infectious diseases be regarded as containable in one nation or locality – in practice they are global (meeting condition 2) and furthermore, they are clearly global problems requiring global solutions (meeting condition 1).

Taken together these five examples, of global governance, global research, global IP regimes, medical tourism and global health threats, show that scientific and medical practice and research are already global and therefore that the bioethics framework we must adopt, in at least most instances, is global. As we have laid out, medical and scientific research and practice fit the three conditions for global ethics clearly: first, at least some medical and scientific problems need global solutions; disease is no respecter of borders. Second, medical and scientific practice is global so effective ethics and governance must also be global. Third, exploitation and injustice happens as a direct result of ignoring the interconnections that exist between locations and justifications – shown clearly in the different aspects of medical and reproductive tourism as well as in the examples of research and IP regimes.

When we consider global health, all three conditions of global ethics are met and therefore any form of effective bioethics must be global for at least some aspects of ethical deliberation. This is not to claim that there must be a single, one size fits all, practice. Nor is it to claim that all health policies should be homogenized or standardized: policy and practices must be implemented locally and be context-specific and appropriate. However, we do claim that the framework within which locally appropriate practices are implemented must be global and take the needs of others beyond the local into account for effective ethics and governance. Moreover, the examples show how strong the claims are for a global understanding of both global health and global ethics. It is simply absurd to think that health research could be local; that laws and governance procedures can be separate; or that disease and health care can be local. Given the strength of the reasons for adopting a global ethical approach, then it seems strange that chapters like this still need to be written. Why this is still the case we consider in the next section.

56   Paul Farmer, *Infections and Inequalities: The Modern Plagues* (Berkeley, CA: University of California Press, 1999), 23.
57   NHS Choices, 'SARS (Severe Acute Respiratory Syndrome)', *NHS Choices* (2010), www.nhs. uk/conditions/SARS/Pages/Introduction.aspx.
58   NHS Choices, 'What Is Swine Flu (H1N1)?', *NHS Choices* (2011), www.nhs.uk/chq/ Pages/2886.aspx?CategoryID=5&SubCategoryID=5.
59   Andrew T. Price-Smith, *The Health of Nations: Infectious Disease, Climate Change, and Their Effects on National Security and Development*, (Cambridge, MA: The MIT Press, 2002), 4.

Why the local/global debate continues

As we have seen the conditions for global ethics are overtly met in the health debate; undoubtedly then a global ethical approach is required. Given this, should we not move directly to ensuring the appropriateness and robustness of a global approach? However, as is so often the case, it is not quite so simple, as it is still a live debate whether we should be seeking global ethics or bioethics at all. For example, proponents of the Asian Values Movement argue that western, individualist values are contradictory to eastern, communitarian norms, as a result of the incompatibility of the two sets of values, a truly global ethics or bioethics is impossible;[60] further, as noted above, proponents of 'western' ethical approaches have also made similar arguments.[61] The argument of this chapter is that to continue in the debate of whether to have a global ethics is to ignore the reality of medical and scientific research and practice. As we have seen, there are overwhelming reasons – both practical and ethical – to adopt a global framework. But before moving to explore how this can be done we first revisit this debate to consider why the arguments set out above, despite their strength, seem not to have been heeded as one might expect. Especially, as shown in condition 3, not to recognize the reality of the need for global ethics, is to fail to address global exploitation – something which is particularly obvious when global standards are not applied in scientific research or in the practices of medical tourism. To fail to develop global standards allows exploitation to continue; moreover, to refuse to develop a global ethical response does nothing to prevent the onward march of global scientific and medical practice. It simply means that we have inadequate ethics and governance tools to address these. Given this, why then are ethicists sincerely arguing against developing global ethical tools?[62] Clearly they are not doing it because they wish to encourage injustice, therefore they must have reasons they believe to be good.

The most common reason that people argue against global ethics is not because they reject the notion of global ethical norms per se, but rather because they worry about the type of global ethics that would be presented. This argument has been made by those who are worried that any global ethics, would essentially be a western and individualistic ethic – one which they believe is unrepresentative and fails to protect individuals and groups. Such arguments have been presented most robustly by a number of Asian and African thinkers – something which has been addressed in detail elsewhere – therefore for the purposes of this chapter a brief overview will suffice.[63]

---

60   Heather Widdows, 'Is Global Ethics Moral Neo-Colonialism? An Investigation of the Issue in the Context of Bioethics', *Bioethics*, 2007, 21: 306–7; Heather Widdows, 'Western and Eastern Principles and Globalised Bioethics', *Asian Bioethics Review*, 2011, 3: 15.

61   Engelhardt, 'Critical Care'.

62   Ibid.

63   Widdows, 'Is Global Ethics Moral Neo-Colonialism?'

Perhaps the strongest voice against global ethics comes from the Asian values movement; again something which has been discussed in more detail in previous work.[64] This movement is primarily associated with Singapore and Malaysia but elements have spread across the Asian world and indeed to much of the developing world. For instance, it is endorsed by Chinese scholars – and even some African scholars.[65] Those who promote this view not only argue that there are 'different' Asian values, but they are also very critical of 'western values';[66] values which, importantly they believe, would be the values promoted by any global ethical approach. The Asian values movement is contentious and we do not wish to enter the debate about its status and validity here, as to do so would be to merely reproduce earlier work.[67] Rather we only introduce it to show the views of those who reject 'global ethics' because they believe that 'global' in this context is merely a euphemism for 'western', and the Asian values movement is fairly representative of those who claim that global, 'Western' ethics is incompatible with 'Eastern' ethics.

64   Particularly vocal in the proposal of Asian values are leaders of Malaysia and Singapore, especially Lee Kuan Yew, former PM of Singapore and Dr Mahathir bin Mohamad, former PM of Malaysia. See for example, Khoo Boo Teik, *Beyond Mahathir: Malaysian politics and its discontents* (London: Zed Books, 2003) and Chandra Muzaffar, *Rights, Religion, and Reform: Enhancing Human Dignity through Spiritual and Moral Transformation* (London: Routledge, 2002). The Asian values movement argues that western values (most particularly those implied in human rights) are alien to the values of Asian countries and communities who endorse not western individual values, but communitarian values which support the political and religious order, which emphasize hard work and thriftiness, which are linked to business and government and which promote loyalty to the family and the wider community. Asian values are especially associated with Malaysia and Singapore, although they have also been endorsed more broadly in the non-western world, by thinkers and politicians across Asia and Africa; for example, Michael D. Barr, *Cultural Politics and Asian Values: The Tepid War* (London and New York: Routledge, 2002); Joanne R. Bauer and Daniel A. Bell, *The East Asian Challenge for Human Rights* (Cambridge: Cambridge University Press, 1999). See also Widdows, 'Is Global Ethics Moral Neo-Colonialism?', Widdows, 'Localized Past, Globalized Future' and Widdows, 'Western and Eastern Principles'.

65   The concept of Asian values has spread across the developing world to, for example, China where Confucianism has been seen as the source of such values and invoked 'as the native cultural ground on which to reject human rights concepts as alien, culture-bound, western impositions' (Widdows, 'Western and Eastern Principles', 22).

66   Mahathir has not only praised Asian values but has been a staunch critic of contemporary 'western values'. According he states that in the West 'the community has given way to the individual and his desires. The inevitable consequence has been the breakdown of established institutions and diminished respect for marriage, family values, elders, and important customs, conventions, and traditions. These have been replaced by a new set of values based on the rejection of all that relates to spiritual faith and communal life': (Mahathir cited in Barr, *Cultural Politics and Asian Values*, note 3, 3). For further details on how the Asian values movement has been received in the countries of its creation see Muzaffar, *Rights, Religion and Reform*, and Teik, *Beyond Mahathir*.

67   See, for example, Widdows, 'Is Global Ethics Moral Neo-Colonialism?'; Heather Widdows, 'Conceptualising the Self in the Genetic Era', *Health Care Analysis* 2007, 15: 5–12, and Widdows, 'Western and Eastern Principles'.

As discussed in previous papers, those who espouse the 'neo-colonialism' argument,[68] claim that the West endorses broadly individual moral values – those of autonomy, freedom and choice – and that the East endorses broadly communal values – respect for community, relationships and family and the 'good life' rooted in community.[69] To give a caricature of this debate, the moral agents who exhibit these values are diametrically opposed. The 'western' moral agent is an autonomous, isolated, free, choosing individual and the Asian moral agent is a connected, community-defined, relational-being. So different are these persons that they could almost be different species.

This divide is clearly false; something that has previously been argued in more detail.[70] Western individuals are not these isolated beings making choices in a vacuum. To present western individuals as making judgements outside their culture and background is to simply ignore the historically and socially constructed nature of all human beings. It is almost impossible to imagine this isolated moral agent and certainly they are not human. The Eastern picture – of an amalgamated creature, conjoined to relations and family with no distinguishable personhood or identity, is no better. Such a person would be entirely passive and lack any sense of self, preference, decision-making and would even lack the ability to form relationships – again not a realistic picture of human being.

Therefore, at most there is a spectrum with a tendency for some ethical systems to prioritize some values and for others to prioritize other values. However, all ethical systems must – if they wish to represent real human beings and their decisions – take into account both the communal and individual aspects of human agency. Hence arguments made elsewhere about the need to ensure that ethical models take into account group and communal goods as well as individual goods for effective ethics and bioethics.[71] Likewise, it is also not accurate to suggest that all western ethics has such a strong focus on autonomy and the individual, indeed to dismiss western ethics on these grounds is to ignore the richness of western ethical discourse. This is again an argument that has been made elsewhere in terms of ethical theory; for instance, it has been argued previously that virtue ethicists and feminist ethicists do not fit this caricature.[72] Virtue ethicists are concerned with character and not individual action and they are particularly critical of focusing on 'individual

---

68 Widdows, 'Is Global Ethics Moral Neo-Colonialism?', 305.

69 Ibid., 306; Widdows, 'Western and Eastern Principles', 15.

70 Widdows, 'Is Global Ethics Moral Neo-Colonialism?', 306. Widdows, 'Western and Eastern Principles', 15.

71 Heather Widdows and Sean Cordell, 'Why Communities and Their Goods Matter: Illustrated with the Example of Biobanks', *Public Health Ethics* 2011, 4: 14–25, 16–19, 22–3.

72 See for example Widdows, 'Conceptualising the Self', 5–12. Widdows, 'Is Global Ethics Moral Neo-Colonialism?', 306, 309–11, and Rosmarie Tong, 'Towards a Feminist Global Bioethics: Addressing Women's Health Concerns Worldwide,' *Health Care Analysis*, 2001, 9: 229–46.

choice'. Moreover, they focus on human flourishing understood in relational, historical and communal terms. Increasingly virtue theories, such as those suggested by Iris Murdoch,[73] Rosalind Hursthouse,[74] Phillippa Foot,[75] and Virginia Held,[76] are mainstream either as theories in their own right or as they influence and change other mainstream ethics, such as utilitarianism and Kantianism.[77] Likewise, feminist ethicists critique the dominant, highly individualist, western construction of ethics.[78] They emphasize the importance of difference and promote the values of social justice over individual choice.[79] And almost all feminists (including liberal feminists) suggest that, at the very least, the over-individualist liberal (and feminists would argue male) model needs supplementing and reforming. There are also more practical examples, for instance, and very obviously, the one we considered earlier of environmental ethics as a response to climate change. In the environmental ethics debate it is overtly communities and common goods – for example, access to natural resources such as clean water, fertile land, energy and food – which are the focus of the debate. Obligations to future generations are also central to the

73   Iris Murdoch, *Metaphysics as a Guide to Morals* 1st edn (New York: Allen Lane, Penguin Press, 1993), 241; Iris Murdoch, 'Vision and Choice in Morality', in *Existentialists and Mystics: Writings on Philosophy and Literature* (New York: Allen Lane, Penguin Press, 1998), 87.

74   Rosalind Hursthouse, 'Virtue Theory and Abortion', *Philosophy & Public Affairs*, 1991, 20(3): 223–46; Rosalind Hursthouse, *On Virtue Ethics* (Oxford: Oxford University Press, 2001).

75   Phillipa Foot, *Virtues and Vices and Other Essays in Moral Philosophy*, (Berkeley, CA: University of California Press, 1978); Philippa Foot, 'Utilitarianism and the Virtues', *Mind*, 1985, 94: 196–209.

76   Virginia Held, 'Care and Justice in the Global Context', *Ratio Juris*, 2004, 17: 143; Virginia Held, *The Ethics of Care: Personal, Political, and Global*, (Oxford: Oxford University Press, 2006).

77   Utilitarians and Kantians have welcomed many of the critiques of virtue ethics at least as a reminder that key areas of moral philosophy have been ignored and should be reassessed and virtue ethics is often regarded as an addition to the dominant theories rather than an alternative theory in itself. For example, Marcia Baron states that 'much of what most virtue ethicists want is actually part of Kant's ethics . . . in instances where it lacks some valuable elements of a virtue approach, many contemporary Kantians (myself included) see many of the virtue ethicists' criticisms as helpful suggestions that Kantians can utilize as they press forward with the Kantian project' (Marcia Baron, Philip Pettit and Michael A. Slote, *Three Methods of Ethics: A Debate* (Malden, MA: Blackwell Publishers Ltd, 1997), 33). See also Marcia Baron, *Kantian Ethics Almost without Apology* (Ithaca: Cornell University Press, 1995).

78   Jean Hampton, *Political Philosophy*, (Boulder, CO: Westview Press, 1997), 169–72, 182.

79   See for example, Anne Donchin and Laura Purdy, *Embodying Bioethics. Recent Feminist Advances* (Oxford: Rowman & Littlefield Publishers, 1999); Susan M. Okin, 'Mistresses of Their Own Destiny: Group Rights, Gender and Realistic Rights of Exit', *Ethics*, 2002, 112: 205–30; Ayelet Shachar, 'Group Identity and Women's Rights in Family Law: The Perils of Multicultural Accommodation', *Journal of Political Philosophy*, 1998, 6: 285–305; Tong, 'Towards a Feminist Global Bioethics', 229–46; Susan Wolf, *Feminism and Bioethics: beyond Reproduction* (New York: Oxford University Press, 1996).

debate on climate change. For example, Attfield discusses the role that current generations have in determining which future generations will come to live and the resources that they will have access to.[80] Again, this shows that groups (both current and future) and common, as well as individual, goods are not unimportant in western ethics.

Accordingly, for both ethical reasons – that 'western ethics' is not a wholly individualist, autonomy focused theory – and for practical reasons – that shared and communal goods are important in both the East and West – the criticisms of any global ethics should be dismissed. This does not mean that some examples of global ethics should not be criticized, but rather that to dismiss all global ethics, irrespective of what the ethic endorses makes no sense. Worse, it has bad consequences as it ignores reality and fails to do the ethical work necessary to ensure just practice. For the very pressing reasons laid out in the first section of this chapter we must not indulge in this local/global debate.[81] Rather, practically, because medical and scientific practice is already global, and for ethical reasons, because individuals and groups and the goods which accrue to them need protection, ethics must be global, comprehensive and representative and flexible. There are many ways in which this could be done, and we touched on some of these earlier; for instance, Human Rights approaches, minimal standards and capability approaches. Moreover, all of these have merits and could be used, together or separately, and to greater and lesser extents in different models.

A global ethics approach

The final section of the chapter will suggest one way in which these different models can be brought together and in a way which meets at least some of the concerns of those who object to global ethics for fear of the promotion of a 'western ethics'. This global ethics approach is one where global ethics is not simply about overtly international issues, where the ethical issues happen to stretch beyond borders, rather it requires a fundamental commitment to including global concerns in *all* ethical reasoning and decision-making. This is a recognizable approach which increasingly those who work in global ethics share and it adopts a broad but identifiable methodology – a very simple one – one which does not prioritize the interests of one group over another. Broadly

---

80   Robin Attfield, 'Ecological Issues of Justice', in Heather Widdows and Nicola J. Smith (eds), *Global Social Justice: Rethinking Globalizations* (London and New York: Routledge, 2011), 82–9.
81   Miltos Ladikas and Doris Schroeder, 'Too Early for Global Ethics?', *Cambridge Quarterly of Healthcare Ethics*, 2005, 14: 404–15, make a similar claim when they argue that normative ethics must be global.

speaking, those in this group include many cosmopolitan political theorists (including, Thomas Pogge,[82] Henry Shue,[83] Simon Caney,[84] Gillian Brock[85] and Darrel Moellendorf);[86] as well as moral philosophers working on global justice and applied ethics (Onora O'Neill and Peter Singer are perfect examples).[87] As well those working on development and capability approaches (most obviously, Amartya Sen and Martha Nussbaum),[88] and in global health (Pogge again, for instance in the proposals for a 'Health Impact Fund',[89] Norman Daniels is also a prominent example).[90]

This is not to suggest that our intention is to suggest a particular global ethic, it is not, or that these thinkers are engaging in a particular disciplinary approach. Rather it is simply to recognize that there are some very broad themes emerging which characterize global ethical approaches. These themes share three characteristics or elements, and together these broadly constitute conditions for global ethics; first, its frame is global, second, it is multidisciplinary and third, it combines theory and practice.[91] This said, global ethics is a broad school and while there are recognizably shared traits, they cover an exceptionally large range of positions and commitments. Thus the phrase 'global ethics' is meant as a general frame – to distinguish fully global from merely local approaches

82   Pogge, *World Poverty and Human Rights*.
83   Shue, *Basic Rights*.
84   Caney, 'Cosmopolitan Justice'; Caney, *Justice Beyond Borders*.
85   Brock, *Global Justice*.
86   Darrel Moellendorf, *Cosmopolitan Justice*, (Boulder, CO: Westview Press, 2002); Darrel Moellendorf, *Global Inequality Matters* (Houndmills, Basingstoke, UK: Palgrave Macmillan, 2009).
87   Onora O'Neill, 'Justice, Capabilities and Vulnerabilities', in Martha Nussbaum and Jonathan Glover (eds), *Women, Culture, and Development: A Study of Human Capabilities* (Oxford: Clarendon Press, 1995), 140–52; Onora O'Neill, *Civic and Cosmopolitan Justice* (Kansas: Department of Philosophy, University of Kansas, 2000); Onora O'Neill, *The Bounds of Justice* (Cambridge, UK: Cambridge University Press, 2000); Peter Singer, 'Famine, Affluence, and Morality', *Philosophy and Public Affairs*, 1972, 1: 229–43.
88   Sen, 'Development as Capabilities Expansion'; Amartya Sen, *Development as Freedom* (New York: Knopf, 1999); Martha Nussbaum, *Women and Human Development: The Capabilities Approach* (Cambridge: Cambridge University Press, 2000); Nussbaum, 'Capabilities as Fundamental Entitlements'; Nussbaum, 'Creating Capabilities'.
89   Hollis and Pogge, 'The Health Impact Fund'; Bannerjee, Hollis and Pogge, 'The Health Impact Fund'.
90   Norman Daniels, *Just Health Care* (Cambridge: Cambridge University Press, 1985); Norman Daniels, 'Social Responsibility and Global Pharmaceutical Companies', *Developing World Bioethics*, 2001, 1: 38–41; Norman Daniels, *Just Health: Meeting Health Needs Fairly* (Cambridge: Cambridge University Press, 2008); Norman Daniels, 'Is There a Right to Health Care and, if so, What Does It Encompass?', in Helga Kuhse and Peter Singer (eds), *A Companion to Bioethics*, (Oxford, UK: Wiley-Blackwell, 2009), 362–72; Norman Daniels and James E. Sabin, *Setting Limits Fairly: Learning to Share Resources for Health Second Edition*, (New York, USA: Oxford University Press, 2008).
91   Heather Widdows, *Global Ethics: An Introduction* (Durham: Acumen, 2011), 6.

which are applied to global questions (again this is something that is set out in more detail elsewhere).[92]

First, the global ethics approach has a global scope – the area of ethical concern is not limited by national boundaries, and the rights and interests of all are significant. Thus when any ethical dilemma is considered the needs of all must be recognized even if they cannot all be addressed in the response. The global scope of global ethics is not something new to applied ethics, however; while applied ethics *can* be global in scope (e.g. as Onora O'Neil's work often is, see *Faces of Hunger: An Essay on Poverty, Justice, and Development*),[93] there are many examples where in fact 'narrow scope' or 'local' ethics is biased and limited. Such limitations may be caused either by specific concerns – for instance, for national or professional interests (as in many professional ethics) – or because priority is given to the needs of a particular ethnic, geographical or simply a wealthy or powerful group – to the detriment of those non-members who are vulnerable.[94] There are two ways in which the 'global in scope' criterion is evident in global ethics: it necessitates a global framework and it requires that the actions and obligations of individuals, associations and institutions, irrespective of location are taken into account.

In terms of framework – ethical frames, within which decision-making occurs, must be global. In any ethical analysis, it is the global that constitutes the sphere of concern and thus the needs and perspectives of all global actors are relevant. Given this, not surprisingly, many global ethicists are cosmopolitan (though some do deny cosmopolitanism), while others are 'weak' cosmopolitans (who recognize only some global duties). What is important is that the needs of all – rather than one locality or group – are considered as relevant to the ethical discussion. In this way the global scope of ethical discourse is recognized and the rights and interests of those not directly the focus of discussion are not forgotten. This does not mean that it is always possible to meet the needs of all or necessarily to give them equal weight. The best possible solutions may be less than perfect and it is of course justified to work practically in a particular locality, but it does mean that the needs of all must be visible. The second

---

92 Ibid.

93 Onora O'Neill, *Faces of Hunger: An Essay on Poverty, Justice, and Development* (London: G. Allen & Unwin, 1986).

94 Gillian Brock's example, mentioned above, of wealthy countries recruiting health care workers from poor countries that cannot afford to lose them is illuminating (*Global Ethics*, 199–203); in this case, locally ethically acceptable practice has severe negative effects at the global level. From a local perspective, such practices could be seen as ethically sound, in virtue of their egalitarian hiring practices for example. However, as noted above, by failing to take into account the impact that the emigration of (expensively trained) health care workers can have on poor countries, those wealthy governments which benefit from international recruitment, justified on local ethical grounds, are causing harm to people living in countries from which health care workers migrate (Ibid., 201–2).

consequence of the global scope condition is that the duties of individuals, associations and institutions are all relevant. Therefore, just as the rights and interests of all must be considered in analysing any dilemma so all actors and their duties must be considered in the solution – ethics cannot just be about the actions of individuals *or* just about systems it must account for both.

The second criterion of global ethics – which fits bioethics well – is that it is multidisciplinary. This is an obvious requirement of any ethics which wishes to engage with contemporary dilemmas. Moral or political-philosophical analysis on its own is clearly insufficient to engage with contemporary ethical problems. We require expertise from across the spectrum: from economists, lawyers, scientists, sociologists, as well as from the practitioner arenas of activists and policy-makers. If we take seriously the global frame of ethics then the need for multidisciplinary expertise is obvious – this clearly is the *only* effective way to do global ethics and governance.

The third distinctive constituent of global ethics is the insistence that theory and practice are interrelated, again well suited to bioethics. Ethicists must take seriously the 'real world' work of policy-makers, practitioners and activists, combining the analysis of practical case studies with rigorous theoretical examination. Theory and practice must be seen as necessary parts of the same pursuit rather than separable endeavours to be conducted in separate spheres and disciplines. If the goal of global ethics is to effect change, effective global ethics cannot remain isolated in an ivory tower of pure philosophical theory.

Taken together these three elements define the emerging area of global ethics. Furthermore, while global ethics does not endorse a single global ethic its three identifiable characteristics of being global in scope, multidisciplinary and connecting theory and practice do suggest a broad commitment to justice and a general bias towards the poor and vulnerable (something that is not always obvious in much of applied ethics, and arguably particularly lacking in bioethics). By considering the needs of all, global ethics results in foregrounding the needs of the worst off and highlighting the often desperate plight of those who are disadvantaged, economically, socially, politically and culturally.

Conclusion

This chapter has shown that practically and ethically there are strong reasons for thinking that bioethics must be global and that if it is not it will be inadequate at best and at worst will permit, or even encourage, injustice (particularly to those who are most vulnerable and not part of a group with status and power). In addition, it has sought to show that the need to address such injustices and for bioethics to be global is strong enough to overturn claims that we should not attempt to engage with global bioethics. There certainly are questions about what global ethics and bioethics should be, but to deny the need of a global framework is simply to fail to engage in the debate, and worse, to permit injustice. The final section of the chapter introduced a global ethics approach which may be of some use in rethinking global bioethics.

4

Needs, Obligations and International Relations for Global Health in the Twenty-First Century

Solomon R. Benatar

There is a crisis in the world today, now felt even by those of us who enjoy the power and privilege at the top of the world. There is a crisis of violence, . . . There is a crisis of misery, and threat of poverty . . . There is a crisis of repression, and threat of repression of all human rights . . . There is a crisis in the environment . . . At the root of the crises is not resource scarcity or price increases or population pressure, but the world structure.[1]

Introduction

Global health has increasingly become a major focus of interest in recent years. The context is a world that, while greatly transformed by spectacular advances in science and medicine and major growth of the economy, is characterized by widening disparities in health, well-being and the achievement of human rights.[2] Such a world, shaped by powerful social, economic and political forces (particularly over the past 30 years through economic polices associated with neo-liberal ideology) that have benefited a small proportion of the world's population maximally and the rest minimally (if at all), is now under severe threat.

This is evidenced by several longstanding trends, most recently the global economic crisis, that have serious implications for health. Inadequate constraints on financial and other trading processes, excessive consumption within a consumerist way of life associated with endless entitlements and economic policies that are designed to ensure accumulation of wealth by a few have

1 Johan Galtung, *True Worlds* (New York: Free Press, 1981).
2 Solomon R. Benatar, 'Global Disparities in Health and Human Rights: A Critical Commentary', *American Journal of Public Health*, 1998, 88: 295–300; Solomon R. Benatar, 'Millennial Challenges for Medicine and Modernity', *J Roy Coll Phys Lond*, 1998, 32: 160–5; Solomon R. Benatar and Gillian Brock (eds), *Global Health and Global Health Ethics* (Cambridge: Cambridge University Press, 2011).

entrenched and exacerbated widespread poverty and poor health for many.[3] Almost 50 per cent of all people in the world lack access to even the most basic health care, and live under conditions of severe poverty and environmental degradation in both rural and urban contexts.[4] People of color, females and the very young are heavily overrepresented among the global poor.

Disparities in health and well-being at a global level

Wide disparities in quality of life, health and access to health care can be succinctly illustrated with a few statistics: (i) life expectancy at birth ranges from about 40 years in such countries as Sierra Leone, Angola and Afghanistan to over 80 years in others such as Japan, Switzerland and Australia; (ii) mortality in children under 5 years of age ranges from less than 5:1,000 live births to over 180:1,000 live births; (iii) maternal mortality is a high of 1 in 7 pregnancies in Somalia and as low as 1 in 11,000 pregnancies in Canada; (iv) annual per capita expenditures on health care is below $15 in many poor countries, over $8,000 in the United States, and averages about $4,000 in many countries.

Africa is the region most severely afflicted by poverty, infectious diseases and premature deaths. Of over 800,000 deaths globally from malaria each year 91 per cent are in Africa, with 85 per cent of such African deaths in children under 5 years of age. Five million African children under 5 years old die each year of preventable diseases. Of 33 million people who were living with HIV in the world in 2008, 22 million were in Africa. Of the estimated 536,000 annual maternal deaths globally, 99 per cent occur in developing countries. Eighteen million deaths each year (one-third of all deaths) are due to poverty-related causes with 50 per cent of these deaths in children under 5 years of age.[5] Chronic diseases are also increasing globally bringing new challenges to health systems in both rich and poor countries.[6]

Disparities within countries are also striking. So, for example, in the United States, CEO earnings compared to average workers have increased from 25-fold in the 1970s to 90-fold in 2,000 and to 500-fold in 2004. Between 1980 and 2006, the wealthiest 1 per cent of Americans tripled their after tax per cent of national income, while the share of the bottom 90 per cent dropped

3   Solomon R. Benatar, Stephen Gill, Isabella Bakker, 'Global Health and the Global Economic Crisis', *American Journal of Public Health*, 2011, 101(4): 646–53.
4   Global Health Watch, *Global Health Watch 2005–2006* (London: Zed Books, 2007).
5   See many chapters in Benatar and Brock (eds) *Global Health and Global Health Ethics*, for these and other factual data on disparities.
6   Abdallah S. Daar, Peter A. Singer, Deepa Leah Persad, Stig K. Pramming, David R. Matthews, Robert Beaglehole, et al., 'Grand challenges in chronic non-communicable diseases', *Nature*, 2007, 450: 494–6.

by 20 per cent. Between 2002 and 2006, 75 per cent of national economic growth went to the top 1 per cent who own 70 per cent of national wealth. Four hundred US billionaires own more than 155 million Americans combined. The US health care system is the most expensive in the world, yet 50 million citizens are without health care, and the United States ranks thirty-seventh in health status in the world. Almost one-and-a-half million Americans filed for bankruptcy in 2009, a 32 per cent increase from 2008. Medical bankruptcies accounted for 60 per cent, and 75 per cent of these were filed by people with health insurance.[7]

Global health

Interest in global health has developed against a background of longstanding involvement in international health that has its focus on health across regional or national boundaries and on the provision of health care assistance in one form or another by health personnel or organizations from some areas or nations (usually wealthy) to other (usually poorer) people or nations.[8] As Ross Upshur and I have described elsewhere, global health goes beyond this. While its scope remains contested, it can be thought of as:

> the science and art of preventing disease, prolonging life and promoting physical and mental health through organized global efforts for the maintenance of a safe environment, the control of communicable disease, the education of individuals and whole populations in principles of personal hygiene and safe living habits, the organization of health care services for the early diagnosis, prevention and treatment of disease, and attention to the societal, cultural and economic determinants of health that could ensure a standard of living and education for all that is adequate for the achievement and maintenance of good health.[9]

In the chapter referred to above we have also suggested that paraphrasing Richard Lewontin in his book 'Biology as Ideology'[10] allows a view of global health as:

> a social concept about which there is a great deal of misunderstanding, even among those who are part of it. Those who work on global health view the topic through a lens that has been moulded by their social experience.

7   David DeGraw, 'The Economic Elite Have Engineered an Extraordinary Coup, Threatening the Very Existence of the Middle Class', 2010, www.alternet.org/economy/145667.
8   Paul K. Drain, Stephen A. Huffman, Sara E. Pyrtle and Kevin Chan, *Caring for the World: A Guidebook to Global Health Opportunities* (Toronto: University of Toronto Press, 2009).
9   Solomon R. Benatar and Ross Upshur, 'What is Global Health?', in Benatar and Brock (eds) *Global Health and Global Health Ethics*.
10   Richard C. Lewontin, *Biology as Ideology* (New York: Harper Collins, 1991).

David Stuckler and Martin McKee have described five metaphors that could be applied to global health.[11] *Global health as foreign policy* (here the motive is political and relates to strategic interests and economic growth); *Global health as security* (where the primary aim is to protect against infectious diseases and bioterrorism); *Global health as charity* (emphasizes 'victims' and the consequences of poverty and disempowerment); *Global health as investment* (based on the idea that improving health is a major factor in maximizing economic growth). Finally and perhaps most plausibly, *Global health as public health* has the purpose of decreasing the global burden of disease, and most especially those diseases that make up the largest proportion of this burden. These authors acknowledge considerable overlap between the attitudes that lie behind these perspectives and that powerful nations will differ on which they consider to be their dominant priority.

Processes contributing to widening disparities in health

It is interesting to recall that improved health and life-expectancy for many were achieved during the industrialization era in 'developed countries' (through improvements in the social conditions of life) long before modern medical treatments became available. For example, with better nutrition and living conditions in the United Kingdom the annual mortality rate from tuberculosis fell from 500 per 100,000 people in 1750 to 50 per 100,000 in the early 1940s before anti-tuberculosis medications were discovered.

Between 1945 and 1970, a second wave of improvements in health and well-being followed through reconstruction of a global economy that had been severely compromised by the Great Depression and two World Wars. Job creation, widespread use of innovative technology, regulation of banking and other financial activities, appropriate redistributive mechanisms and strengthening of essential social and community services such as access to education and health care all contributed to narrowing of disparities.

This is the background against which modern medical advances could be effectively applied to facilitate the eradication of many epidemic infectious diseases. Much was achieved in wealthy countries by the 1970s, as exemplified by further reduction in the annual death rate from tuberculosis to about 2 per 100,000 in the United Kingdom.

However, since the late 1970s, neo-liberal economic policies (now acknowledged as based on flawed economic theory and dogma) stimulated economic growth and improved medical care largely for the benefit of the top

11   David Stuckler and Martin McKee, 'Five Metaphors about Global-Health Policy', *The Lancet*, 2008, 372(9633): 95–7.

20 per cent of the global population. For the remaining majority, post-war trends towards improvement in wealth and health began to reverse under such policies. The extent to which these policies aggravated the impact of HIV/AIDS in poor countries has been well-documented.[12] It should be noted that in South Africa apartheid policies largely limited economic and health advances to white people, and it is not surprising that multi-drug-resistant tuberculosis, and the emergence and spread of HIV became additional markers of the longstanding poor health of the black majority, despite the availability of modern drug treatments.

John Kenneth Galbraith, in his mid-twentieth-century books identified individualism, unlimited wants, self-interest and 'rationality' (characterized as dominated by calculating and measuring) as the myths underlying mid-twentieth-century economics.[13] Charles Taylor described individualism, the primacy of instrumental reason (mathematical calculation of the most economical means to ends, and loss of the sense of sacredness), together with restriction of choices by the politics of a technical industrial society, as the three malaises of modernity.[14] Among others, Robert Heilbroner[15] and Ursula Franklin[16] have expressed similar concerns about the implications of a mechanical and technologically dominated trajectory of progress.

I concur with these authors that distorted values lie at the heart of global disparities and portend a potentially bleak future. Hyper-individualism, unlimited wants, narrow and short-term self-interests and restricted conceptions of freedom, rationality and rights, described very synoptically here, are prominently exhibited by those of us who are the most privileged.

Hyper-individualism

Hyper-individualism can be defined as taking to an extreme the hard won achievement of much valued (and now highly vaunted) freedom of the individual. A focus on the 'anomic' self (minimally connected to community or society), results in the erosion of a sense of solidarity and of connection to others and society, and loss of a sense of awe about life and our natural environment. There is also significant lack of moral imagination regarding the plight of so many fellow creatures, and of our complicity in creating and

12 Rick Rowden, *The Deadly Ideas of Neoliberalism: How the IMF Undermined Public Health & the Fight against AIDS* (London & New York: Zed Books, 2009).

13 John K. Galbraith, *The Affluent Society* (Boston: Houghton Mifflin, 1958); John K. Galbraith, *The New Industrial State* (Boston: Houghton Mifflin, 1976).

14 Charles Taylor, *The Malaise of Modernity* (Toronto: House of Anansi Press, 1991).

15 Robert Heilbroner, *An Inquiry into the Human Prospect* (New York, NY: W. W. Norton, 1974).

16 Ursula M. Franklin, *The Real World of Technology* (Massey Lectures 1989), Revised Edition (Toronto: House of Anansi Press, 1999).

sustaining systems that ignore and aggravate the plight of the less fortunate.[17] It is interesting to reflect on the asymmetry between intense interest in the sanctity of life when abortion and the use of stem cells are debated, as compared with the minimal value seemingly accorded to the (in)dignity and suffering of children already born who are neglected, hungry and die prematurely of preventable disease.

Narrow concept of freedom and of self-interest

A narrow concept of freedom associated with hyper-individualism emphasizes freedom 'to' do what whatever one wishes (liberty), over the concept of freedom 'from' want of basic survival needs (e.g. food and water) and freedom from oppression. The addition of *narrow self-interest* further eclipses notions of duty, obligation and commitment to others and society and allows short-term considerations to trump longer-term interests.

Market and consumerist ideology

A market and consumerist ideology that increasingly pervades all aspects of life encourages *unlimited wants* as the norm. Consequently many individuals and nations, who view the accumulation of wealth and material possessions as the major goals of life, become deeply indebted while living beyond their means, often in pursuit of frivolous goals. In such a world the acquisition of private (consumer) goods overshadows much-needed attention to the essential public goods (education/healthcare) required to hold societies together and nurture the next generation. Exponential consumption, dominance of corporate goals in health care,[18] greed and seemingly insatiable personal wants/entitlements overshadow the notion of at least some degree of austerity as an important value for a good life and a good society. The professions have not escaped such trends, and there is widespread evidence of the erosion of professionalism.[19]

Restricted notion of rationality

A restricted notion of rationality focusing on calculable and measurable outcomes is associated with the view that 'science' offers *the* solutions to

---

17   Solomon R. Benatar, 'Moral Imagination: The Missing Component in Global Health', *Public Library of Science Medicine*, 2005, 2(12): e400.

18   Eliot Freidson, *Professionalism, The Third Logic* (Chicago: University of Chicago Press, 2003); William H. Wiist, 'Public Health and the Anticorporate Movement', *American Journal of Public Health*, 2006, 96(8): 1370–5.

19   Anthony T. Kronman, *The Lost Lawyer: Failing Ideals of the Legal Profession* (Cambridge: Harvard University Press, 1993); Hebert M. Swick, 'Academic Medicine Must Deal with the Clash of Business and Professionalism', *Academic Medicine*, 1998, 73: 741–55; Matthew K. Wynia, 'The Short History and Tenuous Future of Medical Professionalism: The Erosion of Medicine's Social Contract', *Perspectives in Biology & Medicine*, 2008, 51(4): 565–78.

all problems. While it is not disputed that science and medical advances are necessary, it is surely problematic to consider these to be sufficient. Much is lost when the quest for new knowledge is valued more than old knowledge, and when all knowledge is valued more than wisdom in the application of knowledge. Moreover, spiritual and 'compassionate rationality', and the value of caring are not easy to measure and are therefore undervalued in a world in which monetary value and technological practices dominate over inter-personal caring skills.

Narrow conception of human rights

A narrow conception of human rights that emphasizes civil and political rights tends to ignore social, economic and cultural rights (even though all the rights listed in the UDHR are supposed to be indivisible and inalienable). Such a conception of rights also eclipses the reciprocal responsibilities that form part of the conceptual logic of rights, and avoids identification of the bearers of such reciprocal duties. While we focus our attention on individual perpetrators of human rights abuses within nations, and fail to see the world moving towards a post-Westphalian conception of global interdependence, inadequate attention is directed to the powerful *systems forces* that undermine human rights across national boundaries at the level of whole populations.[20]

As a general result of all of the above there is disjunction between economic growth, advances in science, technology and medical care and the ability to use these to improve health more equitably within nations and more widely.[21] A specific result is the erosion of our capacity to reproduce the caring social institutions (health, education, child nurturing) so essential for healthy societies.[22] When countries like the United States do not seem to respect their own citizens sufficiently to provide universal access to health care more equitably, and the pursuit of increasing wealth for a minority takes place at the expense of the basic needs of majority, there is a need to be profoundly sceptical of the reigning value system.[23] 'Inequality is corrosive. It rots societies from within.'[24] It has also been previously argued that:

> substantial improvements in global health will depend on acknowledging that poor health at the level of whole populations reflects systemic dysfunction in a complex world . . . (and that improving global health) will require greater moral

---

20 Solomon R. Benatar and Len Doyal, 'Human Rights Abuses: Balancing Two Perspectives', *International Journal of Health Services*, 2009, 39(1): 139–59.
21 Benatar, 'Global Disparities in Health and Human Rights'.
22 Stephen Gill and Isabella Bakker (eds), *Power, Production and Social Reproduction* (London: Zed Books, 2003).
23 Tony Judt, *Ill Fares the Land* (New York: Penguin Books, 2010).
24 Cited in ibid., 21.

imagination (the ability of individuals and communities to empathize with others) to break the impasse we currently face in improving global health.[25]

A world in entropy

A composite evaluation of these trends reveals what Stephen Gill has called a 'global organic crisis', made up of multiple, deep and interlinked crises that include crises in many aspects of human security – healthcare, education, energy, food, governance, territory and information.[26] Other manifestations of a world undergoing entropy include recrudescence of infectious diseases (when it was thought that these had been largely vanquished), clashes of civilizations, the global economic crisis and environmental degradation.[27]

The health and lives of billions of people are being, and will continue to be affected by climate change – through direct long-term effects on water security, food chain integrity, population migration and displacement, redistribution of vector borne diseases and significant short-term health impacts from catastrophic extreme climatic events.[28]

There are also significant environmental health concerns globally that are not directly associated with climate change such as the cruel manner in which humans 'farm' animals in mass production facilities, and contaminate food and water supplies with cumulative amounts of toxic industrial agents.[29] These are all global in nature, but may have differential local health impacts worsened by systematic, often remediable, disadvantaging of whole populations. Climate change, together with competition for resources, marginalization of the majority of people in the world and global militarization are arguably major potential threats to world peace.[30]

Obligations

The potential foundations for international obligations to improve health globally could be conceptualized through a range of overlapping 'lenses'. Rather

25 Benatar, 'Moral Imagination'.
26 Stephen Gill and Isabella Bakker, 'The Global Crisis and Global Health', in Benatar and Brock (eds) *Global Health and Global Health Ethics*.
27 Solomon R. Benatar, 'Millennial Challenges for Medicine & Modernity', *Journal of the Royal College of Physicians of London*, 1998, 32: 160–5.
28 Sharon Friel, Colin Butler and Anthony McMichael, 'Climate Change and Health Risks and Inequities,' in Benatar and Brock (eds), *Global Health and Global Health Ethics*.
29 David Benatar, 'Animals, the Environment and Global Health,' in Benatar and Brock (eds) *Global Health and Global Health Ethics*.
30 Solomon R. Benatar, 'War, or Peace and Development: South Africa's Message for Global Peace and Security', *Medicine, Conflict and Survival*, 1997, 13: 125–34.

Table 4.1 Moral lenses through which to view international obligations

Historical	Retributive and compensatory justice
Social justice	Distributive justice
Self-interest and security	Medium- and long-term mutual advantage
Ecological	Preserving the environment for future generations
Human rights	Comprehensively understood and applied
Needs	As distinct from rights
Solidarity	Humanitarian obligations of global citizens
Finite resources	Duty to set priorities explicitly
Moral global economy	Fairness in accumulation and distribution
International professional standards	Virtue in professionalism
Global crises	Facing complexity

than attempting to provide detailed arguments from each of these perspectives, only a brief taxonomy and synopsis is provided here (Table 4.1).

Historical

Viewing the distal, upstream causes of wealth distribution around the world through the lens of slavery, colonialism and other forms of exploitation (e.g. racism in apartheid South Africa) enables us to see that arguments for retributive justice have the powerful potential to sensitize us to the obligations of those beneficiaries of practices that have had a deep and sustained adverse impact on many generations of people in affected countries. Good arguments for compensation to victims of the Holocaust and to those who appealed to the Truth and Reconciliation Commission in South Africa provide some examples of moral justification for retributive justice.[31]

Social justice

While there may be disagreement among philosophers and others about exactly what social justice means and how it could be achieved, there is surely no disagreement that when access to the basic needs for a minimally decent human existence are denied to so many, both within wealthy nations and across the globe, there is moral urgency to at least begin to diminish such injustice.[32]

Madison Powers and Ruth Faden provide guidance on how to think about health inequalities within an approach that views social justice as

---

31 Martha Minow, *Between Vengeance and Forgiveness: Facing History after Genocide and Mass Violence* (Boston: Beacon Press, 1998).

32 Jonathan Glover, 'Poverty, Distance and Two Dimensions of Ethics', in Benatar and Brock (eds), *Global Health and Global Health Ethics*.

the foundation of public health and public health policy.[33] Gillian Brock's cosmopolitan account of global justice defends the equal moral worth of every person globally without ignoring all considerations such as nationality or other identities.[34] Following a review of criticisms and defenses of Rawls's Law of Peoples, she provides a theoretical account of cosmopolitanism and some practical suggestions for reducing gross global injustices through protection of individual liberties, reduction in poverty and protection of public goods.

Norman Daniels and James Sabin, noting as many others have done that there is no agreement on any substantive account of distributive justice, have described a procedurally fair process ('accountability for reasonableness') for setting priorities in the allocation of health-care resources.[35] While many see this as an acceptable means of setting priorities in the context of limited resources,[36] Richard Ashcroft has chastised bioethicists for taking this 'easy way' out of a persisting dilemma.[37] While agreeing with him that tough issues should continue to be pursued intellectually, within the current globally dominant economic system no country, regardless of how wealthy, can provide all that medicine could offer to everyone all the time. Therefore, setting priorities is a pragmatic reality that must be faced. With constructive changes to the global economy (see below), the resources available for providing more health care could be greatly increased, with resulting less stringent need for setting priorities.

With regard to pursuing social justice in relation to the global distribution of resources for health, there are also no easy answers. I suggest that making progress here would be dependent on a series of changes. These would include wealthy and powerful nations accepting the need for, and working towards less social injustice within their own borders, some changes to the way in which the global economy functions to reverse widening disparities in the accumulation of wealth, and imaginative approaches to redistribution that would require some constraints on 'casino-like' economies.[38]

---

33 Madison Powers and Ruth Faden, *Social Justice: The Moral Foundations of Public Health and Public Health Policy* (New York: Oxford University Press, 2006).

34 Gillian Brock, *Global Justice: A Cosmopolitan Account* (Oxford: Oxford University Press, 2008).

35 Norman Daniels and James Sabin, *Setting Limits Fairly: Can We Learn to Share Medical Resources?* (Oxford: Oxford University Press, 2002).

36 Douglas K. Martin and Solomon R. Benatar, 'Resource Allocation: International Perspectives on Resource Allocation', in Kris Heggenhougen and Stella Quah (eds) *International Encyclopedia of Public Health. Vol 5.* (San Diego: Academic Press, 2008).

37 Richard Ashcroft, 'Fair Process and the Redundancy of Bioethics: A Polemic', *Public Health Ethics*, 2008, 1(1): 3–9.

38 Benatar, Gill and Bakker, 'Global Health and the Global Economic Crisis'; Jeffrey Sachs, *The Price of Civilization* (New York: Random House, 2011); Solomon R. Benatar, 'Justice and Priority Setting in International Health Research,' in Richard Ashcroft, Angus Dawson, Heather Draper and John R. McMillan (eds), *Principles of Health Care Ethics*, 2nd edn (Chichester: John Wiley and Sons, 2007).

Self-interest and security

The emergence and rapid spread globally of many new infectious diseases (HIV, SARS and Avian flu having the highest contemporary profile) are stark reminders of the major threats to individual and population health posed by emerging infectious diseases.[39] Increasing resistance to drugs used to treat many diseases (e.g. tuberculosis, malaria and HIV) pose additional global threats. Moral arguments favouring expenditure on reducing the emergence and spread of such diseases are supported by the potential for saving many lives.[40] Arguably, those with knowledge and resources have at least some responsibility to prevent such tragedies in the future. Human security is similarly threatened in the medium- and long-term by food, water and shelter insecurity.[41] These not only lead to immediate harms for many but also have the potential to lead to mass migration, increased numbers of refugees living under desperate conditions and wars of redistribution associated with reciprocal devaluation of lives.

Ecological

Considerations of the current impact of climate change and environmental degradation and of the ongoing implications for health of future generations as such change escalates provide a moral basis for taking preventive actions.[42] Excessive consumption of meat, the production of which is less food energy efficient than production of vegetable forms of protein, enhances environmental damage and should provide motivation for preventive action that could considerably improve global health.[43]

Human rights

The Universal Declaration of Human Rights of 1948 (UDHR) and all the energy devoted to attempting to ensure that such rights are widely satisfied have not met with the extent of success many have long hoped for.[44] Nevertheless,

39 Solomon R. Benatar, 'The Coming Catastrophe in International Health', *Canadian Journal of International Affairs*, 2001, 56(4): 611–31.
40 Michael Selgelid, 'Justice, Infectious Diseases and Globalization', in Benatar and Brock (eds), *Global Health and Global Health Ethics*.
41 Anne-Emanuelle Birn, 'Addressing the Societal Determinants of Health: The Key Global Health Ethics Imperative', in Benatar and Brock (eds), *Global Health and Global Health Ethics*; Lynn McIntyre and Krista Rondeau, 'Food Security and Global Health', in Benatar and Brock (eds), *Global Health and Global Health Ethics*.
42 Friel, Butler and McMichael, 'Climate Change and Health: Risks and Inequities'.
43 Benatar, 'Animals, the Environment and Global Health'.
44 Solomon R. Benatar, 'Global Health and Human Rights: Working with the 20th Century Legacy', Annual Human Rights Lecture, University of Alberta 2011, www.uofaweb.ualberta.ca/humanrightslecture/.

the language and motives of the human rights endeavour are potentially powerful means of promoting improvements in health and well-being globally.[45]

Extending the discourse on human rights beyond the popular rhetoric of civil and political rights to include all the indivisible and inalienable rights proclaimed in the UDHR will require attention to systems forces that promote human rights abuses in addition to seeking out and punishing and/ or educating individual perpetrators.[46] The Declaration of Human Duties and Responsibilities, which could have a role in extending the reach of the UDHR, also deserves a higher profile.[47]

Needs

The extent of unmet basic human needs is revealed by the statistics provided earlier. These are augmented by a few additional facts: two-and-a-half billion people lack access to basic sanitation, 2 billion lack access to essential medicines, 1.6 billion lack electricity, 1.02 billion are chronically undernourished, 924 million have inadequate shelter, 884 million do not have access to safe water, 774 million adults are illiterate and 218 million children are child labourers.[48]

Few would contest that health could be defined as the ability and the opportunity to utilize one's natural endowments to achieve the potential to live a full and satisfying life. Achievement of health requires attention to the social and societal needs that so powerfully influence health and disease. A lifelong supportive environment is required, and should include good pre-natal care, safe childbirth, a nurturing childhood, adequate education, prevention of avoidable diseases and opportunities to flourish physically, socially and intellectually. Modern health services, over and above such social forces, should provide access to affordable, effective health care with recognition of the limits of medicine, particularly at the end of long lives or in the face of irremediable prolonged suffering, where alleviation of pain and comfort care may be the most appropriate.

45 Jonathan Wolff, 'The Human Right to Health,' in Benatar and Brock (eds), *Global Health and Global Health Ethics*; Stephanie Nixon and Lisa Forman, 'Exploring the Synergies between Human Rights and Public Health Ethics: A Whole Greater than the Sum of Its Parts', *BMC International Health and Human Rights*, 2008, 8(2); Gurcharan Bhatia, John O'Neill, Gerald L. Gall and Patrick D. Bendin (eds), *Peace, Justice and Freedom: Human Rights Challenges for the New Millennium* (Alberta: University of Alberta Press, 2000).

46 Benatar and Doyal, 'Human Rights Abuses'; Solomon R. Benatar, Abdallah S. Daar and Peter A. Singer, 'Global Health Ethics: The Rationale for Mutual Caring', in Benatar and Brock (eds), *Global Health and Global Health Ethics*.

47 M. C. Patricia Morales, *The Declaration of Human Duties and Responsibilities: From Human Rights to Responsibilities of the Global Community*. Available at www.onlineunesco.org/conferencias/tele6/human%20duties%20and%20responsibilities.ppt#256,1.

48 Thomas Pogge, 'The Health Impact Fund: How to Make New Medicines Accessible to All', in Benatar and Brock (eds), *Global Health and Global Health Ethics*.

Distinction between needs and rights

The UDHR has led to 'Human Rights' as a 'new standard of civilization' for judging nations.[49] This Declaration, supported by growing legislation to promote and enforce rights, has achieved many successes and it is widely acknowledged that both the concept and the language of rights are powerful. However, as noted by Michael Ignatieff:

> Rights language can meet some needs but not all ... For example the need for respect and consideration, fraternity, love and belonging that engender a sense of worth ... Rights language offers a rich vernacular for the claims an individual may make on or against the collectivity but it is relatively impoverished as a means of expressing the individual's need for the collectivity. It is because fraternity, love, belonging, dignity and human gestures which confer respect, cannot be bought, nor rights guarantee them as entitlement, that any decent society requires a public discourse about ... human needs.[50]

Anne Robertson has proposed that a language of need provides a moral discourse for promotion of health and the common good – 'a moral economy of interdependence' that is more appropriate to the notion of common good. She argues that such language goes beyond an individualistic oriented 'political economy', accounts for the inherently 'political nature of need' and situates the definition and adjudication of needs within community life. Notions of reciprocity are also incorporated that go beyond the dichotomy of dependence and independence.[51]

Len Doyal and Ian Gough argue on moral grounds that the freedom to develop one's potential must be coupled to 'freedom from want' of basic needs. They view security of the person and access to first-order biological needs (food, clean water and shelter) as some of the essentials for decent lives. They also contend that a sense of empowerment and control over ourselves is essential for human flourishing. Human flourishing requires respect for the basic needs and dignity of others, respect for the full range of human rights, belief in the rule of just law, the willingness to take responsibility for one's actions and societal well-being, deriving satisfaction from work well done, contributing to new knowledge and the freedom to develop one's full potential. Twelve broad categories of 'intermediate needs' that define how the need for physical health and personal autonomy are fulfilled are described by them: adequate nutritional food and clean water; adequate protective housing; a safe environment for working; a supply of clothing; a safe physical environment; appropriate health care; security in childhood; significant primary relationships with others;

---

49   Jack Donnelly, *Universal Human Rights in Theory and Practice* (London: Cornell University Press, 1989).
50   Michael Ignatieff, *The Needs of Strangers* (New York: Viking Press, 1984).
51   Ann Robertson, 'Critical Reflections on the Politics of Need: Implications for Public Health', *Social Science and Medicine*, 1998, 47(10): 1419–30.

physical security; economic security; safe birth control and child-bearing; and appropriate basic and cross-cultural education. Determination of how needs should be satisfied requires rational identification of needs using the most up-to-date scientific knowledge, the use of the actual experience of individuals in their everyday lives and democratic decision-making.[52]

As rights alone are insufficient, more attention must be focused on needs, for example the needs of children. Declarations of the rights of children are potentially powerful but realistically only become relevant when the basic duties of care and affection that parents and societies should have towards the needs of children are failing (duty here is a conceptually different notion from the duties reciprocal to rights). Moreover, rights cannot guarantee love, a sense of belonging and of being valued for one's existence and potential. Meeting these needs is of crucial importance, as eloquently stated by Michael Ignatieff (see page 75).

Solidarity

Solidarity as global citizens, supported by valid moral arguments,[53] is widely expressed through the efforts of many humanitarian endeavours. Solidarity can be considered as:

> [A]ttitudes and determination to work for the common good across the globe in an era when interdependence is greater than ever and in which progress should be defined as enhancing capabilities and social justice ... Without solidarity it is inevitable that we shall ignore distant indignities, violations of human rights, inequities, deprivation of freedom, undemocratic regimes, and respect for the environment. If a spirit of mutual caring could be developed between those in wealthy countries and those in developing countries, we see constructive change as being possible.[54]

Finite resources

Given that endless economic growth in not feasible and that our planetary resources are finite, there is a great need to foster better understanding of the limits of our entitlements, and what our societies 'owe' us. Setting priorities is an unavoidable feature of life, in the context of limited resources. When priorities are set through transparent, explicit and accountable processes that involve representatives of all relevant stake-holder groups, and opportunities for appeals and revision are built into the process, setting priorities within

---

52 Len Doyal and Ian Gough, *A Theory of Human Need* (London: McMillan, 1991).
53 Peter Singer, *One World: The Ethics of Globalization* (New Haven: Yale University Press, 2001); Glover, 'Poverty, Distance and Two Dimensions of Ethics'.
54 Solomon R. Benatar, Abdallah S. Daar and Peter A. Singer, 'Global Health Ethics: The Rationale for Mutual Caring', *International Affairs*, 2003, 79(1): 107–38.

achievable limits could be more easily accepted and applied. Some recent examples in health care show the way.[55]

Moral global economy

Dissatisfaction with the way the global political economy operates to the disadvantage of the majority of the world's people has been the subject of debate over many decades.[56] The outcome of seminars on social progress in Copenhagen was acknowledgement that the forces of economic globalization are erosive of democracy, and that good reasons could be mounted for developing a more moral economy.[57] More recently John Kenneth Galbraith,[58] Stephen Gill,[59] Justin Fox,[60] Jeffrey Sachs[61] and Tony Judt,[62] among others, have written eloquently of the serious shortcomings in economic theory and practice that led to the still unfolding economic crisis – confirming what Galbraith had predicted many decades ago, and that is now becoming obvious to more people:

> The present age of contentment will come to an end only when and if the adverse developments that it fosters challenge the sense of comfortable well-being. As well as the strong and successful political appeal to the disadvantaged I have already mentioned, there are three other plausible possibilities as to how this will happen. They are: widespread economic disaster, adverse military action that is associated with international misadventure, and eruption of an angry underclass.[63]

Reflection on the fact that the United States has spent $1 trillion on the war in Iraq, and that this is equal to 30 years of US foreign development aid reveals the potential dividend for alternative uses of resources. The implications of the 'Occupy Wall Street' movement, as one form of long pursued 'globalization

55   Douglas K. Martin, Peter A. Singer and Mark Bernstein, 'Access to ICU Needs for Neurosurgery Patients: A Qualitative Case Study', *J Neurology, Neurosurgery and Psychiatry*, 2003, 74(9): 1299–303; Jens Mielke, Douglas K. Martin and Peter A. Singer, 'Priority Setting in Critical Care: A Qualitative Case Study', *Critical Care Medicine*, 2003, 31: 2764–8; Samia A. Hurst, Nathalie Mezger and Alex Mauron, 'Allocating Resources in Humanitarian Medicine', in Benatar and Brock (eds), *Global Health and Global Health Ethics*.
56   Susan George, *A Fate Worse than Debt* (London: Penguin Books, 1988).
57   *Building a Global Community. Globalization and the Common Good* (Copenhagen: Royal Danish Foreign Ministry for Foreign Affairs, 2000).
58   John K. Galbraith, *The Economics of Innocent Fraud: Truth for Our Time*, (Boston: Houghton Mifflin, 2004).
59   Stephen Gill, *Power and Resistance in the New World Order*, 2nd edn (New York: Palgrave MacMillan, 2008).
60   Justin Fox, *The Myth of the Rational Market: A History of Risk, Reward, and Delusion on Wall Street* (New York, NY: Harper Business/Harper Collins, 2009).
61   Jeffrey Sachs, *The Price of Civilization* (New York: Random House, 2011).
62   Judt, *Ill Fares the Land.*
63   John K. Galbraith, *The Culture of Contentment*, (New York: Houghton-Mifflin Company, 1992), 156–7.

from below'[64] is another example of the relevance of Galbraiths's perspicacity. Guidance is also available from Adam Smith:

> No society can surely be flourishing and happy, of which the far greater part of its members are poor and miserable.[65]

International professional standards

Many deeply held values within the health-care professions and in the scientific community are believed to be universal. For example, within the medical profession these include respect for human dignity, empathy and compassion, dedication to excellence, the desire not to harm and to do good, seeking equity in the delivery of health care and pursuit of new knowledge without exploiting the vulnerable.[66] In science, simplicity and elegance of theory, internal consistency, predictive value, the potential for unifying diverse observations, good judgement, curiosity, intuition and creativity are universal values.[67] Commitment to widespread propagation of these standards could add to the force with which the view through the other lenses described above may be implemented.

Global crises

The complex organic crisis, to which Stephen Gill has referred,[68] and the implications of such for the future of our planet and of all life provide yet another lens through which to perceive some of the moral obligations (based on their access to knowledge and resources) for wealthy nations to accept and act on their role to ameliorate the human condition and improve the future. Arguments from an understanding of a systems perspective[69] and of the interactions of technology and society[70] become relevant here.

What can be done? Some practical considerations

While it is utopian to consider that equity can be achieved in such a world, the future looks bleak if we do not soon embark on measures that could at least

64   Jeremy Brecher, Tim Costello and Brendan Smith, *Globalization from Below: The Power of Solidarity* (Cambridge, MA: South End Press, 2000).
65   Cited in Judt, *Ill Fares the Land*, 12.
66   Ros Levinson, Steve Dewar, Susan Shepherd, *Understanding Doctors: Harnessing Professionalism* (London: King's Fund, 2008).
67   Committee on the Conduct of Science, *On Being a Scientist*, US National Academy of Sciences, 1989, available at www.pnas.org/content/86/23/9053.full.pdf.
68   Stephen Gill (ed.), *Global Crises and the Crisis of Global Leadership* (Cambridge: Cambridge University Press, 2011).
69   Anatol Rapoport, *General System Theory* (Tunbridge Wells: Abacus Press, 1986).
70   Franklin, *The Real World of Technology*.

begin to reverse some of these seemingly inexorable trends. It is credible to suggest that 'business as usual' will not work and that innovative social ideas and action are required to achieve meaningful progress in health and human rights in the twenty-first century. John Kenneth Galbraith reminds us that it is not utopian to pursue achievable goals.[71]

We should begin with some introspection to allow re-evaluation of our current paradigm of thought, entitlements and actions. I shall not reiterate here the arguments for the examined life, but the need for each of us, and especially those who are privileged, to accept this, is surely unquestionable. Second, we need to promote the development of a global state of mind about our interdependence as global citizens, and enhanced moral imagination regarding the interconnectedness of all life. These ideas have been described more fully elsewhere.[72]

The next focus of attention should be the global political economy, which has been described as *'the result of a combination of negligence, hubris and wrong economic theory'*.[73] It has now become an imperative to strive actively to achieve wider public acknowledgement that the global economy is based on a flawed economic paradigm and policies. As the economic crisis is a manifestation of a world made more unstable in part by (exponential) patterns of consumption that deplete resources, the inevitability needs to be widely accepted that doing better with less will be one of the characteristics of progress. Privatization of profits and socialization of losses can no longer continue to be the norm.[74] The massive recent losses that have profoundly affected health and well-being of many globally should be addressed by short-term, medium-term and long-term restructuring of the global political economy with social justice foremost in our minds.[75]

These tasks require re-shaping of public conversations, a more responsible media and new social attitudes to life. It is reasonable to claim that it is not beyond human ability to modify the 'free-market' through reasonable constraints and improved accountability. Tax avoidance, tax evasion and international taxation all need to be reviewed.[76] In addition, trade rules that have been locked into place over recent decades in line with neo-liberal economic policies and the 'new constitutionalism' could be modified in a constructive manner.[77]

---

71 John K. Galbraith, *The Good Society* (Boston: Houghton Mifflin, 1996).
72 Benatar, Daar, Singer, 'Global Health Ethics'; Benatar, 'Moral Imagination'.
73 Stephen Gill and Isabella Bakker, 'The Global Crisis and Global Health', in Benatar and Brock (eds), *Global Health and Global Health Ethics*.
74 Benatar, Gill S. and Bakker, 'Global Health and the Economic Crisis'.
75 Ibid.
76 Gillian Brock, 'Taxation and Global Justice: Closing the Gap between Theory and Practice', *Journal of Social Philosophy*, 2008, 39(2): 161–84.
77 Meri Koivusalo, 'Trade and Health: The Ethics of Global Rights, Regulation and Redistribution', in Benatar and Brock (eds), *Global Health and Global Health Ethics*.

A 'new common sense' to achieve this would include measures to 'bolster the social commons ... in ways that are consistent with greater democracy, social justice and social and ecological sustainability'.[78] Achieving this would require, inter alia, a more equitable broad-based tax-system where capital and ecologically sustainable consumption are taxed more than labour. How to best achieve such goals should become the goal of a multi-disciplinary research thrust.

Finally there is a need to set moral examples. The example of South Africa's peaceful transition from apartheid to democracy in the early 1990s, with the development of a model constitution, is one such example of a visionary compromise when facing the abyss.[79] While many mistakes have been made by the new government, few would contend that South Africa would have been better off if the negotiated political transition had not been made in 1994. As difficult as it was to achieve that transition, and as complex as the ensuing steps required to lead to a more socially just society may be, such complexity is no excuse for not trying.[80]

Conclusions

I conclude by reiterating the recommendation previously made by Anne-Emanuelle Birn that the lead taken by some to fund ambitious programmes to develop vaccines for AIDS, malaria and tuberculosis should be matched by the formulation and pursuit of several alternative Grand Challenges aimed at finding solutions to some of the problems outlined in this chapter.[81] In the same way that a multitude of ambitious researchers from diverse fields of biology and science have come together to address complex scientific challenges, so it would seem to me that a range of committed and adequately funded scholars in the social sciences could work together in a productive manner to seek and find imaginative and workable solutions to the humanly constructed social complexities we face in the twenty-first century. New ways of thinking could assist us in breaking away from the current impasses to achieve meaningful human progress.[82]

---

78   Isabella Bakker and Stephen Gill, 'Towards a New Common Sense: The Need for New Paradigms of Global Health', in Benatar and Brock (eds), *Global Health and Global Health Ethics*.

79   Allister Sparks, *Tomorrow is Another Country* (New York: Hill and Wang, 1995).

80   Solomon R. Benatar, 'South Africa's Transition in a Globalizing World. HIV/AIDS as a Window and a Mirror', *International Affairs*, 2001, 77(2): 347–75; John K. Galbraith, *The Socially Concerned Today* (Toronto: University of Toronto Press, 1998); Judt, *Ill Fares the Land*.

81   Anne-Emanuelle Birn, 'Gates' Grandest Challenge: Transcending Technology as Public Health Ideology', *The Lancet*, 2005, 366(9484): 514–19.

82   Solomon R. Benatar, 'Global Leadership, Ethics and Global Health: The Search for New Paradigms', in Stephen, *The Global Crisis and the Crisis of Global Leadership* (Cambridge: Cambridge University Press, 2011).

5

Just Health, from National to Global: Claiming Global Social Protection

Gorik Ooms and Rachel Hammonds

Introduction

Out of every thousand children born in Sierra Leone, 262 will die before their fifth birthday; out of every thousand children born in San Marino, two will die before their fifth birthday.[1] Global health inequalities like this are so appalling that merely considering that they may not be inequities – 'inequalities which are judged to be unfair and unjust'[2] – may seem outrageous. Yet that is exactly what Norman Daniels does in the final chapter of 'Just Health: Meeting Health Needs Fairly', when he tries to move his concept of justice in health from the national to the global level, and with disarming honesty admits that he has no straightforward answers to the many questions this transition raises.[3]

To qualify global inequalities as inequities requires a concept of global justice. We could use a rather straightforward concept of global justice: all humans should enjoy fair equality of opportunity, or, as Darrel Moellendorf argues, global justice demands a situation in which 'a child growing up in rural Mozambique would be statistically as likely as the child of a senior executive at a Swiss bank to reach the position of the latter's parent'.[4] To have the same chance to become a senior executive at a Swiss bank, all children of the world would first of all need to have the same chance of surviving to their fifth birthday. That would require, among other things, that all the world's women enjoy the same access to quality education, adequate nutrition, safe water and quality health care including emergency obstetric care. Under the current global system ensuring that all children have the same chance of surviving to their fifth birthday would require such massive transfers of financial resources that many of the present social protection efforts within the wealthier countries

---

1   World Health Organisation, *World Health Statistics 2009* (Geneva: World Health Organisation, 2009), 40–3.
2   Hilary Graham, *Unequal Lives: Health and Socioeconomic Inequalities* (Berkshire: McGraw-Hill Open University Press, 2007), 3.
3   Norman Daniels, *Just Health. Meeting Health Needs Fairly* (Cambridge, UK: Cambridge University Press, 2008), 335.
4   Darrel Moellendorf, *Cosmopolitan Justice* (Boulder: Westview Press, 2002), 49.

may become unaffordable. At this point the logical consequences of applying Moellendorf's principles of global justice run into conflict with principles of national justice advanced by other thinkers including David Miller. If one supports Miller's contention, 'that nations are indeed communities of the kind that can support special obligations',[5] just as family members have special obligations towards each other, then the special obligations of inhabitants of wealthier countries towards each other can trump obligations they may have towards inhabitants of poorer countries.

Whether or not we agree with the position that demands of national justice trump demands of global justice, such thinking is in line with present political reality. Whatever inhabitants of a country feel they owe to each other will likely trump whatever they are willing to provide to inhabitants of other countries. On top of being a political reality, this position is in line with the principle of state sovereignty, which has been challenged but remains a building block of international law.[6]

The first section of this chapter focuses on the dichotomy between Rawls' principles of national and global justice. It draws on the work of Daniels, Moellendorf and Miller that addresses John Rawls' 'Theory of Justice',[7] and his reluctance in 'Law of Peoples',[8] to expand his principles of justice to the global level. We go in the opposite direction, moving an elaborated version of Rawls' first principle of global justice back to the national level, and argue that it would undermine his second principle of (national) justice. Then we examine the objections that Rawls may have raised towards applying his first principle of global justice at the national level, and argue that these objections are equally valid at the global level.

The second section of this chapter proposes an alternative set of principles of justice that allow for special obligations towards compatriots, but nonetheless demands similar less intense obligations towards inhabitants of other countries. Our principles draw no fundamental distinction between obligations towards compatriots and obligations towards those living in other countries, only a difference in their intensity. We also try to address what we believe was Rawls' main fear in extending his principles of justice from the national to the global. Finally we discuss how a global-level, low-intensity social protection mechanism is both practically feasible and does not conflict with Rawls' first principle of national justice.

5   David Miller, *National Responsibility and Global Justice* (Oxford: Oxford University Press, 2007), 34.
6   David P. Forsythe, *Human Rights in International Relations* (Cambridge: Cambridge University Press, 2006), 20.
7   John Rawls, *A Theory of Justice. Revised Edition* (Cambridge, MA: The Belknap Press of the Harvard University Press, 1999).
8   John Rawls, *The Law of Peoples* (Cambridge, MA: Harvard University Press, 2001).

Principles of national and global justice

Rawls' 'Theory of Justice' proposes a concept of national justice – for communities of people sharing a government. It is based on two principles:

1 *Each person has the same indefeasible claim to a fully adequate scheme of equal basic liberties, which scheme is compatible with the scheme of liberties for all.*

2 *Social and economic inequalities are to satisfy two conditions: first, they are to be attached to offices and conditions open to all under conditions of fair equality of opportunity; and second, they are to be to the greatest benefit of the least-advantaged members of society (the difference principle).*[9]

In applying this theory to the global level in 'The Law of Peoples', Rawls proposes fundamental adjustments. The idea of distributive justice cannot be transformed into 'distributive justice among peoples', or so argues Rawls. Peoples must be allowed to take their own decisions and then should bear the consequences of their choices. For Rawls, there is a 'duty of assistance' between peoples, but this duty is less demanding than (national) distributive justice: 'The crucial point is that the role of the duty of assistance is to assist burdened societies to become full members of the Society of Peoples and to be able to determine the path of their own future for themselves.'[10]

To illustrate his point, Rawls provides the following example.[11] Two different countries 'provide the elements of equal justice for women', however, 'the first happens to stress these elements and its women flourish in the political and economic world', while the second 'because its prevailing religious and social values, freely held by its women, does not reduce the rate of population growth and it remains rather high'. Then, 'some decades later, the first society is twice as wealthy as the second'.[12] Can the first country now be obliged in any way to support the latter? No, or so argues Rawls, without providing much explanation except that 'this latter position seems unacceptable'.

But what exactly is unacceptable about this position? Examining Rawls' principles of global justice – 'Principles of the Law of Peoples' – it is the first that seems to explain best why the position is unacceptable: 'Peoples are free and independent, and their freedom and independence are to be respected by

---

9 John Rawls, *Justice as Fairness: A Restatement* (Cambridge, MA: The Belknap Press of the Harvard University Press, 2001), 42.

10 Rawls, *Law of Peoples*, 118.

11 In fact, Rawls provides two examples, but the essential arguments are the same. The other example compares two countries, one investing heavily in industrialization, the other 'preferring a more pastoral and leisurely society'.

12 Rawls, *Law of Peoples*, 117–18.

other peoples.'[13] Applied to the example above, it leads to two similar but different arguments:

1 The second country is presumed to be responsible for its relative poverty – its destitution is due to the choices its people freely made. It may have been affected by choices made by other countries or by people living in other countries, but as it is independent, it could have kept those negative influences out, so even if its destitution could be attributed to external factors, the country is still responsible for letting these external factors influence its prosperity. This we call the 'self-containment' argument. If countries are self-contained, or could be self-contained if they wanted, then ultimately the responsibility for the well-being of the inhabitants of a country rests within that country.

2 The first country may not want to support the second country and that opinion may be the result of the conscientious judgements and values freely held by its inhabitants. If we were to confirm a principle of global justice that obliges the first country to support the second, which would overrule the decision freely taken by the first country; then it would no longer be free. Furthermore, if the first country were nonetheless obliged to support the second, it should at least be allowed to demand that the second country adopt the policies that allowed the first country to become wealthier (otherwise the first country will have to support the second forever). Then global justice would overrule the conscientious judgments and values held by the inhabitants of the second country. This we call the 'autonomy' argument.

Similar arguments can be made against Rawls' second principle of (national) justice. Within a state, different individuals, different families and different communities make different choices. Some parents encourage their children to develop their commercial talent, others encourage their children to develop their scientific or artistic talent – and these choices and preferences may lead to differences in income and wealth. At the national level, the self-containment argument would suggest the following with regard to obligations of support to others. Person A would have no obligation of support to destitute person B unless we can demonstrate that person A is responsible somehow for the destitution of person B, and that the influence of person A on person B's destitution was beyond the control of person B. The autonomy argument would suggest that free and equal people have different values about solidarity and individual responsibility, so any principle obliging person A to provide support against his or her will would undermine the autonomy of person A.

13 Ibid., 37.

Further, any requirement that the persons receiving support would be obliged to try harder to support themselves would undermine their autonomy.

What would that mean in practice? All member states of the Organisation for Economic Co-operation and Development (OECD) have developed social protection schemes; schemes through which more than 20 per cent of the Gross Domestic Product (GDP) is collected and re-distributed.[14] Inhabitants of OECD countries are not free to decide individually how much they will contribute. They may have a right to vote in favour or against the policies, or for the politicians that decide the policies, but everyone has to comply with the decisions taken on their behalf, or face the consequent fines or prison. Similarly, people are not entirely free to exercise their autonomy when it comes to their claims for social protection: people who refuse to work may be excluded from some social protection efforts, for example. With the self-containment argument in mind, we should wonder why OECD countries are doing this. If every person is responsible for the consequences of his or her choices, why would they collectively decide to re-distribute 20 per cent or more of their income? With the autonomy argument in mind, we should question the legitimacy of taxation and the legitimacy of conditions imposed upon those benefitting from social protection.

Social protection efforts started to emerge long before Rawls developed his theory of justice, so we cannot hold him accountable. But we know that he approves of such solutions. So how would he deal with the self-containment and autonomy arguments, if used against social protection at the national level?

Let us start with the autonomy argument. Have people who comply with national tax obligations or conditions that come with social protection benefits lost their autonomy? On the contrary, Rawls would argue, people who comply with the principles of justice are truly autonomous: 'by acting from these principles persons are acting autonomously; they are acting from principles that they would acknowledge under conditions that best express their nature as free and equal rational beings.'[15] But what about individuals who truly disagree, and who are nonetheless forced to comply? For Rawls, 'it is not true that the conscientious judgments of each person ought to be respected; nor is it true that individuals are completely free to form their moral convictions.'[16] In other words: when we know what justice demands, we should not be protective of those who would prefer to act unjustly. If autonomy were understood as freedom to behave exactly how one wants to behave, it would lead to anarchy. The real challenge is to find out what justice demands: 'How do we ascertain that their conscience and not ours is mistaken . . .?'[17]

14   Willem Adema and Maxime Ladaique, *How Expensive is the Welfare State? Gross and Net Indicators in the OECD Social Expenditure Database (SOCX)* (Paris: Organization for Economic Cooperation and Development, 2009).
15   Rawls, *Theory of Justice*, 452.
16   Ibid., 452–3.
17   Ibid., 453.

If that is what personal autonomy means, then the autonomy argument can be invalidated at the global level too. The real challenge is to find out what global justice demands. If some states prefer to behave unjustly, we should not – or at least not as a matter of principle – condone their desire to behave unjustly. That concept can be easily understood when we think about states desiring to invade other states. And if we were to find that justice demands that states not only leave each other in peace, but also support each other, then a state that prefers not to support others should not expect to meet with approval for such unjust behaviour. The same can be argued for a state that may be willing to accept support, but unwilling to make certain choices that would reduce its need for support: if justice demands that states make those choices, the autonomy argument does not turn unjust reluctance into just behaviour. In fact, the autonomy argument does not add much to the debate about the demands of global justice, but it does highlight a procedural challenge: how do we ascertain what the true demands of global justice are, in the absence of a global government where states' representatives can deliberate and decide? We return to this challenge in the second section of this chapter.

To be sure, we do not consider global justice as a matter of states' rights and duties towards each other; we are convinced that it is fundamentally tied to individuals' rights and duties towards each other across borders. For now, we stick to Rawls' paradigm for a 'Society of Peoples'. The autonomy argument is easier to counter when used to deny the existence of a duty between individuals to support each other across borders. If that is what justice demands, than a state that refuses to support others is to be seen as a collective of individuals of which the majority prefers to behave unjustly, and their autonomy does not justify their unjust collective preferences.

We countered the autonomy argument, using Rawls' own counter-arguments, both at national and global level. But we have not yet dealt with the self-containment argument: in as much as the destitution of some countries is – or should be considered as – a consequence of their own choices, the relatively richer countries should not be obliged to support the poorer. Again, this argument can be transposed to the national level. In a country where people are free to decide the level of energy and resources they invest in their education and that of their children, are free to move around and look for a better job, are free to decide how hard they really want to work, should individuals or families not then be considered self-contained units too? If so, then why should richer individuals or families be obliged to support poorer individuals or families? If richer individuals earned their income and wealth in an honest manner, should we not then agree with Robert Nozick that '[t]axation of earning from labor is on par with forced labor'?[18]

---

18   Robert Nozick, *Anarchy, State and Utopia* (New York: Basic Books, 1974), 169.

Rawls would answer that we cannot attribute the relative poverty of individuals entirely to the choices they made, and that we cannot exonerate the relatively wealthy from having contributed to the relative poverty of others. Within a competitive environment, some are unable to make full use of their talents and commitment because others with fewer talents and less commitment have more opportunity – for example because their parents where richer and able to pay for private education. Rawls acknowledges that problem, and argues that 'background institutions must work to keep property and wealth evenly enough shared over time to preserve the fair value of the political liberties and fair equality of opportunity over generations'.[19] The problem Rawls refers to is what Gunnar Myrdal calls 'cumulative causation': centres of economic growth – families, clans, cities – investing their gains in future competitive advantages and becoming even stronger, while the periphery of these centres undergoes a 'backwash effect' and becomes even weaker.[20] To illustrate that his theory of cumulative causation really is common sense, Myrdal refers to Matthew's Gospel,[21] and later the phenomenon that became known in economics as the 'Matthew Effect'.[22] More than 50 years ago Myrdal predicted that if less developed countries would open up to a global market, they would not benefit but instead would become relatively poorer. Contemporary economists find that indeed a globalizing economy allowed a Matthew Effect to happen. One of these economists, Branko Milanovic, calls the problem 'bad inequality' or inequality that 'provides the means to preserve acquired positions', as opposed to 'good inequality' or inequality that 'is needed to create incentives for people to study, work hard, or start risky entrepreneurial projects'.[23]

Whenever we compare two individuals, living in the same country, who acquired very different levels of personal wealth, we find a wide range of potential explanations: uneven intelligence, uneven commitment to hard work, uneven willingness to take risks, uneven luck and uneven opportunity. For Rawls, the plausibility of inequality of opportunity as one of the causes of wealth inequality, and the reality of wealth inequality as a cause of inequality of opportunity, are sufficient arguments to claim measures like taxation and re-distribution of income – not limited to a single generation, not to create a level playing field once, but continuously, over generations. It is important to understand that these arguments are sufficient for Rawls (at the national level): one

---

19   Rawls, *Justice as Fairness*, 51.
20   Gunnar Myrdal, *Rich Lands and Poor: The Road to World Prosperity* (New York: Harper and Row, 1957), 12.
21   'For to the one who has, more will be given, and he will have an abundance, but from the one who has not, even what he has will be taken away.' Matthew 13:12, English Standard Version of the Bible.
22   Daniel Rigney, *The Matthew Effect: How Advantage Begets Further Advantage* (New York: Columbia University Press, 2010).
23   Branko Milanovic, *Worlds Apart: Measuring International and Global Inequality* (Princeton and Oxford: Princeton University Press, 2005), 12.

does not have to demonstrate that those who are supposed to contribute are somehow guilty of enjoying excessive opportunity and therefore responsible for unfairly outcompeting others, nor does one have to demonstrate that those who are supposed to benefit from re-distribution are somehow victims of the excessive opportunity of others. Taxation of income and re-distribution of income is not a correction for identifiable harm done.

If distributive justice is not a matter of correcting for identifiable harm done, what is it then? What moral arguments can we develop to argue that a person has to give up part of his or her income to support another person, if the first is in no identifiable way responsible for the destitution of the second? We can imagine at least two:

1 The functionality of a society in the long run should be everyone's concern. Inequality of income and inequality of opportunity are mutually self-amplifying and lead, if uncorrected, to a situation in which a part of society will refuse to cooperate. Therefore, all should contribute to keeping inequality of income and opportunity within acceptable ranges.

2 A society can be understood as a huge web of cooperation, composed of an endless network of interactions that connect all members and through which all members have some impact on all other members. For example, when a person takes a taxi in New York, he or she pays the taxi driver, and indirectly the bank that gave the driver a loan to buy his car, and the factory where the car was made. The taxi driver then buys a pizza and indirectly pays the farmer who grew the tomatoes. And so on. This endless web of cooperation produces benefits and the benefits are shared, but unevenly. The unevenness can be fair – for example, if workers at the factory where the car was made do not take as much risk as the factory owner – or unfair – for example, if the factory owner only earns more because he or she inherited the factory. The uneven sharing of the benefits of cooperation can exacerbate pre-existing unfairness, amplifying inequality of opportunity – the factory workers are so poorly paid that they cannot send their children to school, and their children will never have a chance to become engineers; the factory owner can purchase the most expensive private education for his or her children, even if they never make any serious effort, they will still end up in very comfortable positions. At this point, we can argue that harm is being done to those who are arrested in their underprivileged positions. But it is not easy to attribute the responsibility for the harm done. We can blame the owner of the car factory. But he or she will blame the taxi driver, who wants the cheapest car. The taxi driver will blame the client who does not want to pay more for a 'fair taxi ride'. In the end, the client who wanted a ride

at a reasonable price may have contributed to the very low salaries of undocumented migrants at a tomato farm in Fresno. Within a society that agreed to leave the distribution of the benefits of cooperation entirely to market forces, cooperation will do harm, but a lot of the harm done would be unintended, unidentifiable and unforeseeable. Any cooperation carries with it the risk of unintended harm-doing, for which correction is needed. We cannot be sure, but we can assume that those who obtain the bigger shares of the benefits of cooperation are those who contributed most to the good of cooperation but also those who contributed most to the bad of cooperation. We do not need to suspect them of having enjoyed and sustained excessive opportunity; we can assume that they are or should be willing to finance an insurance policy against their unintended, unidentifiable and unforeseeable contribution to the harm done by the cooperation.

Both arguments can be used to challenge Nozick's characterization of taxation as on par with forced labour. On the basis of our above analysis we would argue that a just person understands that she or he has a contribution to make to a functional society. Also, a just person understands that a society that leaves the distribution of the benefits of cooperation entirely to market forces will do harm, and therefore a just person will agree to underwrite an insurance policy against his or her unintended, unidentifiable and unforeseeable contribution to the harm done. Rawls explicitly endorses the first argument, for example when he writes: 'To ensure stability men must have a sense of justice or a concern for those who would be disadvantaged by their defection, preferably both.'[24] The second argument comes from Rawls too, but we have to acknowledge that we may have pushed the logic further than he intended. However, we find support in his comments that '[t]he social system is to be designed so that the resulting distribution is just however things turn out' and that '[w]ithout an appropriate scheme of these background institutions the outcome of the distributive process will not be just',[25] which we can turn around to argue that in a society that does not contain the necessary corrective policies, those who benefit the most have the highest at risk of contributing to the injustice done to those who received least.

To conclude this section, we argue that both arguments are valid at the global level too. Today, a vast majority of the world's people are connected in a global society and engaging in the global system of cooperation. All people are in some way connected. The taxi driver of our example may not only buy a pizza, he may also buy a cup of coffee for which the beans where grown in Kenya, or a shirt that has been made in a factory in China. By taking a taxi in

24   Rawls, *Theory of Justice*, 435.
25   Ibid., 243.

New York, the client contributes to the distribution of benefits in Kenya and China and so on.

If distributive justice is a matter of contributing to a functional society, can we not argue that the global society needs distributive justice too? Is our global society, as currently structured, dysfunctional as Jean Ziegler warns in 'La Haine de l'Occident' or 'Hate for the West'?[26] In our opinion, 'hate' may be too strong a word, but a 'grudge' towards the global West is a reality.[27] The fact that the global West continues to reject responsibility for extreme human suffering in other parts of the world is deeply problematic for the functionality of global society.

Furthermore, present global inequalities far exceed the point where one may have real doubts about whether they may contain at least some bad or self-amplifying inequality. Any cooperation carries with it a risk of unintended, unidentifiable and unforeseeable harm-doing and that risk is very high for cooperation between a person living in a high-income country and a person living in a low-income country. Those who benefit most from the benefits of global cooperation should therefore also contribute most to a form of insurance to mitigate unintended, unidentifiable and unforeseeable contributions to harm-doing.

Global justice and the governance problem

Simon Caney is not alone in attributing Rawls' rejection of distributive justice beyond borders to his perception of states as 'reasonably self-contained systems of cooperation'.[28] This perception of self-containment creates a dichromatic picture. If two people live in the same state, they belong to a single system of cooperation, and they should support each other (to support the functionality of the cooperation in the long run, or because the impact of cooperation is assumed to contain a risk of harm-doing). If two people live in different states, they belong to different systems of cooperation and they should not support each other (they have no common system of cooperation to sustain, and they have no significant inevitable impact on each other), or that is what the dichromatic picture suggest.

This dichromatic picture is insufficiently sensitive to accurately represent present political reality within states, let alone present economic reality. In the current political reality, people do not belong to a single self-contained system

---

26 Jean Ziegler, *La Haine de l'Occident* (Paris: Editions Albin Michel, 2008).

27 Gorik Ooms, 'Why the West is Perceived as Being Unworthy of Cooperation', *Journal of Law, Medicine & Ethics*, 2010, 38(3): 594–613.

28 Simon Caney, *Justice Beyond Borders: A Global Political Theory* (Oxford: Oxford University Press, 2006), 108.

of cooperation; they belong to many systems or layers of cooperation. And they support each other in each of those systems or layers, in accordance with the estimated level of intensity of cooperation that happens within each layer. For example, the average inhabitant of a member state of the European Union pays taxes and participates in social protection at the level of the city he or she lives in. In many European Union member states, there are taxes at the sub-state level ('communities' or 'regions' in Belgium; 'länder' in Germany). The largest amount of tax is levied at the state or national level. Finally, all member states of the European Union contribute financially to the running of the European Union, which now contains some mutual social protection, albeit very modest.

Within the United States of America, the situation is similar. Most people pay taxes at the municipal level, that is to the city in which they live, at county level, at the state level (e.g. as income tax or sales tax) and then at the federal level.

Obviously, there are historical reasons that explain the multiple layers of social support schemes. But perhaps they are more than just legacies from the past. They may reflect the existence of different layers of society, each of them requiring a different intensity of mutual social protection to remain functional. In a very wealthy city, the minimum level of well-being to be guaranteed to all inhabitants in order to keep the city functional may be higher than the minimum level of well-being to be guaranteed to all inhabitants of the state for the state to remain functional.

The multiple layers may also reflect how geographical proximity is accepted as an indicator of the level of intensity of cooperation, and therefore as an approximation of the risk of unintended, unidentifiable and unforeseeable harm-doing, and therefore an approximation of the level of social protection required to correct harm-doing. Two people living in the same city are presumed to cooperate intensely, and therefore are presumed to have an intense and inevitable impact on each other's well-being, thus, the risk they may be harming each other is high. Consequently, they should support each other more intensely than two people living in different cities should.

Multiple layers of social protection may reflect two implicitly accepted principles of justice, the first based on a political duty to contribute to the functionality of the societies one belongs to, the second based on the duty to avoid or correct unintentional, unidentifiable and unforeseeable harm to others. These are two different but related principles. Both are derived from the inherent unjustness of the results of the market-based distributive process that amplifies pre-existing inequality of opportunity: the first acknowledges that if uncorrected the self-amplification of inequality of opportunity will break down a society, the second acknowledges that if uncorrected the self-amplification of inequality of opportunity will put those who receive the biggest shares of the benefits of cooperation in a position where they are involved in unintentional, unidentifiable and unforeseeable harm-doing.

We believe that these principles are equally applicable to cooperation beyond state borders. There is a global society that urgently needs to become one which serves the interest of all people, but the current inequality of opportunity in global society is staggering and self-amplifying and a lot of so-called cooperation continues only because the less powerful partners have, thus far, no alternative. For the inhabitants of countries to which the vast majority of the benefits of global cooperation accrue, it has become almost impossible to avoid the risk of unintentional, unidentifiable and unforeseeable harm-doing. When we, inhabitants of one of those countries, buy a pound of coffee, we can buy one with a 'fair trade' label. This label tells us that the farmer who grew the beans received a fair price, whatever that means – other than that the price the farmer would normally receive is hugely unfair. What we do not know is where all the other persons whose services we purchase buy their coffee – if they prefer 'unfair' coffee, we indirectly support that, whether we like it or not. Furthermore, the fair trade certification process exists for only a few of the goods we consume. In a world without global standards for minimum decent wages, and a global market economy that relentlessly drives consumer prices as low as possible, making sure that we do not unintentionally harm others has become an impossible task. Those who value global justice should be willing to pay for insurance against unintentional harm-doing, in the form of a global mutual social support scheme.

And therefore, the burning questions – excluding those harking back to the times in which states were truly self-contained systems of cooperation; the 'good old times' that never existed – are not about whether we should develop a global low-intensity layer of mutual social support, but about how to develop, manage and govern it. It is not difficult to imagine a multi-layered social protection scheme with a global low-intensity layer, as Figure 5.1 illustrates, but it would be difficult to govern it.

Our principles of global justice flow from those proposed by Thomas Pogge in 'World Poverty and Human Rights', which are focused on 'human rights deficits that are *causally traceable to social institutions*', on 'those who *actively cooperate* in designing or imposing the relevant social institutions' and on 'compensatory duties to the amount of harm one is responsible for by cooperating in the imposition of an unjust institutional order'.[29] We are in agreement with Pogge that a lot of the present human rights deficits in low-income countries are due to past and present global social institutions that caused and cause harm in intentional, identifiable and foreseeable ways (think the slave trade, colonialism, modern-day agricultural export subsidies). However, with Daniels we agree that:

> International harming is complex in many ways. The harms are often not
> deliberate; sometimes benefits were arguably intended. Harms are often mixed

29   Thomas Pogge, *World Poverty and Human Rights: Cosmopolitan Responsibilities and Reforms: Second Edition* (Cambridge: Polity Press, 2008), 26.

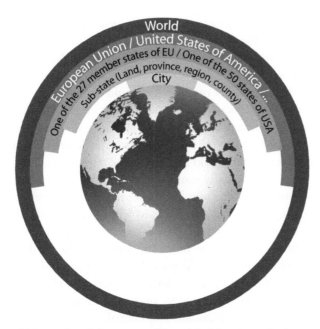

Figure 5.1 Multi-layered social support with a global low-intensity layer

with benefits. In any case, great care must be taken to describe the baseline in measuring harm. Such a complex story about motivation, intentions, and effect might seem to weaken the straightforward appeal of the minimalist strategy, but the complexity does not undermine the view that we have obligations of justice to avoid harming health.[30]

We could presume that those who obtain the greatest share of the benefits of global cooperation are probably contributing most to the harm that is being done. But this line of debate often involves complex discussions relating to causation. For our purposes all we need to presume is that those who obtain the greatest share of the benefits of global cooperation are most at risk of being involved in unintended, unidentifiable and unforeseeable contributions to harm-doing, and therefore are obliged to contribute most to an insurance to mitigate against unintended harm-doing.

If the justification of a claim to global social protection lies in the dual assumption that cooperating individuals should support each other to keep global society functioning and that cooperating individuals should be willing to underwrite insurance against unintended, unidentifiable and unforeseeable involvement in harm-doing, that claim would logically aim for a mechanism to which all individuals contribute, under agreed conditions, and from which all individuals receive support, again under agreed conditions. That is what

---

30 Daniels, *Just Health*, 340.

Milanovic proposes: 'creating a global body (Agency) that would be financed by a tax raised from the rich in rich countries (i.e. a tax on goods or activities with very high income elasticity) and which would transfer these funds to poor *individuals* in poor countries.'[31]

For practical and political reasons, we would propose a scheme that builds on the existing national social support institutions and enables 'cross-subsidies' between states. We imagine a fund that would collect contributions from national social protection schemes and transfer them to national social protection schemes. What would such a scheme require?

First, states as representatives of their inhabitants would have to agree on what a global social protection scheme should cover (and what it should not cover). Then, they would have to agree to what extent states should provide this coverage themselves, and to what extent they can rely on support from other states. Once we know how much support would be needed, states would have to agree which states should provide the support and how that burden will be shared. Finally, states would have to agree on a mechanism. These are exactly the questions we are trying to answer as members of the Joint Action and Learning Initiative on National and Global Responsibilities for Health.[32] We do not want to pre-empt the answers to these questions here, but we do need some preliminary answers to illustrate the practical feasibility of the proposal and to address what may have been Rawls' primary concern – that any form of global distributive justice would negatively affect his first principle of (national) justice.

When it comes to health, the World Health Organisation (WHO) estimates that US$65 per person per year is needed to provide 'Universal Health Coverage' of essential health-promoting and health-protecting goods and services.[33] This estimate includes private health expenditure of about $15 per person per year in low-income countries, on average; meaning that governments of low-income countries should be in a position to spend $50 per person per year – for health only. Even the poorest countries of the world are able to generate some domestic government income; we assume that domestic government revenue equivalent to 20 per cent of GDP is within reach of all countries, and that all countries can allocate 15 per cent of domestic government revenue to health.[34] Combining those estimates with the present GDP of countries, we estimate that

31   Branko Milanovic, *Global Income Inequality: What It Is and Why It Matters* (Washington, DC: World Bank, 2006), 29.

32   Lawrence O. Gostin, Eric A. Friedman, Gorik Ooms, Thomas Gebauer, Narendra Gupta, Devi Sridhar, Wang Chenguang, John-Arne Røttingen and David Sanders, 'The Joint Action and Learning Initiative: Towards a Global Agreement on National and Global Responsibilities for Health', *PLoS Medicine*, 2011, 8: 5.

33   World Health Organisation, *The World Health Report: Health Systems Financing: The Path to Universal Coverage* (Geneva: World Health Organisation, 2010).

34   Gorik Ooms, Rachel Hammonds, 'Taking up Daniels' Challenge: The Case for Global Health Justice', *Health & Human Rights*, 2010, 12(1): 29–46.

about $40 billion per year would be needed to cover the gap between the aim of public health expenditure at $50 per person per year and realistic domestic government income for health. As the combined GDP of the members of the OECD stands at about $40 trillion per year, and only 0.1 per cent of that amount would provide $40 billion per year, the easiest solution would be to ask these high-income countries to share the burden among themselves. However, we are also exploring more inclusive schemes, under which all countries would contribute and receive. Finally, we are looking at the Global Fund to fight AIDS, Tuberculosis and Malaria (Global Fund) as one of the models that could be used. The Global Fund was originally created to collect and distribute $10 billion per year. It has yet to reach that level of distribution, but it nonetheless is a multi-billion dollar non-profit foundation, governed by its own by-laws and the law of Switzerland.[35] It has a board comprised of 20 voting members: richer countries have eight voting members and two other voting members (one representing the private sector and the other representing private foundations) and are considered as being on the side of richer countries; poorer countries have seven voting members, and the three voting members representing civil society organizations are considered to be on the side of the poorer countries.

The current structure and modus operandi of the Global Fund are controversial and it is obvious that if it ever were to be transformed into a global social protection scheme, several of its present features would have to be changed. The purpose here is not to critically analyse the Global Fund in its current form as an efficient or effective instrument for development assistance, but to critically analyse from a philosophical angle, whether its governance structure can stand the test of Rawls' first principle of (national) justice, according to which '[e]ach person has the same indefeasible claim to a fully adequate scheme of equal basic liberties, which scheme is compatible with the scheme of liberties for all'.[36]

To be functional, a global social protection scheme would require reliable contributions; contributions that do not depend on purely discretionary decisions by contributing states. A solution needs to be found that seriously constrains the discretionary character of the contributions. Even if we set aside the practical problems this raises for a while – about how to make a reluctant state contribute – there is a philosophical problem: would any imaginable solution not inevitably lead to a situation in which the liberties of the inhabitants of the contributing states are negatively affected, because they would no longer be in a position to vote for a policy that ends the contributions? Furthermore, a global social protection scheme would impose certain conditions on recipient states, if only to make sure that transfers are used in ways supported by the

---

35 Global Fund to fight AIDS, Tuberculosis and Malaria, *By-laws, as Amended 21 November 2011* (Geneva: Global Fund to fight AIDS, Tuberculosis and Malaria, 2011).
36 Rawls, *Justice as Fairness*, 42.

contributing states.[37] No matter how strict or flexible these conditions are, they would affect the liberties of the inhabitants of the states receiving support negatively.

To some extent, we have already discussed this problem when we countered the autonomy argument. If we know what justice demands, then we should not defer to those who prefer to behave unjustly (even if their opinion is shared by a majority in the country where they live). If it were possible to oblige all states to contribute, whether a majority of inhabitants agrees or not, this would not in our opinion create a conflict with Rawls' first principle of (national) justice, as that principle does not condone unjust preferences.

The real challenge is how to ascertain what global justice demands exactly. If it is relatively easy to argue that present global inequalities demand a degree of global social support, it is far more difficult to obtain a consensus on what exactly it should entail. Can a board comprised of 20 persons be entrusted with this task?

Let us return to the national level. When people disagree on what justice demands, how can we 'ascertain that their conscience and not ours is mistaken . . .?'[38] In 'Political liberalism', Rawls expresses his lukewarm trust in 'deliberative democracy': parliamentary democracy as we know it, but enhanced or 'pimped' with additional features. To name only two: deliberative democracy 'limits the reasons citizens may give in supporting their political opinions to reasons consistent with their seeing other citizens as equals', and calls for 'public financing of elections, and the providing for public occasions of orderly and serious discussion of fundamental questions and issues of public polity'.[39] Not many 'real life' parliamentary democracies live up to these standards.

If parliamentary democracies as we know them are not good enough, what can we say about a board comprised of 20 persons? On the one hand, we can argue that a board comprised of 20 persons designated by a multitude of platforms of which none lives up to the ideal of deliberative democracy, can never be trusted to ascertain what global justice demands. On the other hand, we can argue that if we can live with imperfect solutions at the national level, we should not aim for perfection at the global level.

We could aim for an international agreement based on consensual answers to the questions above (what global mutual social support should cover; what individual states should cover themselves; how the burden of international

---

37 Depending on the design, many or all states could be contributing and receiving at the same time. That would overcome the contributor-recipient dichotomy, but raises the problem that inhabitants of states could no longer vote for policies that are incompatible with the requirements of global social protection.

38 Rawls, *Theory of Justice*, 453.

39 John Rawls, *Political Liberalism. Expanded Edition* (New York: Columbia University Press, 2005), 448–9.

support will be shared; and what mechanism will be created to manage global mutual support). Then no person would be expected to comply with something his or her government – democratically elected or not – does not agree to. Rawls' second principle of global justice holds that '[p]eoples are to observe treaties and undertakings' and his third that '[p]eoples are equal and are parties to the agreements that bind them'.[40] In other words, there is no contradiction between individuals having rights to participate in collective decisions and states adhering to treaties and international undertakings that reduce the future scope of collective decision-making. The international agreement could take the form of an international convention, or the form of an international common undertaking like a global fund: whatever the form it does not negatively affect Rawls' first principle of (national) justice as long as it is based on an agreement to which states voluntarily adhere. Then a board composed of 20 persons could perhaps be trusted enough to fine-tune and implement the prior agreement.

The real problem with this approach is that it will be limited to what the most powerful countries are willing to commit themselves to. And that is likely to be less than what global justice demands. So Thomas Nagel may have been right when he speculated that 'the most likely path toward some version of global justice is through the creation of patently unjust and illegitimate global structures of power that are tolerable to the interests of the most powerful current nation-states'.[41] The context in which a global social protection scheme has to be negotiated faces a legitimacy problem. The most powerful states will at best embrace a scheme that is far too modest to be called just. But we have to be clear about where the injustice lies: not in constraining the discretionary character of states' decisions about international solidarity, but in insufficiently constraining states' discretion for want of a more representative platform. We therefore disagree with Nagel's conclusion that 'the global scope of justice will expand only through developments that first increase the injustice of the world': moving from the present situation of no global social protection towards some global social protection would not increase global injustice, it would decrease global injustice.

Conclusion

A critical analysis of Rawls' rejection of the application of his principle of distributive justice at the global level allows us to develop two arguments: an argument flowing from self-containment (countries can determine their own

40   Rawls, *Law of Peoples*, 37.
41   Thomas Nagel, 'The Problem of Global Justice', *Philosophy & Public Affairs*, 2005, 33(2): 113–47.

future path and therefore there should not be an obligation of support between countries) and an argument based on autonomy (it is preferable that countries make their own decisions). Both arguments can be used at the national level and would undermine Rawls' principle of distributive justice. In defence of his distributive justice principle, Rawls may have argued that individuals and families are not self-contained but rely on cooperation, that to prevent cooperation from becoming unfair or harmful wealth must be sufficiently evenly shared to ensure equality of opportunity, and that personal autonomy cannot be used as an argument to condone individual unjust behaviour.

We transpose these arguments to the global level and argue that any cooperation between individuals, within or across state borders, contains a risk of unintended, unidentifiable and unforeseeable harm-doing, and therefore requires correction in the form of social protection. The intensity of the correction required (or the intensity of social protection required) depends on the intensity of the cooperation. It is therefore justifiable that inhabitants of the same country protect each other more than they protect inhabitants of other countries, but global justice requires that people protect each other across borders too.

A global social protection scheme is feasible in the form of cross-subsidies between national social protections schemes, and it does not conflict with the principle that inhabitants of a state ought to be allowed to participate in decisions about contributions or about policies that make them eligible for support. The price for such a solution, however, is to accept the political reality that global mutual social support is only feasible if the world's most powerful countries are supportive of its establishment, and this will probably result in an insufficiently ambitious global layer. Nonetheless, if all other factors hold constant, it would not increase global injustice, it would decrease global injustice.

PART TWO

Practical Challenges in Global Health Governance

6

Righting Climate Change Wrongs? The Human Right to Health as Accountability Mechanism for the Health Impacts of Climate Change

Keith Syrett

Introduction

If the premise that health constitutes a global public good, which 'affect[s] all countries and regions, which may have intergenerational impacts, which all may share and from which none may be excluded' is accepted,[1] it becomes imperative for the international community to take steps to address the consequences of climate change. While the consequences for human health have, in the past, tended to be somewhat overlooked by comparison with the widely known (albeit, often not fully understood) environmental impacts,[2] there is an evolving consensus that climate change represents a significant challenge for the health of all populations. Indeed, one influential account has contended that 'climate change is the biggest global health threat of the 21st century'.[3] Furthermore, since the effects of climate change tend to amplify existing risks to health,[4] poor and disadvantaged populations in the global South bear a burden of disease which is grossly disproportionate to the extent of their contribution to the problem.[5] Climate change therefore exacerbates existing health inequalities

---

1   Graham Lister, 'Interdependence' in Marshall Marinker (ed.), *Constructive Conversations about Health: Policy and Values* (Abingdon: Radcliffe Publishing, 2006) 142.
2   See for example Edward Maibach, Matthew Nisbet, Paula Baldwin, Karen Akerlof and Guoqing Diao, 'Reframing Climate Change as a Public Health Issue: An Exploratory Study of Public Reactions' *BMC Public Health*, 2010, 10: 299, reporting survey results which indicate that 'the human health consequences of climate change are seriously underestimated and/or poorly understood, if grasped at all'.
3   Anthony Costello, Mustafa Abbas, Adriana Allen, Sarah Ball, Sarah Bell, Richard Bellamy, et al., 'Managing the Health Effects of Climate Change', *Lancet*, 2009, 373: 1693.
4   Ibid., 1712. See also Sharon Friel, Michael Marmot, Anthony McMichael, Tord Kjellstrom and Denny Vågerö, 'Global Health Equity and Climate Stabilisation: A Common Agenda', *Lancet*, 2008, 372: 1677.
5   See for example Jonathan Patz, Holly Gibbs, Jonathan Foley, Jamesine Rogers and Kirk Smith, 'Climate Change and Global Health: Quantifying a Growing Ethical Crisis', *EcoHealth*, 2007, 4: 397.

between developed and developing nations, and between rich and poor. As such, it raises profound and difficult problems of justice.

The goal of this chapter is to explore the potential for the human right to health to play a role as a space within which accountability for the injustices caused by climate change may be critically interrogated and, potentially, secured. The focus is upon accountability through judicial or quasi-judicial human rights mechanisms. Of course, various other modes of accountability exist in this context: Potts additionally enumerates administrative, political and social means through which answerability for acts and omissions in respect of the right to health may be realized,[6] and these may well be germane to the climate change context. However, a concentration upon judicial/quasi-judicial forms may be justified on a number of bases.

First, while a human right carries hugely significant normative and political weight, and functions discursively as a particular means of 'framing' an issue within political and civil society,[7] an argument for legal enforcement lies at the core of a rights claim. Indeed, it is, in part, the obstacles to legal enforcement which have led some to contend that human rights are inapplicable to health and/or health care.[8] Following from this, and secondly, judicial (and to a somewhat lesser extent, quasi-judicial) mechanisms constitute interesting subjects of study *precisely because* accountability through such means is problematic. In this respect, the central objective of the subsequent analysis is to explore readings of accountability which might render judicial and non-judicial mechanisms more helpful in the context of the health impacts of climate change than has sometimes been supposed. Thirdly, and most specifically, the notion that legal modes form the primary means through which the human right to health can be articulated, and accountability for the health impacts of climate change thereby realized, appears to have currency with the Office of the High Commissioner for Human Rights (OHCHR) at the United Nations. The report upon the linkages between human rights and climate change which was issued by the OHCHR in 2009 forms the foundation of the critical analysis offered in this chapter.[9] While its conclusions cannot be regarded as determinative of the

---

6   Helen Potts, *Accountability and the Right to the Highest Attainable Standard of Health* (Colchester: University of Essex Human Rights Centre, 2008), 17.

7   The value of 'framing' is explored at length in Karen O'Brien, Asunción Lera St Clair and Berit Kristoffersen, 'The Framing of Climate Change: Why It Matters', in Karen O'Brien, Asunción Lera St Clair and Berit Kristoffersen (eds), *Climate Change, Ethics and Human Security* (Cambridge: Cambridge University Press, 2010).

8   For discussion, see for example Brigit Toebes, 'Towards an Improved Understanding of the International Human Right to Health', *Human Rights Quarterly*, 1999, 21: 661; Imre Loefter, '"Health Care is a Human Right" Is a Meaningless and Devastating Manifesto', *British Medical Journal*, 1999, 318: 1766; Philip Barlow, 'Health Care Is Not a Human Right', *British Medical Journal*, 1999, 319: 321; Theodore Dalrymple, 'Is There a "Right" to Health Care?', *Wall Street Journal*, 28 July 2009.

9   Report of the Office of the United Nations High Commissioner for Human Rights on the relationship between climate change and human rights (A/HRC/10/61) (15 January 2009).

position in international human rights law, they are nonetheless likely to prove highly influential – especially within the United Nations human rights system – as they amount to the first statement made by an international human rights body on the relationship between climate change and human rights.[10]

The subsequent discussion is structured as follows. First, the implications of climate change for population health are briefly outlined. The analysis then turns to consider the prospects for securing accountability for the consequences of climate change by means of invocation of the human right to health in judicial and quasi-judicial fora, with particular reference to the views expressed by the OHCHR on this matter. Next, an argument is advanced for an expanded conception of the meaning of accountability. It is contended that this may render human rights adjudication a more useful vehicle through which the health impacts of climate change, and the means selected to address them, may be articulated, debated and scrutinized. The final section of the chapter explores the manner in which the human right to health is best construed if concerns as to the suitability and scope of judicial and quasi-judicial activity at the climate change/health interface are – at least to some extent – to be allayed.

The human health impacts of climate change

The impacts of climate change on human health have usefully been classified as being either direct or indirect in character.[11] Direct effects include those which arise from thermal stress at either end of the temperature scale (heatwaves and winter cold), other extreme weather events (floods, storms, droughts) and increases in certain air pollutants and aeroallergens (spores and moulds). In certain countries, there may be beneficial aspects to these developments (e.g. milder winters in temperate countries may reduce mortality), but the expectation is that the impacts will be predominantly negative. Importantly, however, 'the extent of change in the frequency, intensity and location of extreme weather events due to climate change remains uncertain'.[12]

Effects which manifest themselves in more indirect ways include those upon the transmission of infectious diseases, such as those borne in water (e.g. cholera), vector organisms (e.g. dengue fever and malaria) or food (e.g. salmonella), and on regional food productivity (particularly cereal grains, which account

10 See John Knox, 'Linking Human Rights and Climate Change at the United Nations', *Harvard Environmental Law Review*, 2009, 33: 477.
11 See A. McMichael, 'Global Climate Change and Health: An Old Story Writ Large', in A. McMichael, D. Campbell-Lendrum, C. Corvalán, K. Ebi, A. Githeko, J. Scheraga and A. Woodward (eds), *Climate Change and Human Health: Risks and Responses* (Geneva: World Health Organization, 2003), 11.
12 Ibid.

for some two-thirds of global food energy).[13] In addition, climate change is likely to impact upon a range of social, economic and political structures, with deleterious consequences for human health. For example, decreases in food productivity or geographical distribution of fish stocks may trigger malnutrition, migration (often to already overcrowded urban areas) and conflict, leading in turn to increased pressure on health-care resources and other social services, and to mental health problems.

Given uncertainties in modelling, quantification of the precise extent of these impacts is problematic.[14] Campbell-Lendrum et al. estimate that 5.5 million disability-adjusted life years were lost in 2000 as a consequence of climate change, a figure which is expected to increase progressively over time (in contrast to some other threats to health, such as tobacco use, which – while contributing more to the overall global burden of disease – are decreasing in incidence).[15] There is, however, general agreement that the effects will exacerbate existing inequalities in health between developing and developed nations.[16] For example, it has been estimated that poor African populations will suffer 500 times greater loss of healthy life years than their European counterparts as a consequence of global environmental change, including climate change.[17] A number of factors explain such variation, including differing rates of incidence, existing underlying vulnerabilities (both health-related and social, economic and political) and adaptive capacity. As Smith has graphically stated, the consequence is that 'the rich will find their world to be more expensive, inconvenient, uncomfortable, disrupted, and colourless – in general, more unpleasant and unpredictable, perhaps greatly so. The poor will die'.[18]

The (f)utility of human rights? The OHCHR report

In his report to the United Nations General Assembly of August 2007, the Special Rapporteur on the right of everyone to the enjoyment of the highest

---

13   Ibid.
14   See Anthony McMichael, Rosalie Woodruff and Simon Hales, 'Climate Change and Human Health: Present and Future Risks', *Lancet*, 2006, 367:859, 864.
15   D. Campbell-Lendrum, C. Corvalán and A. Prüss-Ustün, 'How Much Disease Could Climate Change Cause?', in McMichael, Campbell-Lendrum, Corvalán, Ebi, Githeko, Scheraga and Woodward (eds), *Climate Change and Human Health*.
16   See for example Costello, Abbas, Allen, Ball, Bell, Bellamy, et al., 'Managing the Health Effects'; Friel, Marmot, McMichael, Kjellstrom and Vågerö, 'Global Health Equity'; Patz, Gibbs, Foley, Rogers and Smith, 'Climate Change and Global Health'; Report of the Office of the United Nations High Commissioner for Human Rights, 32–3.
17   A. McMichael, S. Friel, A. Nyong and C. Corvalán, 'Global Environmental Change and Health: Impacts, Inequalities and the Health Sector', 336 *British Medical Journal*, 2008, 336: 191.
18   Kirk Smith, 'Introduction: Mitigating, Adapting and Suffering: How Much of Each?', *Annual Review of Public Health*, 2008, 29: 11, 11.

attainable standard of physical and mental health, Paul Hunt, issued some brief observations on the relationship between climate change and health in the context of a discussion of water, sanitation and the human right to health. Referring to the 'disturbing trends' of increased frequencies of droughts and floods and the consequent impact upon vector-borne diseases, diseases arising from polluted water supplies, drowning and malnutrition arising from flooding, the Special Rapporteur claimed that 'the international community has not yet confronted the health threats posed by global warming. The failure of the international community to take the health impact of global warming seriously will endanger the lives of millions of people across the world'.[19] Accordingly, he called upon the Human Rights Council to 'urgently study the impact of climate change on human rights generally and the right to the highest attainable standard of health in particular'.[20] In response, the Council passed a Resolution which expressed concern that climate change posed 'an immediate and far-reaching threat to people and communities around the world and [that it] has implications for the full enjoyment of human rights' and called upon the Office of the High Commissioner for Human Rights (OHCHR) to conduct a detailed analytical study of the relationship between climate change and human rights.[21]

The resulting report was published on 15 January 2009. The OHCHR observed that global warming, which it regarded as synonymous with climate change, might potentially carry implications for the full range of human rights,[22] but it identified six which were likely to be most severely affected, including the right to health.[23] Describing the health impacts of climate change, the report observed that individuals and communities with low adaptive capacity – particularly those already suffering from poor health or malnutrition – were most vulnerable, and noted that 'comprehensive measures', including education, health care and public health initiatives, would be necessary to address such vulnerability.[24]

The OHCHR reached the perhaps unsurprising conclusion that climate change 'has generally negative effects on the realisation of human rights',[25] including the right to health. More striking and contentious was its argument that 'it is less obvious whether, and to what extent, such effects can be qualified

---

19   Report of the United Nations Special Rapporteur on the right of everyone to the enjoyment of the highest attainable standard of physical and mental health (A/62/214) (8 August 2007), 102.

20   Ibid., 107.

21   United Nations Human Rights Council, Resolution 7/23, 'Human Rights and Climate Change' (28 March 2008).

22   Report of the Office of the United Nations High Commissioner for Human Rights, 20.

23   The other rights listed were the right to life, the right to adequate food, the right to water, the right to adequate housing and the right to self-determination.

24   Ibid., 33–34.

25   Ibid., 69.

as human rights violations in a strict legal sense',[26] and – still more bluntly – that 'the physical impacts of global warming cannot easily be classified as human rights violations'.[27] Despite this conclusion, the OHCHR was at considerable pains to indicate that 'legal protection remains relevant as a safeguard against climate-change-related risks and infringements of human rights resulting from policies and measures taken at the national level to address climate change'.[28] Its reasoning here appears to have rested upon the familiar tripartite typology of obligations which exist, *inter alia* under the International Covenant on Economic, Social and Cultural Rights, to respect, protect and fulfil human rights.[29] On the basis of this classification, it can be seen that the OHCHR was of the opinion that enforceability of the obligation to *respect* those human rights which might be affected by climate change could not be achieved through legal means ('it is doubtful . . . that an individual would be able to hold a particular State responsible for harm caused by climate change'),[30] but that some degree of accountability through judicial and quasi-judicial mechanisms could be achieved through enforcement of the obligation to *protect* against an individual's 'home' state ('in such cases, it would appear that the matter of the case would rest on whether the State through its acts or omissions had failed to protect an individual against a harm affecting the enjoyment of human rights').[31]

The OHCHR identified a number of obstacles to legal enforcement of the obligation to respect human rights in the climate change context.[32] First, there is a problem of attribution of responsibility. Given that all countries have – albeit to varying extents – contributed to global warming through the emission of greenhouse gases, it is impossible to connect a particular impact upon human rights to the actions of a given state. Secondly, there are problems of causation. The direct cause (in so far as it occupies the same spatiotemporal field) of the impaired right may be a heatwave, flood or vector-borne disease, etc.; that

26   Ibid., 70.
27   Ibid., 96.
28   Ibid.
29   See Report of the Special Rapporteur on the right to adequate food of the UN Sub-Commission on Prevention of Discrimination and Protection of Minorities, *The Right to Adequate Food as a Human Right* (E/CN.4/Sub.2/1987/23) (7 July 1987). The Committee on Economic, Social and Cultural Rights has endorsed this typology in the context of the right to health: see General Comment No.14, *The Right to the Highest Attainable Standard of Health* (E/C.12/2000/4) (11 August 2000), 33. For a discussion of the evolution of this typology, see Magdalena Sepúldeva, *The Nature of the Obligations under the International Covenant on Economic, Social and Cultural Rights* (Antwerp: Intersentia, 2003), 157–64.
30   Report of the Office of the United Nations High Commissioner for Human Rights, 72. Note also Knox's view that the conclusion reached by the OHCHR was influenced by political factors; that is, that assigning liability to powerful states (such as the US) for violations of human rights as a consequence of greenhouse gas emissions would render future negotiations towards a climate agreement considerably more awkward: 'Linking Human Rights and Climate Change', 489–90.
31   Ibid., 73.
32   Ibid., 70.

event *may* have been caused by climate change, but achieving the standard of legal proof of causality necessary to establish this is likely to be impracticable. Thirdly, the OHCHR refers to the problem of future harm, noting that the Human Rights Committee has indicated that, for an act or omission to be characterized as a violation of rights, it is necessary that the adverse impact should already have taken place or be imminent.[33] Demonstrating this will frequently prove problematic in the climate change context, as is the case with many other forms of environmental harm.

In addition to the impediments acknowledged by the OHCHR, other factors militate against securing accountability for the impacts of climate change upon health through imposition of a legal obligation to respect human rights. First, there is the difficulty that international law does not normally permit litigants to bring actions alleging that a state has interfered with the enjoyment of human rights beyond its own national boundaries. This precludes citizens of, for example, the United States from seeking legal redress for harms caused to (say) populations living in sub-Saharan Africa as a consequence of the former state's greenhouse gas emissions. This is problematic because those who are most likely to activate judicial and quasi-judicial mechanisms tend to reside in those countries which are least affected by climate change. Secondly, even if the subject-matter of a legal challenge is harm done within the aspiring litigant's own jurisdiction, there may well be problems of *locus standi*. That is, an individual (or, where the applicable legal framework permits this, a representative organization) may find it difficult to show that he/she is sufficiently and directly harmed by climate change to a degree greater than other residents of that state (as frameworks for the protection of human rights generally require), given that many of its effects – including those upon human health – tend to be geographically and temporally highly diffuse in character. Finally, there are familiar arguments relating to the non-justiciability of the right to health. These centre upon its lack of definitional clarity; the collective nature of at least some of the actions which may need to be taken to give it effect; the fact that it frequently gives rise to positive obligations on the part of states to expend resources; and the fact that, as a right which is subject to an obligation of progressive realization on the part of the state, it may be said to possess a 'programmatic' character. These last two arguments, in particular, speak to concerns as to possible violation of the separation of powers and the democratic legitimacy of judges which may be said to render questions of the right to health more suitable for enforcement and accountability through political mechanisms than legal.[34]

33   See *Aalbersberg v The Netherlands*, No. 1440/2005.
34   For a critical analysis of these latter two objections to justiciability, see Roberto Gargarella, 'Dialogic Justice in the Enforcement of Social Rights: Some Initial Arguments,' in Alicia Yamin and Siri Gloppen (eds), *Litigating Health Rights* (Cambridge, MA: Harvard University Press, 2011), 232.

As the OHCHR suggests, certain of these obstacles can be overcome if one construes the legal obligation which is placed upon the state in the climate change context as being one of protecting individuals against threats arising from climate change which may interfere with the enjoyment of human rights. In particular, the problems of attribution and causation do not arise, because the claim which is made is not that the state bears responsibility for causing or contributing to climate change (i.e. that its emissions of greenhouse gases trigger events which impact upon human health), but rather that it has *failed to take steps to ensure that individuals are secure from the harm which climate change may bring about.* In such circumstances, also, there is no risk of impermissible transboundary litigation, since the legal action turns upon the measures which the state has taken (or, more frequently, failed to take) to address harms which may eventuate to those residing within its borders – albeit that, as noted above, this is likely to afford little protection to those populations who must suffer the worst consequences of climate change at a global level. Furthermore, the temporal reach of the litigation is likely to be reduced since a legal obligation upon the state will only arise in respect of those harms which are foreseeable.

However, the requirement to demonstrate the foreseeability of events which threaten to harm human rights may itself prove problematic. This is because (as previously discussed) there is uncertainty as to the *degree* to which climate change will increase the frequency of events such as heatwaves, floods or the incidence of infectious diseases, with the consequence that it is unclear how far the state's legal obligations to take adaptive measures to protect the right to health can be said to extend. When set alongside continued difficulties relating to *locus standi* (it being difficult for an individual to demonstrate that he/she is more adversely affected than the rest of the population by the state's failure to take steps to protect against the impacts of climate change) and ambivalence regarding justiciability, it becomes apparent that there remain limited prospects of securing accountability in judicial and/or quasi-judicial mechanisms for the health impacts of climate change through invocation of an obligation to protect the human right to health, notwithstanding the views of the OHCHR.

Towards a re-reading of 'accountability'

If the preceding analysis is accepted, a plausible response would be for those who would seek to secure accountability for the health impacts of climate change to abandon any attempt to utilize judicial and quasi-judicial human rights mechanisms for the purpose. It is submitted that this would be a regrettable course of action. Such mechanisms have value, particularly in so far as the authority which attaches to a statement of the legal position is likely to be highly influential in shaping future debate (whether at state level, or in the international arena) about the consequences of climate change and the most appropriate means to address these. Furthermore, the existence of legal precedent, even in situations in which – as is the case with many international legal frameworks – there is an absence of effective sanction for violation, may serve to set parameters as to the actions which, at least as a matter of politics, are regarded as acceptable in this context. Thus, as Osofsky notes in a study of the value of climate litigation in both domestic (United States) and international law, 'these cases help to bring attention to the regulatory options and debates, and push policymakers to address more nuances of the problem in the process'.[35]

The argument which is advanced here is that it is not necessary to jettison this mode of accountability, even assuming that it may be possible to sever it from other mechanisms.[36] Rather, what is required is the adoption of a broader perspective as to the meaning and function of accountability than that which is taken in the OHCHR report discussed in the preceding section. This, in turn, can inform a more nuanced approach on the part of judicial and quasi-judicial institutions albeit that – as will subsequently be discussed – this may prove no easy task.

It was not inevitable that the OHCHR should have read the notion of accountability as being predominantly legal in character, focused upon the attribution of responsibility for violations of rights. This much is apparent from the work of Paul Hunt, which – as noted previously – was highly instrumental in prompting the United Nations to consider the relationship between climate change and human rights. In his first interim report to the General Assembly in 2004, the then Special Rapporteur sought to build awareness of the existence of a wider range of institutional mechanisms for the realization of accountability for the right to health, on the basis that 'in relation to a human right as complex as the right to health, a range of accountability mechanisms is required and the form and mix of devices will vary from one State to another'.[37] However, of more significance for the present analysis, he also called for a broader understanding of the meaning of the concept, contending that 'all too often, "accountability" is used to mean blame and punishment. But this narrow understanding of the term is much too limited. A right to health accountability

---

35 Hari Osofsky, 'The Continuing Importance of Climate Change Litigation', *Climate Law*, 2010, 1: 3, 29.

36 Potts, *Accountability*, 27 argues that 'while it is principally the judicial accountability mechanism that provides the final platform for government accountability (for the right to health), this is a mechanism that rarely operates in isolation from other mechanisms. Frequently, recourse to judicial mechanisms arises from and feeds back into other accountability mechanisms'.

37 Report of the United Nations Special Rapporteur on the right of everyone to the enjoyment of the highest attainable standard of physical and mental health (A/59/422) (8 October 2004), 38.

mechanism establishes which health policies and institutions are working and which are not, and why, with the objective of improving the realization of the right to health for all'.[38] Elsewhere, reiterating his rejection of an approach rooted purely in the assignment of blame and attendant sanctions, Hunt has stated that accountability 'is a process that helps to identify what works, so it can be repeated, and what does not, so it can be revised. It is a way of checking that reasonable balances are fairly struck'.[39]

On this approach, accountability is not profitably viewed as a one-off win or lose scenario in which the successful 'victor' assigns blame to the 'loser' for deficiencies in their performance (in this case, those which amount to violations of the right to health). Rather, it is a continuous,[40] educative process which contributes to the enhancement of institutional performance and future decision-making. As Diane Longley has argued in the context of the accountability of health services, legal mechanisms (such as courts) will play a role in such an exercise, in so far as there will be a need for some form of guidance and structuring to ensure that the objectives of the process are realized:

> Accountability is an ongoing evaluative process which should provide a vehicle for improvement and change. Such a focus might preclude the provision of any easy answers, but it should frame the questions that could lead to a better understanding of contending issues. Accountability is thus fundamental to an organisation's learning. For this to become a possibility some external direction is required . . . The techniques and processes of law can assist in providing that external direction.[41]

In order for this form of accountability to exist, it is necessary for there to be 'open discussion of priorities and objectives before decisions reach a stage in which there is no real choice'.[42] Longley therefore characterizes the components of accountability as follows:

> The central prerequisite for genuine accountability is clearly openness, a transparency which needs to embrace all decision-making from policy-setting, through implementation to monitoring. A commitment to openness is of prime importance in order to counteract any tendency to control or distort information which might in turn prevent issues being the subject of proper debate and reduce capacity for reasoned choices to be made . . . The same commitment also implies an obligation on the part of decision-makers to give explanations and justifications for their activities.[43]

38 Ibid., 37.
39 Paul Hunt and Gunilla Backman, 'Health Systems and the Right to the Highest Attainable Standard of Health', *Health and Human Rights,* 2008, 10: 81, 89.
40 See further Potts, *Accountability,* 13.
41 Diane Longley, *Public Law and Health Service Accountability* (Buckingham: Open University Press, 1993), 104–5.
42 Ibid., 104.
43 Ibid., 7–8.

When viewed from this angle, accountability takes on a quite different character from that envisaged in the OHCHR report. It entails the presentation of reasoned arguments, evidence and explanation for activities and decisions with a view not to the attribution of blame, but rather to the development of public understanding and social and institutional learning. The process therefore attains a deliberative or dialogic character which has been well captured by Schedler:

> The norm of accountability continues the Enlightenment's project of subjecting power not only to the rule of law but also to the rule of reason. Power should be bound by legal constraints but also by the logic of public reasoning. Accountability is antithetical to monologic power. It establishes a dialogic relationship between accountable and accounting actors.[44]

Rights adjudication and accountability

How might human rights adjudication fit within this expanded notion of accountability? Guidance in this regard may be found in contemporary analyses of judicial approaches to socioeconomic rights, including the right to access healthcare services, with a particular emphasis being given to those rights which are protected by the Constitution of South Africa.[45] It has been argued that cases such as *Government of the Republic of South Africa v Grootboom*[46] and *Minister of Health v Treatment Action Campaign (No. 2)*[47] illustrate a willingness on the part of the Constitutional Court of South Africa to adopt a *deliberative* or *dialogic* conceptualization of the function of rights litigation. In these cases, judicial evaluation of the lawfulness of state action against a standard of 'reasonableness' functions as a means of requiring 'that the State explain and justify to the court, and therefore to the litigants and the public more generally, the grounds of its decisions and the reasons for the selection of particular means'.[48] Although the court's judgment is determinative of the issue in front of it, it does not foreclose further deliberation within the political branches and civil society in general, that is 'the decision remains part of a process of continuing revisability, whether through Parliament, case law or public discourse'.[49] Indeed, the publicity attendant upon a judicial

---

44   Andreas Schedler, 'Conceptualising Accountability' in Andreas Schedler, Larry Diamond and Marc Plattner (eds), *The Self-Restraining State* (Boulder: Lynne Rienner, 1999), 15.

45   For discussion, see Sandra Fredman, *Human Rights Transformed* (Oxford: Oxford University Press, 2008); Keith Syrett, *Law, Legitimacy and the Rationing of Health Care* (Cambridge: Cambridge University Press, 2007), especially Chapter 8.

46   (2001) (1) SA 46.

47   (2002) (5) SA 721.

48   Fredman, *Human Rights*, 108.

49   Ibid., 109.

pronouncement, especially one issued by a supreme or constitutional court, serves as a *catalyst* for further public dialogue on the issue which forms the subject-matter of the litigation. Understood in this manner,

> Rights should not be regarded as simply overriding the will of the democratic majority or trumping policy considerations. Rights are not fixed immutable boundaries, but are standards of justification, the content and meaning of which alter with shifts in the social context . . . Rights cannot be considered brightline boundaries between the spheres of individual freedom and legitimate state power, but rather constitute a social practice and an occasion for deliberation on vital social issues.[50]

While the constitutional entrenchment of socioeconomic rights (as exists in South Africa) undoubtedly serves to facilitate judicial adoption of this deliberative approach, the key to rereading the nature of accountability lies in the adoption of a conception, which runs as a thread through this jurisprudence, of 'law as justification'.[51] On this understanding, litigation functions as a means by which decision-makers are obliged to explain and rationalize their choices using arguments which can be accepted – or, at least, comprehended – by all. It therefore serves to build public understanding and to provide the foundation for a broad societal debate upon problems and their purported solutions. This function is not exclusively performed in instances where justiciable socioeconomic rights are in play. Rather, it is an inherent (albeit, not always clearly articulated) feature of the judicial role in all cases in which the exercise of state power is at issue. As Dyzenhaus argues, 'what justifies all public power is the ability of its incumbents to offer adequate reasons for the decisions which affect those subject to them . . . The courts' special role is as an ultimate enforcement mechanism for such justification'.[52]

Interestingly, both the narrow and broader conceptions of accountability discussed here can be discerned at play in one well-known instance of climate change litigation. In 2005, the Inuit Circumpolar Conference lodged a petition at the Inter-American Commission on Human Rights in which it alleged that the acts and omissions of the government of the United States had contributed to climate change which, in turn had affected the enjoyment by the Inuit peoples of various human rights, including the right to health.[53] The quasi-judicial Commission, adopting an approach similar to that of the OHCHR discussed

---

50 Johan van der Walt and Henk Botha, 'Democracy and Rights in South Africa: Beyond a Constitutional Culture of Justification', *Constellations*, 2000, 7: 341, 343–4.

51 Ibid., 344 commenting on Etienne Mureinik, 'A Bridge to Where? Introducing the Interim Bill of Rights', *South African Journal of Human Rights*, 1994, 10: 31.

52 David Dyzenhaus, 'The Politics of Deference: Judicial Review and Democracy', in Michael Taggart (ed.), *The Province of Administrative Law* (Oxford: Hart, 1997), 305.

53 Petition to the Inter-American Commission on Human Rights seeking relief from global warming caused by acts and omissions of the United States, 7 December 2005, available at http://inuitcircumpolar.com/files/uploads/icc-files/FINALPetitionICC.pdf.

previously, declined to entertain the case on the basis that it had insufficient information to determine whether the alleged facts would tend to characterize a violation of the rights protected by the American Declaration on the Rights and Duties of Man, although a subsequent hearing on the linkages between climate change and human rights did take place. However, the petitioner construed the function of the litigation in a much more deliberative manner than did the Commission, viewing it as a means of catalysing a debate on an issue which, for reasons of US domestic politics, had not proved possible in other, political, arenas. This is clearly apparent from the statement made by the Chair of the Conference, Sheila Watt-Cloutier:

> A declaration from the Commission may not [be] enforceable, but it has great moral value. We intend the petition to educate and encourage the United States to join the community of nations in a global effort to combat climate change . . . This petition is our means of inviting the United States to talk with us and to put this global issue into a broader human and human rights context. Our intent is to encourage and inform.[54]

As Osofsky observes, the dialogic character of the petition, which informs Watt-Cloutier's remarks, should give us cause to reconsider the traditional 'win-lose' model of litigation,[55] which – it is argued – underpins the OHCHR's conclusions as to the prospects of securing accountability for the impacts of climate change via human rights adjudication. On this broader, more deliberative reading of accountability, judicial and quasi-judicial mechanisms function to some extent independently of the outcome of the litigation. That is, they represent valuable means of catalysing a debate on climate change issues within civil society and the political branches of government (both domestically and internationally), even if the affected parties fail to demonstrate a violation in law of the obligation either to respect or protect human rights, such as the right to health.

Proceduralization of the right to health?

The preceding discussion has sought to outline the manner in which accountability might be reconceptualized in order that rights adjudication through judicial and quasi-judicial mechanisms might make a useful contribution to a wider process of democratic debate as to the nature of the

---

54   Sheila Watt-Cloutier, *Presentation to Eleventh Conference of Parties to the UN Framework Convention on Climate Change,* 7 December 2005, available at www.inuitcircumpolar.com/index.php?ID=318&Lang=En.
55   Hari Osofsky, 'The Inuit Petition as a Bridge? Beyond Dialectics of Climate Change and Indigenous Peoples' Rights', *American Indian Law Review,* 2007, 31: 675, 696.

impacts of climate change (including those on human health) and how best
these should be managed. However, although it is suggested that realization
of the broader form of accountability should be viewed as intrinsic to the
judicial/quasi-judicial function when called upon to regulate exercises of
state power, it does not follow that adoption of such a reading will necessarily
prove to be a straightforward task.

The difficulty lies in the fact that judges and others who bear responsibility
for operation of these institutions may themselves be rooted in the narrower
conception, in which litigation amounts to a zero-sum game and accountability
connotes blame and the attendant visitation of sanctions. The influential
Dworkinian account of rights as 'trumps',[56] overriding other types of reasons
for decisions, actions, policies or omissions which are advanced by the
state, tends to reinforce this more limited perspective on the nature of legal
accountability. And while the South African example demonstrates that such
an understanding, while dominant, is not inevitable, the particular character of
constitutional rights jurisprudence in that state, which connects closely to its
recent history,[57] needs to be recognized. That is, the prospect of transplantation
to other legal orders, whether domestic, regional or international, must be read
in light of the socio-political context of the system within which this approach
to accountability has evolved.[58]

With regard to the subject-matter of this chapter, this problem is exacerbated
by continuing ambivalence as to the justiciability of the right to health for the
reasons previously identified. Persuasive arguments have been advanced within
the academic literature 'that judicial intervention in cases involving health
rights in particular and social rights in general can be perfectly justifiable'.[59]
Nonetheless, the inherent conservatism of the judiciary, especially that which
operates within domestic legal systems with no tradition of entrenchment of
socioeconomic rights, is likely to limit willingness to articulate the broader
vision of accountability for the health impacts of climate change which is
argued for here.

For these reasons, courts and cognate institutions may remain reluctant
to entertain cases in which individuals or groups seek to argue that rights to

---

56   See for example Ronald Dworkin, 'Rights as Trumps', in Jeremy Waldron (ed.), *Theories of Rights* (Oxford: Oxford University Press, 2004).

57   Mureinik, 'A Bridge to Where?', 32 argues that the shift to a 'culture of justification' reflected a desire to build a political order based upon persuasion rather than the coercion which had characterized the apartheid regime.

58   Although note that the deliberative or dialogic reading of rights adjudication has not solely been identified as operating within the South African context; for example, Fredman refers extensively to the jurisprudence of the Indian Supreme Court: *Human Rights*, Chapter 5. See also Varun Gauri and Daniel Brinks (eds), *Courting Social Justice* (Cambridge: Cambridge University Press, 2008), analysing rights litigation in Brazil, Indonesia and Nigeria, in addition to South Africa and India.

59   Gargarella, 'Dialogic Justice', 243. See also Yamin and Gloppen (eds), *Litigating Health Rights*, generally; Syrett, *Law, Legitimacy*, especially Chapter 9.

health have been violated as a consequence of climate change. If this is so, then a possible way forward may be for judicial and quasi-judicial bodies to focus attention upon the *procedural* dimensions of the right to health, rather than being drawn into evaluation of whether the *substance* of the right has been violated or not. Such an approach would limit the scope of judicial encroachment on the territory of the political branches of government (since there would be no question of prescribing a particular substantive outcome and consequent allocation of resources). Yet it would still afford an opportunity for affected individuals and groups to articulate the health impacts of climate change in a public forum, with a view to contributing to a process of social learning about those impacts and catalysing a public debate about how they might best be addressed.

A model for this type of procedural reading has evolved in recent years in the wider context of adjudication, especially by regional human rights institutions in Europe, of rights which are impacted by various forms of environmental harm and degradation. Of particular importance here has been the influence of the Aarhus Convention on Access to Information, Public Participation in Decision-Making and Access to Justice in Environmental Matters (1998) which, as its title indicates, obliges state parties to guarantee certain procedural rights to the public in respect of environmental matters, including those which impact upon health and wellbeing. The Convention has informed the jurisprudence of the European Court of Human Rights on Article 2 (the right to life) and Article 8 (the right to respect for private life, family, home and correspondence) of the European Convention on Human Rights. The Court has ruled that failure of a state to provide information on the severity of an environmental threat,[60] or to provide opportunity for participation in a fair decision-making process on the issuing of authorization for activities which gave rise to environmental damage,[61] constitute grounds for determination of cases in favour of applicants. Similarly, the quasi-judicial European Committee of Social Rights has concluded that the right to health (protected by Article 11 of the European Social Charter) entails provision of information, processes of consultation and education policies designed to involve local communities in environmental impact assessment and health policy debate regarding a particular industrial activity which had caused harm to the environment (in this case, lignite mining).[62]

Although this line of jurisprudence does not specifically address the health impacts of climate change, there seems no reason why it could not, in principle, apply in that context. Of course, there remain certain limitations. In particular, the cases noted above are focused upon provision of information and

---

60 *Öneryildiz v Turkey*, 2004-XII 41 Eur. Ct. H.R. 20.
61 *Taskin v Turkey*, 2004-X 42 Eur. Ct. H.R. 50.
62 *Marangopoulos Foundation for Human Rights v Greece*, No.30/2005, 37, 103.

opportunities for participation in decision-making to those who are themselves directly affected by the harm. By contrast, in the case of the health consequences of climate change, the state in which the deficiencies in democratic procedure arise will, most probably, be one in which those impacts are minimal. Although the Aarhus Convention is applicable 'without discrimination as to citizenship, nationality or domicile',[63] populations in countries affected by climate change may lack the resources necessary to pursue human rights litigation, while those in defaulting nations may lack the necessary motivation or may face difficulties of *locus standi*, given the absence of impact upon *their* interests.

Conclusion

In light of these continuing hurdles, the modest assessment advanced by Paul Hunt (in a wider context), that 'courts [and quasi-judicial mechanisms] are not a panacea ... Nonetheless as one form of accountability, [they] have a significant role to play in the promotion and protection of health-related rights',[64] would seem to be highly apposite to the climate change case.

The argument advanced here is that, in order to fulfil their potential to play such a role, courts and quasi-judicial mechanisms need to adopt a conception of accountability which moves beyond simple attribution of blame and which instead situates rights adjudication within a broader democratic, deliberative arena. This can enable litigation to act as an impetus for social and institutional learning about, and as a catalyst for public debate upon, the health impacts of climate change and the most appropriate means to address these. The most fruitful avenue by which this objective might be achieved would appear to be *via* articulation of procedural rights at the climate change/health interface, since this is likely to minimize judicial concerns as to intrusion on the territory of the political branches of government. Instead, the latter are left free to respond to the effects of climate change upon population health in whatever manner they see fit, provided that they have respected certain democratic procedural obligations when adopting the measures which they consider suitable.

Alan Boyle has contended that:

> As the internationalization of the domestic environment becomes more extensive, through policies of sustainable development, protection of biodiversity, and mitigation of climate change, the role of human rights law in democratizing national decision-making processes and making them more rational, open and legitimate will become more and not less significant.[65]

63   Article 3(9).
64   Report of the United Nations Special Rapporteur on the right of everyone to the enjoyment of the highest attainable standard of physical and mental health (A/HRC/4/28) (17 January 2007), 88.

The analysis presented in this chapter would tend to support such a view. If the global good of population health is to be upheld, as far as possible, in the face of the significant challenges presented by climate change, it may well be necessary to exert pressure upon recalcitrant states through means other than 'traditional' politics. Rights adjudication, if approached in the manner outlined here, presents an opportunity to circumvent political channels which may be blocked by unsympathetic governments.[66] It is not a substitute for inclusive and informed debate and decision-making, but it nonetheless possesses the capacity to function as a valuable input into, and stimulus for, such democratic activities.

---

65   Alan Boyle, 'Human Rights or Environmental Rights: A Reassessment', *Fordham Environmental Law Review*, 2007, 18: 471, 510.
66   For a discussion of this, and other forms of 'blockage', see Varun Gauri and Daniel Brinks, 'Introduction: The Elements of Legalization and the Triangular Shape of Social and Economic Rights', in Gauri and Brinks (eds), *Courting Social Justice*, especially 26–7.

7

Genetically Modified Organisms: An Ethical and Sustainable Way to Food Security?

Lisbeth Witthøfft Nielsen

Introduction

The problem of anthropogenic climate change and the challenges it poses to agriculture and food production in general has brought up the question about application of GMOs (genetically modified organisms)[1] as part of a climate adaptation strategy to food security. A report published by the Royal Society, United Kingdom, in 2009, argues that there is an urgent need for a sustainable intensification of agriculture, where crop production can be increased; without expansion of land-use; and without causing adverse impact on human health and the environment (including the atmosphere) and without compromising economic development and socio-economic equity.[2] The report mentions potential for development of GMOs with improvements to the nutritional value of plants or with resistance towards particular pests or fungi, ensuring optimal yield outcome in storage and cultivation. Another report published in 2009 by the National Research Council, United States, argues that use of GMOs in agriculture can benefit food production and the environment, but warns against overuse.[3] While both reports argue in

---

1 In this chapter, I use the term GMOs within the narrow context of agricultural crop production for food production. GMOs refer to *plants* whose genetic material has been modified artificially, as opposed to conventional crops, based on naturally occurring variations developed through targeted breeding of plants with desirable characteristics. See European Food Safety Authority (EFSA), 'Genetically Modified Organisms', available at www.efsa.europa.eu/en/gmotopics/topic/gmo.htm and European Commission, 'Genetically modified Food and Feed – What are GMOs?', available at http://ec.europa.eu/food/food/biotechnology/gmo_En.htm.

2 The Royal Society, '*Reaping the Benefits – Science and the Sustainable Intensification of Global Agriculture*', 2009, available at http://royalsociety.org/Reapingthebenefits/.

3 National Research Council of the National Academies, 'Impact of Genetically Engineered Crops on Farm Sustainability in the United States', report by the Committee on the Impact of Biotechnology on Farm-Level Economics and Sustainability, Board on Agricultural and Natural Resources (BANR) and Earth and Life Studies (DELS) 2010, available at www.nap.edu/openbook.php?record_id=12804&page=1, summary, 4, 6, 8, 14.

favour of GMOs as part of a sustainable development in agriculture and food production, they also emphasize that GMOs alone cannot be the solution to food security. GMOs have been widely used for the past 20 years; yet consumer scepticism remains strong, especially among citizens within the European Union. The ethical concerns brought forward in the GMO debate have focused on the impact of GMOs on the natural environment and issues around environmental justice.

In this chapter, I examine the ethical concerns about GMOs in light of the problem of anthropogenic climate change and discuss the ethical foundation for application of GMOs as a mode of agricultural adaptation for food production in response to global climate change. In the first section I outline the ethics of sustainability in the context of anthropogenic climate change. I argue that anthropogenic climate change generates an ethical responsibility to ensure a sustainable development by introducing climate-adaptation *and* mitigation strategies in agriculture and food production. I argue that this ethical responsibility is *shared* and must reflect *global interests*; and, that it should include measures aimed at conservation[4] of nature[5] including the atmosphere. In the next section, two of the main ethical concerns about GMOs are examined and evaluated in light of the ethics of sustainability: first, the invasiveness of GMOs to nature and second, concerns about justice with regard to patenting, access and distribution of benefits from green biotechnology in developing countries, to protection of small-scale farmers. It is argued that it is necessary to promote debate about nature conservation in light of the ethics of sustainability of anthropogenic climate change, and that GMOs do not necessarily contradict the idea of nature conservation in this case. Furthermore, it is argued, that if GMOs are to be applied as part of a sustainable development to food security, introduction of policy measures are necessary to ensure justice in development and use of GMOs both locally and globally. This will lead into the identification of four criteria for assessment and application of GMOs that are in line with the ethics of sustainability. Finally, the criteria are discussed in light of the existing international conventions and relevant EU regulations which apply to GMOs. It is argued that it may be necessary to re-evaluate current policies with respect to environmental risk assessment criteria for GMOs; and that it may be necessary to develop new policies for assessment of agricultural methods and crop technologies overall according to their potential for sustainable development and food security.

---

4   Here nature conservation is used as a general reference to the idea of 'management of the Earth's natural resources: plants, animals and the environment to ensure that they survive or are appropriately used': see www.agriculturedictionary.com/definition/nature-conservation. html.

5   In this paper I refer to nature as the sum of the biological systems which includes *all* living organisms *and* the environment in which they function. I argue that the atmosphere should be included in this context due to the interdependence between ecosystems and climate.

The ethics of sustainability of anthropogenic climate change

The United Nations Convention on Climate Change Article 2 commits the Parties to promote a sustainable development in order 'to ensure that food production is not threatened and to ensure economic development to proceed in a sustainable manner'.[6] The principle of sustainable development was first introduced in environmental policy with the World Commissions on Environment and Development report in 1987, which defines a sustainable development as '[A] development that meets the needs of the present without compromising the ability of future generations to meet their own needs.'[7] The principle is an ideal that requires interpretation and concretization.[8] In the following, I argue that the ethics of sustainability of anthropogenic climate change is generated on the basis of three core responsibilities.

(a) First, an *ethical responsibility to compensate for anthropogenic climate change* can be identified on the basis of the idea of corrective justice.[9] In 2007, the Intergovernmental Panel on Climate Change (IPCC) concluded in its Fourth Assessment Report (AR4) that global warming is taking place and that there are causal connections between human emission of greenhouse gases, global warming and past and current climate changes.[10] The application of corrective justice is determined here by the scientific nature of anthropogenic climate change including the uncertainty in regard to the predicted long-term scenarios of its impact. Three aspects are central for determining the extent of the ethical responsibility to compensate. First, it is not possible to trace anthropogenic contribution to climate change to individual countries' emissions of greenhouse gases; it is the sum of contributions, and not the individual contribution that causes the impact on the climate systems. Secondly, contribution to anthropogenic climate change happens over time and with significant delay, thus damage done by present generations may be delayed, affecting future generations instead. Thirdly, the contribution is not limited to the physical area where the emission

---

6 United Nations, '*United Nations Framework Convention on Climate Change (UNFCCC)*', FCCC/Informal/84 (1992). Art. 2, 4, http://unfccc.int/essential_background/convention/items/2627.php.

7 World Commission on Environment and Development, *Our Common Future* (Oxford: Oxford University Press, 1987), 43.

8 Peter Kemp and Lisbeth Witthøfft Nielsen, *The Barriers to Climate Awareness – A Report on the Ethics of Sustainability* (Ministry of Climate and Energy: Copenhagen, 2009), 47.

9 Corrective justice is here applied in a similar way as the 'polluter pays principle', which is implemented in environmental policy and embodied in the Kyoto Protocol. Three approaches to justice are represented in climate change politics: preventive, corrective and compensatory. See Jekwu Ikeme, 'Equity, Environmental Justice and Sustainability: Incomplete Approaches in Climate Change Politics', *Global Environmental Change*, 2003, 13: 95–206.

10 Intergovernmental Panel on Climate Change (IPCC), *Climate Change 2007, Synthesis Report – A Report of the Intergovernmental Panel on Climate Change* (Cambridge: Cambridge University Press, 2007), 30, 39, www.ipcc.ch/publications_and_data/publications_ipcc_fourth_assessment_report_synthesis_report.htm.

takes place. In practice the ethical responsibility to compensate, can be translated into a two-fold responsibility of the present generations to minimize impact now and in the future[11] by: (a) compensation by ensuring adaptation to climate changes are already happening and (b) correcting the current developments by minimizing harm over time through mitigation practices.[12]

(b) Secondly, the ethics of sustainability of anthropogenic climate change includes a *shared responsibility of all countries to take an active role in the effort to ensure adaptation and mitigation*. Anthropogenic climate change is by nature a shared global environmental problem due to the accumulated effect of greenhouse gas emissions from human activities, leading to climate changes in different physical and biological systems worldwide. The problem is, however, that many developing countries are geographically situated in areas which are particularly vulnerable to climate change impacts such as rising sea-levels and severe weather conditions. Bearing this in mind, how do we determine the ethical responsibility to compensate for anthropogenic climate change, in terms of distribution of the burdens and benefits related to adaptation and mitigation, to ensure food security over time?

The climate convention prescribes that the distribution of costs of adaptation and mitigation measures is to be carried out according to 'common, but differentiated responsibilities and respective capabilities'.[13] The objective is to ensure justice, and avoid further inequity between developed and developing countries as a result of the socio-economic burdens related to adaptation and mitigation costs.[14] With reference to Rawls' difference principle,[15] it can be argued that a fair distribution of costs and benefits from a sustainable intensification of agriculture is one that ensures the greatest benefits to the least advantaged members of the global society.

(c) Thirdly, the ethics of sustainability of anthropogenic climate change includes a *responsibility to protect nature including the atmosphere*. The scientific evidence of anthropogenic climate change confirms that the natural

---

11   I refer to present generations but not to past, emphasizing the scientific evidence of anthropogenic climate change as constitutional for the ethical responsibility to ensure adaptation and mitigation.

12   The principle of sustainable development is usually associated with a responsibility towards future generations based on the idea of intergenerational justice. The nature of such a responsibility and what constitutes justice in this context is, however, disputed. Here I maintain that the delayed effect of present greenhouse gas emissions is generating a responsibility to ensure adaptation *and* mitigation because of the uncertainty with respect to when the impact of present emissions sets in.

13   United Nations, *'United Nations Framework Convention on Climate Change'*, Art 3, 1, 4; and Ikeme, 'Equity, Environmental Justice and Sustainability', 200.

14   In this context I refer to justice, understood as distribution of public goods according to standard democratic principles.

15   John Rawls, *Political Liberalism: Expanded Edition* (New York: Columbia University Press, 1993), see 'Basic Elements', 5–6.

environment – including the atmosphere – is not immune to human activity. Combined with a steadily growing world population, climate change is predicted to pose a threat to global food security in 30–40 years.[16] In order to meet the demand for food in 2050, an increase in food production based on current agricultural practices would not only mean an increase in current greenhouse gas emission related to food production, but also involve expansion of land-use.[17] The latter is likely to influence biodiversity negatively, and may contribute further to vulnerability in food production, as the decrease in biodiversity make ecosystems more vulnerable to damage from pests and diseases in crop species.[18] Climate change is also predicted to contribute to changes of specific aspects of nature, including ecosystems or specific species which are of value to humans and included in present nature protection programmes.[19]

Considering the impact of anthropogenic climate change on nature and the value that nature represent to humans, both as a habitat and as a resource, it can be argued that the ethics of sustainability must include a responsibility to ensure conservation of nature. Failing to do so is very likely to cause harm in terms of limiting the availability of natural resources, and in general, have a negative impact on ecosystems and biodiversity. Thus, the ethics of sustainability must include a sustainable development focusing on adapting food production in a way that integrates nature conservation. However, it would be contradictory to claim that the ethics of sustainability generates a responsibility to protect nature if this does not involve an effort to reduce further anthropogenic contribution to climate changes.

In summary, the ethics of sustainability prescribes a shared responsibility of present generations to compensate for anthropogenic climate change.

16 N. V. Fedoroff, D. S. Battisti, R. N. Beachy, P. J. M. Cooper, D. A. Fischhoff, C. N. Hodges, *et al.*, 'Radically Rethinking Agriculture for the 21st Century', 2010, *Science* 327: 833–4. The growing world population requires an increase in existing food production of min 50 per cent if food security is to be established over the next decades. See: The Royal Society, '*Reaping the Benefits – Science and the Sustainable Intensification of Global Agriculture*', 1. Food insecurity is an already existing problem in many countries and regions of the world with an estimated 2 billion people suffering from diseases related to malnutrition and 1 billion people who currently do not have access to sufficient food and water. See Christopher B. Barret, 'Measuring Food Insecurity', *Science*, 2010, 327: 825.

17 The Royal Society, '*Reaping the Benefits – Science and the Sustainable Intensification of Global Agriculture*', 7.

18 Intergovernmental Panel on Climate Change (IPCC), 'Chapter 5: Food, Fibre and Forest Production', in Martin Parry, Osvaldo Canziani, Jean Palutikof, Paul van der Linden and Clair Hanson (eds), *Climate Change 2007: Impacts, Adaptation and Vulnerability* (Cambridge: Cambridge University Press, 2007).

19 IPCC, *Climate Change 2007, Synthesis Report*, topic 2 and 3, 42, 48; The value of nature is here referred to from an anthropocentric approach where the responsibility to ensure nature conservation and protecting the atmosphere is based on human interest and not on an inherent value in non-human nature.

Compensation involves adaptation combined with mitigation measures which includes a responsibility to ensure conservation of nature, including the atmosphere.

GMOs and the ethical concerns for non-human nature: A question about sustainability

GMOs have been debated since they were first introduced in agricultural production in the early 1990s. Scepticism has been particularly strong among citizens of the European Union, and has also influenced the development of the existing EU regulation regarding GMOs.[20] Ethical concerns about the naturalness or invasiveness of GMOs to ecosystems and to biodiversity, together with concerns about justice and equality in application of gene technology in agriculture, have played a central role in the rejection of GMOs by sceptics. This section examines the two types of ethical concerns put forward in the past debate on GMOs, and evaluates them in light of the ethics of sustainability of anthropogenic climate change. On the basis of this examination I discuss what criteria must apply for assessment and application of GMOs, if they are to contribute to a sustainable development to food security, that is in line with the ethics of sustainability.

GMOs and concerns about the 'unnatural'

One of the more profound ethical concerns put forward in the debate about GMOs focuses on their impact on nature. It has been argued that using genetic engineering to alter the genetic make-up of plants (or animals) is a violation of the inherent value of nature; thus suggesting that nature has a superior force which should not be tampered with.[21] Some maintain that genetic

---

20 The latest Eurobarometer assessing European Citizens' attitudes to biotechnology from 2006 shows that more than 10 years after GMOs have been introduced on the market more than 58 per cent of the respondents still oppose GM food. See George Gaskell, Agnes Allansdottir, Nick Allum, Cristina Corchero, Claude Fischler, Jürgen Hampel, et al., 'Europeans and Biotechnology in 2005: Patterns and Trends, Eurobarometer 64.3, Report to the European Commission's Directorate-General for Research', 2006. http://ec.europa.eu/research/press/2006/pdf/pr1906_Eb_64_3_final_report-may2006_En.pdf, 4, 22–3; Yann Devos, Dirk Reheul, Danny De Waele, Linda Van Spreybroeck, 'The Interplay between Societal Concerns and the Regulatory Frame on GM Crops in the European Union', *Environmental Biosafety Research*, 2006, 5(3): 127–49.

21 Wolfgang Wagner, Nicole Kronberger, George Gaskell, Agnes Allansdottir, Nick Allum, Suzanne de Cheveigné, et al., 'Nature in Disorder: The Troubled Public of Biotechnology', in George Gaskell and Martin W. Bauer (eds), *Biotechnology 1996–2000 – The Years of Controversy* (London: Science Museum, 2001), 86–7.

engineering is a violation of species integrity; others refer to it as a violation of an inherent value which lies embedded in natural reproduction; and yet, others see it as a violation of an inherent value embedded in biodiversity or in ecosystems as a whole.

An inherent problem of 'naturalness' concerns lies in defining the value of nature, together with the particular aspect of nature that needs to be protected and why it needs to be protected. One of the more profound ethical concerns towards gene technology applied in crop development is the aspect of 'unnaturalness'. The focus of this type of concern is on the ability to modify specific genes and to transfer gene traits between species, which enables development of new types of organisms which would not occur 'naturally' or through conventional cross-breeding methods.[22] Another major concern is the aspect of irreversibility; once GMOs are introduced in agricultural production, it is difficult to ensure that they will not spread into the 'natural' environment.

The common problem with arguments referring to 'naturalness' or the 'natural environment' is that they link the qualitative distinction with an assumed absolute distinction between what is natural and unnatural, and use this distinction normatively as an argument for rejecting GMOs altogether. Distinctions between 'natural' and 'unnatural' or for that matter between 'natural' and 'artificial' are, however, neither consistent nor absolute, but entirely context dependent.[23] For example, a non-modified species introduced by humans into an environment or an ecosystem where it does not occur naturally, would be considered as unnatural in that environment, regardless of the fact that the species itself is considered as natural, that is belonging to nature.

'Naturalness' concerns can also represent more profound ethical concerns about the way technology in general is forming agriculture and about interfering with natural processes, and in a way that is irreversible.[24] An example of this is the organic farmer's view which argues in favour of agricultural production on nature's own terms. Any technological interference is as such considered problematic. The organic farmer's view is in favour of agricultural production on nature's premises, as opposed to a technology controlled production where nature is alienated from human beings and merely considered as a resource.[25] GMOs are seen as the ultimate symbol of such alienation.

---

22 Claire Marris, 'Public Views on GMOs: Deconstructing the Myths', *EMBO Reports*, 2001, 2(7): 545–8, 546.

23 Gregory Kaebnick, 'It's Against Nature', *The Hastings Centre Report*, 2009, 39(1): 24–6, 24.

24 Marris, 'Public Views on GMOs', 546; Wagner, Kronberger, Gaskell, Allansdottir, Allum, de Cheveigné, et al., 'Nature in Disorder: The Troubled Public of Biotechnology', 86. See also: Henk Verhoog, 'The Reasons for Rejecting Genetic Engineering by the Organic Movement', FORUM TTN, 2003, available at www.ecopb.org/fileadmin/ecopb/documents/reasons_reject_gmo.pdf, 3–4.

25 Verhoog, 'The Reasons for Rejecting Genetic Engineering by the Organic Movement', 10.

Common for 'naturalness' arguments are that they reflect the perception that genetic modification disturbs the equilibrium in nature, and 'pushes nature beyond its limits'.[26] These concerns reflect more profound perceptions on how humans ought to interact with nature which are not to be ignored. The perceptions have an impact on what people consider as sustainable approaches in agriculture and food production. Maintaining that gene technology is inherently bad and should be rejected on the basis of its 'unnaturalness' or with reference to the aspect of irreversibility is, however, problematic from an ethical point of view.

Assessing GMOs with nature conservation in mind and in light of the challenges that anthropogenic climate change poses to agriculture and food production, it seems problematic to maintain that GMOs pose a greater threat to the environment than is conventional agriculture and food production technologies, and to ultimately reject GMOs on this basis.[27] The problem of anthropogenic climate change calls for a rethinking of the existing distinctions between nature and the atmosphere altogether. Concerns about irreversibility and naturalness must be reconsidered in this context. 'Naturalness' arguments against GMOs seem to fall short here, because GMOs may contribute to nature conservation in a wider context where conservation may involve mitigation of climate change. Thus the scenario where GMOs are blankly rejected as inherently bad and in contradiction with nature conservation is to be avoided for this reason. On the other hand, an unconditional acceptance of GMOs without considering biosafety and the potential risks of harm to human health and the environment would, however, be irrational. The same is the case for a food security strategy based on genetic engineering only, and without assessing other options for a sustainable development. Against these scenarios it can be argued that GMOs do not represent a solution on their own, and that introduction of new types of GMOs, as well as use of existing GMOs, should be applied with precaution due to the unknown long-term effects on human and animal health and to biodiversity. Other, and perhaps less-invasive methods to ensure environmentally sustainable solutions to food security have been suggested and could, for example, include changing eating habits

---

26   Marris, 'Public Views on GMOs', 546.
27   This is especially so, because agriculture and food production is already contributing with between 17–32 per cent of the global greenhouse gas emissions. See Jørgen E. Olesen, 'Fødevarernes andel af klimabelastningen', in Danish Council of Ethics, *Vores mad og det globale klima – etik til en varmere klode* (Copenhagen: Det Etiske Raad, 2010) (only available in Danish), 25. Low-input agriculture such as organic farming may be better for the environment and help by reducing use of pesticides. However, it may require de-forestation to expand land use in order to obtain the same crop yield. Expansion of land-use may have a negative impact on existing biodiversity, biological systems, ecosystems and species. See: The Royal Society, *Reaping the Benefits – Science and the Sustainable Intensification of Global Agriculture'*, 7, 47.

towards a less-meat-based diet.[28] However, given the extent of the problem of climate change and the urgency[29] of establishing sustainability in agriculture and food productions on a global scale, it may be argued that GMOs must *at least* be taken into consideration as part of a solution to food security, on a *case-by-case basis*. It is important that naturalness concerns do not become an unjustified moral barrier to climate adaptation strategies, and that lack of consumer support, or specific concerns about nature conservation do not result in discrimination against research and application of specific technologies like genetic engineering of plants.

Considering the remaining scepticism towards GMOs especially among citizens within the European Union it may be time for a renewed debate or re-evaluation of GMOs focusing on the potential benefits for nature conservation. Different ways of assessing individual types of GMOs and their risks and benefits to the environment along with other agricultural methods, and according to the overall aim of climate sustainable production and global food security, may also have to be considered in this context. However, that is not to say that local ethical concerns can be undermined because local interests weigh less than the overall benefit for a greater number of people. Instead, a way forward may be to develop international standards for assessment of GMOs to ensure high level of biosafety as well as nature conservation, globally. Standards could include assessment of GMOs together with other agricultural technologies *in light of the ethics of sustainability* and according to the potential for contributing to sustainable development with the local, regional and global environmental and socio-economic interests in mind.

Environmental justice and vulnerable population groups

Pro-GMO movements' claims that GMOs are *the solution* to food security and that they can contribute to the United Nations Millennium Development Goals[30] of reducing hunger and poverty, have been met with criticism from

---

28 Livestock and meat production involve the highest greenhouse gas (GHG) emission in agriculture and require extensive land-use. Emissions stem from production of animal feed, methane emissions from the animals and other GHG emissions related to transport of animals or meat products. Meat consumption has increased drastically, especially in the developed countries, over the last 20 years. An increase in meat production involves expansion of land-use. See Olesen, 'Fødevarernes andel af klimabelastningen'.

29 The Royal Society highlights that an increase of at least 50 per cent of current food production levels is necessary if food security is to be ensured in 2050. This is based on estimates according to the current population growth. The Royal Society, '*Reaping the Benefits – Science and the Sustainable Intensification of Global Agriculture*', 1.

30 United Nations Millennium Development Goals: www.un.org/millenniumgoals/.

social movements concerned with environmental justice.[31] They criticize the process towards privatization and industrialization of agriculture which GMOs symbolize.

The current GMO market is primarily driven by commercial interests of large agro-biotech companies, who are protecting their technological discoveries and products through patents. A major ethical concern put forward in the past debate is that GMOs may contribute negatively to equality and economic development in poor countries due to priorities of agro-biotech companies.[32] With only few competitors on the market, these multinational biotech companies can potentially continue to increase their prices on crop seeds.[33] This impacts the potential financial gain that a farmer may obtain from a higher crop yield from GM seeds. In particular, poor farmers in third world countries, where food insecurity is already a problem, are exceptionally vulnerable to increases in prices and dependency on private multinational agro-biotech companies.[34] Furthermore, several of these companies produce both GM seeds and herbicides which also contribute to increase dependence on these companies.[35] Patenting of crop types as well as technologies contributes to privatization of seeds and increases the reliance on such companies.

It has been argued that GMOs would not solve the problem of food insecurity in third world countries; for example, patents and high prices of these seeds restrict access of knowledge and technology to developing countries, thereby putting business of local farmers in greater economical jeopardy.[36] Furthermore, research into the potential of gene technology for development of GM crops or GM technologies with limited market interest, is not likely to be carried out at all.

Although the concerns outlined here have elements in them that are specific to agro-biotechnology, several of the problems outlined, such as the concern about lack of research in areas with little or no commercial interests, as well as restricted access to new knowledge and know-how, also apply to the wider debate on environmental justice and sustainability in relation to development of climate adaptation and mitigation measures.

31   Hein-Anton van der Heijden, *Social Movements, Public Spheres and the European Politics of the Environment – Green Power Europe?* (New York: Palgrave Macmillan, 2010), 142.
32   Jonathan Kydd, Janet Haddock, John Mansfield, Charles Ainsworth and Allan Buckwell, 'Genetically Modified Organisms: Major Issues and Policy Responses for Developing Countries', *Journal of International Development*, 2000, 12(8): 1133–45, 1139.
33   Ibid., 1137.
34   Ibid., 1137–38.
35   van der Heijden, *Social Movements, Public Spheres and the European Politics of the Environment – Green Power Europe?* 141.
36   Rikker Bagger Jørgensen, 'GMO: En løsning på ændrede klimaforhold', in Mickey Gjerris, Christian Gamborg, Jøregen E Olesen and Jakob Wolf (eds), *Jorden Braender – Klimaforandringerne i videnskabsteoretisk og etisk perspektiv* (Forlaget: Alfa Frederiksberg, 2009) (only available in Danish), 178–9.

The ethics of sustainability emphasizes that burdens and benefits related to research and development of new GMOs are to be *shared* in a just way; that would reflect the *global* interests in food security and sustainable agriculture and food production. When GMOs were first introduced for commercial use, they were promoted as a possible solution to food insecurity problems in poor countries. There is, however, no evidence to date that the first generation of GMOs has contributed to reduce the problem of hunger or poverty. Only a limited variety of GM crops has been developed, such as Maize, soya, cotton and canola, and the majority of the produced soya is mainly used as animal feed for live-stock in developed countries, and not for human consumption.[37] Within the recent debate about climate change and food security, sceptics have rejected application of GMOs as part of a larger climate adaptation strategy to food security on this basis. The concerns focus on the lack of GM crop types that are specially adapted to local areas. For example, many developing countries suffer from lack of arable land and sufficient water resources, fertilizers and pesticides essential to provide a higher crop yield from existing GMO types. A final concern is that current technology and risk assessment is insufficient in developing countries due to the lack of necessary know-how to properly address biosafety issues.[38]

A crucial element in the aim to obtain a global sustainable development of agriculture and food production methods is to ensure the open exchange of new knowledge and know-how and that research and development of new plant technologies and soil and water management is taking place. The concerns about commercial interests and the potential negative impact of patenting are particularly important in this context. Considering the current market for GMOs, there is a significant risk for the variety of crop development and distribution of know-how and technology necessary for a sustainable development to be inequitably distributed, because private multinational biotech firms have to protect their commercial interests.[39] It is essential to ensure that the climate-adapting and mitigation potentials of GMOs are to be explored even if there is little, or no commercial gain involved, and that developing countries get the necessary access to know-how to develop their own crop industry with locally adapted crops.

If a climate aware strategy to sustainable development of agriculture and food production is to include GMOs, a progressive approach in terms of targeted research supported through public funding and/or more direct governance of the current GMO market may be required.[40] This could, for example, involve

37 van der Heijden, *Social Movements, Public Spheres and the European Politics of the Environment – Green Power Europe?* 124, 142.
38 Jørgensen, 'GMO: En løsning på ændrede klimaforhold', 177–8.
39 The Royal Society, '*Reaping the Benefits – Science and the Sustainable Intensification of Global Agriculture*', 10–11.
40 Ibid., 50.

reservation of public funds or funding from non-commercial organizations to ensure research into agriculture management and crop technologies including gene technology, aimed at benefitting agriculture and food production in particular climate vulnerable areas.[41] Similarly it could involve transfer of tax resources provided from food industry into public research funds to ensure that new agricultural management methods and crop technologies (including GMOs) can be developed and explored where there are few or no commercial interests to be found. Other types of governance could include development of local and international ethical standards for research and application of GMOs which has to be followed by agriculture and food industry. Such standards could involve criteria for patenting; and assessment of individual agricultural management methods' and crop technologies' contribution to a sustainable development in terms of targeting challenges that climate change poses to agriculture and food production in various regions of the world.

In summary, concerns put forward in the past debate about biosafety together with ethical concerns with respect to environmental justice, are equally relevant in the debate about food security strategies and sustainable development in the context of climate adaptation. GMOs in food production must be assessed on a case-by-case basis and applied with precaution to ensure a high level of biosafety. That said, there is a need to rethink the more profound ethical concerns about the naturalness of GMOs in light of the problem of anthropogenic climate change, where nature conservation is seen in a wider context that includes the atmosphere. The evaluation of the ethical concerns suggests four criteria to be taken into account in assessment and application of GMOs, for it to be in line with the ethics of sustainability:

1 Both the risks *and* the benefits *of* GMOs to the environment and to global food security must be assessed. Such an assessment ought to take into account the responsibility to ensure a sustainable development where nature conservation includes the atmosphere.

2 GMOs must be assessed along with other agricultural methods and crop technologies, according to their potential contribution to a sustainable development in agriculture and food production.

3 The socio-economic impact of GMOs must be assessed locally but with a global application perspective in mind. Both the socio-economic risks *and* benefits of GMOs must be assessed.

4 Public funding, local and international governance initiatives are to ensure equal distribution of burdens and benefits in order to reflect the shared responsibility in the ethics of sustainability to ensure global sustainability. This may include the development of international

41 Ibid., 45–6.

standards for risk/benefit assessment focusing on biosafety but also on the potential for GMOs to contribute to a global sustainable development.

The criteria for ethical use of GMOs and the international legal framework

In the previous section, four criteria were suggested for application of GMOs in line with the ethics of sustainability. In the following, I discuss the possibility of meeting these criteria on the basis of existing international conventions and the regulatory framework for deliberate release of GMOs within the European Union. Two international conventions apply to the question of GMOs as part of a climate-adaptation strategy to food security: the United Nations Framework Convention on Climate Change and the United Nations Convention on Biological Diversity. Both conventions are established with view to protecting the natural environment against irreversible damage from human interference. 'Sustainable development' is a key objective in both conventions. According to the ethics of sustainability, protection of climate systems and conservation of biological diversity are two sides of the same coin. This is, however, not necessarily the case in the existing international conventions relevant for the assessment of GMOs as a climate-adaptation strategy to food security.

Implementation and regulation of climate adaptation and mitigation measures are covered under the principles of the Convention on Climate Change including the Kyoto Protocol. Sustainability is here to be seen in the context of the convention's objective of protecting climate systems and the atmosphere from irreversible and undesired changes due to anthropogenic greenhouse gas emissions. A sustainable development is one that ensures stabilization of greenhouse gas emissions, without compromising food production and economic development in general.[42] Use of GMOs in agriculture and food production falls under the principles of the Convention on Biological Diversity and the Cartagena Protocol, which outlines rules for biosafety. The objective of the Convention is to ensure conservation of biological diversity through a sustainable development; to avoid irreversible decline of biological resources in the long term that could compromise future generations' possibility of meeting their needs.[43] It may be argued that the convention on biodiversity indirectly includes climate systems in its aim to protect life-sustaining systems of the biosphere.[44]

---

42 United Nations, 'United Nations Framework Convention on Climate Change', Art.2.
43 United Nations, 'United Nations Convention on Biological Diversity (CBD)' (1992): www. cbd.int/convention/text/, Article 2, 2.
44 Ibid., preamble.

The convention recognizes the potential in modern biotechnology to contribute to human well-being and need for food security, but is also concerned with the potential risks that modern biotechnology may pose to human health and the environment.[45] The Cartagena Protocol on Biosafety lists a set of criteria for risk assessment and management of GMOs.[46] The objective of these criteria is protection of biological diversity against damage from the introduction of GMOs. In this context GMOs are assessed according to their risk to biosafety and to conservation of biological diversity.[47]

The Ethics of sustainability of anthropogenic climate change challenges the existing conventions with respect to the perception of the nature that is to be protected. More specifically, the difference in objectives in the Convention on Climate Change and the Convention on Biological Diversity respectively, challenges the possibility of meeting the first two criteria, identified in section two, for assessment of GMOs according to their contribution to nature conservation and sustainable development. The first two criteria call for an assessment of risks and benefits of GMOs according to the overall aim of nature conservation, including protection of the atmosphere, and for an assessment of existing and new agricultural technologies and methods, according to their potential contribution to global food security. The Cartagena Protocol leaves no room for an assessment of the benefits, that GMOs may represent to nature conservation in terms of their potential for contributing to climate change mitigation. Likewise, it does not leave room for an assessment of GMOs along with other agricultural methods according to their overall contribution to a sustainable development where the risks and benefits to biological diversity, and the atmosphere are taken into consideration. As for the remaining two criteria (3 and 4) regarding just distribution of benefits and burdens involved in the implementation of GMOs as part of a larger climate-adaptation strategy to food security, these may be met in the existing international conventions.

Both the Convention on Climate Change and the Convention on Biological Diversity emphasize that equality and justice in distribution of resources and responsibilities are crucial for a development to be sustainable. The Convention on Biological Diversity and the Nagoya Protocol outlines principles for access and fair and equitable transfer of technology including sharing of financial resources and distribution mechanisms. Patents and intellectual property rights are recognized to have an influence on the implementation of the convention. The convention emphasizes that intellectual property rights must be respected. Development and transfer of technology, however, shall be subject to regulation and policy measures on a national level; it takes into account the aim of ensuring

45   United Nations, 'Cartagena Protocol on Biosafety to the Convention on Biological Diversity, Text and Annexes', 2000, http://bch.cbd.int/protocol/text/, 1, Introduction.
46   Ibid., 1, Introduction.
47   Ibid., 1. Introduction and Art, 11.

the sharing of benefits among governmental institutions and the private sector, without compromising the overall objectives of the convention.[48] According to the criteria (3 and 4) outlined in section two, equal distribution and socio-economic sustainability must be ensured through an assessment of GMOs locally and globally bearing in mind the shared responsibility to ensure sustainbility globally. The question is whether current regional or local regulatory frameworks on GMOs can meet these criteria or if they may represent a potential barrier to climate adaptation in agriculture and food production?

The EC Directive 2001/18/EC on deliberate release of GMOs into the environment reflects the objective of the Convention on Biological Diversity and the requirements for biosafety set out in the Cartagena Protocol on Biosafety. The directive prescribes procedures for risk assessment of new types of GMOs, and for monitoring of their impact on the environment once a specific type of GMO is released. This includes procedures to ensure traceability at all stages involved with the release of GMOs on the market or in food production.[49] According to Devos et al. there is currently no aspect in the EU regulation on GMOs which allows for a wider assessment of the socio-economic benefits and risks in a wider context of sustainability.[50] Member states have the competence, according to the directive, to take into account ethical aspects when GMOs are introduced for deliberate release.[51] This, however, applies to EU member states only, and does not take into account the broader concerns regarding GMOs, and justice in distribution of burdens and benefits between developing and developed countries, and between the private sector and governmental institutions, which plays an important part in the Convention on Biological Diversity.

The EU policy is that release of GMOs into the environment and use of GMOs in food production, must be based on thorough scientific assessment of biosafety.[52] GMOs are assessed on their impact on the surrounding environment such as the compatibility with other cultivated and wild plants in the

---

48   United Nations, 'United Nations Convention on Biological Diversity (CBD)', Art. 1, 16, 1–5 and Art. 20–1.

49   See: 'Directive 2001/18/EC of The European Parliament and of the Council of 12 March 2001, on the deliberate release into the environment of genetically modified organisms and repealing Council Directive 90/220/EEC', *Official Journal of the European Communities* 17 April 2001. The risk assessment of GMOs' impact on the environment is to be carried out in accordance with section 27 and the elements to be assessed are outlined in the Directive's Annex II.

50   Y. Devos, D. Reheul, D. De Waele and L. Van Speybroek, '*The Interplay between Societal Concerns and the Regulatory Frame on GM Crops in the European Union*', *Environmental Biosafety Research* 5 (2007), 18.

51   'Directive 2001/18/EC of The European Parliament and of the Council of 12 March 2001, on the deliberate release into the environment of genetically modified organisms and repealing Council Directive 90/220/EEC.'

52   European Commission: 'GMO Evaluation – EU GMO Policy in a Nutshell': http://ec.europa. eu/food/food/biotechnology/evaluation/gmo_nutshell_En.htm; and: European Commission: 'General Food Law – Principles': http://ec.europa.eu/food/food/foodlaw/principles/index_ En.htm.

area.[53] The European Food Safety Agency's guidelines for risk assessment apply an approach in which GMOs are assessed comparatively to its conventional counterpart.[54] The existing regulations reflect the perceptions that GMOs are qualitatively different from conventional crop. They do not provide any room for assessment of their potential for contributing to a sustainable development in agriculture and food production, where the risks and benefits of GMOs along with conventional crops or agricultural methods can be assessed on an equal basis.[55]

Current regulation within the EU addresses consumer scepticism towards GMOs through requirements with regard to access to and availability of sound scientific information about the environmental impact of GMOs; and through labeling-requirements for products containing GMOs. This is to allow consumers to exercise autonomy as to whether they want to buy such products. Yet, willingness to buy GM food remains low among the consumers in this region. Considering the persistent scepticism within the European Union, a necessary first step towards meeting the challenges that climate change poses to agriculture and food production and the problem of food security may be a renewed debate about GMOs. There is a need for clarification with regard to what nature (or aspect of it) is to be protected in this context. Such a clarification may request for a re-evaluation of the existing policy frameworks for assessment of both risks and benefits of GMOs, according to the ethics of sustainability. This is crucial if the criteria outlined in section two, regarding public funding and governance initiatives are to be met, and if use of public funding for research into development of GMOs is to find acceptance within the EU and beyond.

Conclusion

In this chapter, I have discussed the application of GMOs as part of a larger strategy to ensure a sustainable development in agriculture and food production, that takes into account the challenges that anthropogenic climate change poses to global food security.

---

53 'Directive 2001/18/EC of The European Parliament and of the Council of 12 March 2001, on the deliberate release into the environment of genetically modified organisms and repealing Council Directive 90/220/EEC', Annex III B.
54 European Food Safety Authority (EFSA): 'Scientific Opinion, Guidance on the Environmental Risk Assessment of Genetically Modified Plants, EFSA Panel on Genetically Modified Organisms (GMO), Summary', *EFSA journal*, 2010, 8(11): 1879.
55 Devos, Reheul, De Waele and Van Speybroek, 'The Interplay between Societal Concerns and the Regulatory Frame on GM Crops in the European Union', 18; A sustainability assessment would in this case also involve a comparative assessment of organic agriculture and its contribution to secure a sustainable intensification of agriculture.

For a climate-adaptation strategy to achieve success, it requires public support in terms of willingness to embrace local, regional and global initiatives. This support requires recognition and awareness of the ethical responsibility generated by anthropogenic climate change. The ethics of sustainability of anthropogenic climate change prescribes a shared responsibility to compensate for anthropogenic climate change by developing strategies for climate adaptation and mitigation with a view to ensure sustainable development globally. A sustainable development in this context is one that aims at protecting nature including the atmosphere and distributes the benefits and burdens of the adaptation and mitigation strategies in accordance with principles of justice. With this in mind the biggest challenge to the implementation of GMOs as part of a climate adaption strategy to food security in line with the ethics of sustainability is perhaps the existing moral barriers towards such technologies. Four criteria were suggested for an assessment and application of GMOs, in accordance with the ethics of sustainability. These criteria emphasize the need for assessment of both environmental and socio-economic risks *and* benefits of GMOs, together with a wider assessment of the risks and benefits of agricultural management methods and crop technologies according to their contribution to sustainable development in agriculture and food production, and in light of the ethics of sustainability.

The Convention on Biological Diversity focuses mainly on the risks that GMOs pose to biodiversity and ecosystems in general. The same is the case for regional regulation in the EU. This focus does not allow for an assessment of both risks and benefits of GMOs in the context of nature conservation, where this includes the atmosphere. Bearing in mind the more profound ethical concerns about naturalness and the impact of GMOs on biodiversity brought forward in the past GMO-debate, there is a need for a renewed debate about the potential of GMOs to contribute to nature conservation in a wider context of climate adaptation and mitigation. This is to clarify: (a) the embedded irrationality in 'naturalness' arguments and that nature conservation should include protection of the atmosphere; (b) to prevent such moral concerns from becoming a barrier to implementation of climate-adaptation strategies aiming for a sustainable food production and global food security; and (c) to promote new ways of assessing GMOs and other agricultural methods, including conventional crops and low-input agriculture such as organic farming, according to the overall aim of food security, and through a sustainable intensification of agriculture and food production. Additionally, if GMOs are to be included as part of a sustainable development to food security, it is necessary to ensure just and equitable distribution of knowledge and technology, and development of varieties of GMOs specifically targeting some of the climate challenges in agriculture. In this context, it may be necessary to introduce measures; for example, public funding and governance initiatives, to regulate agriculture and food production towards a sustainable development in line with the ethics of sustainability of anthropogenic climate change. This requires looking beyond regional interests only. Failing to do so may lead to an injustice among population groups or regions. A renewed debate on GMOs is also crucial, if new policies and assessment criteria that take into account the need for assessment of the socio-economic risks and benefits of GMOs on local and global level are to be developed and find support.

Acknowledgement

I am deeply grateful to Theodora Kwok and Syahirah A. Karim, for their insightful comments and constructive corrections. Needless to say, any errors are those of the author. Thanks to Peter Kemp, Benjamin J. Capps, Matthias Kaiser and Gregory Kaebnick for their insightful comments on earlier drafts and ideas for this chapter. Thanks to Sarah Chan, the organizers at the iSEI and the Eugenides foundation for inviting me to present preliminary ideas for this chapter at the conference 'Greening Humanities: Science, Innovation, Ethics and the Green Economy', Athens, October 2010. Finally, thanks to John Harris and to the editors John Coggon and Swati Gola, for inviting me to contribute to this volume.

8

Improving Global Health: Intellectual Property Rights and Alternative Ways of Incentivizing Innovation

Sadie Regmi

Introduction

According to the Universal Declaration of Human Rights, 'everyone has the right to a standard of living adequate for the health and well-being of himself and of his family, including food, clothing, housing and medical care and necessary social services'.[1] Yet millions of people die every year because they cannot afford medicines that already exist.[2] As the high price of medicines is largely due to monopoly rights that are granted to their innovators, and not due to the costs of production, intellectual property rights (IPRs) seem to be at conflict with the right to medical care. In addition, funding for diseases does not correspond to the disease burden in the world, causing tropical diseases prevalent in low- and middle-income countries (LMICs) to be largely ignored. This has also raised questions about whether IPRs and the incentives they provide to only pour research resources into the disease burden of the world's richest minority are reinforcing health disparities.[3]

Lack of incentives for research into neglected diseases (NDs) has been attributed to the loose IPR regimes in LMICs.[4] In 1994, IPRs were globalized through the agreement on Trade-Related Aspects of Intellectual Property Rights (TRIPS), which all member states of the World Trade Organisation (WTO) are bound by.[5] The logic behind this was simple; high-income countries have strict IPRs and their disease burden is not ignored, the disease burden of LMICs

1 United Nations General Assembly, *Universal Declaration of Human Rights* (1948) www.ohchr. org/EN/UDHR/Documents/UDHR_Translations/eng.pdf, [accessed 30 November 2010].
2 Graham Dutfield, 'Delivering Drugs to the Poor: Will the Trips Amendment Help?', *American Journal of Law & Medicine* 34 (2008), 107–24.
3 Solomon R. Benatar, 'Reflections and Recommendations on Research Ethics in Developing Countries', *Social Science & Medicine* 54, no. 7 (2002), 1131–41.
4 Monique F. Mrazek and Elias Mossialos, 'Stimulating Pharmaceutical Research and Development for Neglected Diseases', *Health Policy* 64 (2003), 75–88.
5 WTO, 'Agreement on Trade-Related Aspects of Intellectual Property Rights', in *Marrakesh Agreement Establishing the World Trade Organisation*, ed. World Trade Organisation (1994).

with weak IPRs is ignored, hence implementing stricter IPRs should incentivize research into the disease burden of LMICs with formerly weak IPRs. Yet, in 2007, 12 years after TRIPS was implemented, there was little documented evidence of any improvements in the 90/10 gap, fuelling questions about the motivations behind the globalization of IPRs and the wisdom of the TRIPS agreement.[6]

Margaret Chan, Director-General of the World Health Organisation (WHO), asserts the 'need for a system of intellectual property that rewards innovation in the interest of keeping it sustainable'.[7] Most public policy on drug patents is based on the notion that patents could, overall, be more conducive to public welfare because they incentivize innovation. Awareness of the shortcomings of the current system is a prerequisite of effectively comparing IPRs to the alternatives. The aim of this essay is thus to assess such shortcomings.

The TRIPS agreement

Ever since IPRs and trade were linked by the United States in the 1980s, various attempts have been made to globalize IPRs through bilateral and multilateral trade agreements.[8] Arguably, the most successful of these attempts, at least in terms of making IPRs applicable in many countries, was the 1995 TRIPS agreement.

With regard to pharmaceuticals, TRIPS requires:[9]

- Patents for pharmaceutical products and microorganisms to have a 20-year duration, starting when the inventor files for the patent

- Patent rights of imported products to be upheld

- Patented holders to get exclusive marketing rights until the patent expires.

---

6 Jillian Claire Cohen-Kohler, 'The Morally Uncomfortable Global Drug Gap', *Clinical Pharmacology & Therapeutics* 82 (2007), 610–14. Gaëlle Krikorian, 'New Trends in IP Protection and Health Issues', in *The Political Economy of HIV/Aids in Developing Countries*, ed. Benjamin Coriat (Cheltenham: Edward Elgar, 2008), 52–77.

7 Margaret Chan, 'Strengthening Multilateral Cooperation on Intellectual Property and Public Health', text of presentation at the World Intellectual Property Organisation Conference on Intellectual Property and Public Policy Issues, (2009), www.who.int/dg/speeches/2009/intellectual_property_20090714/en/index.htm [accessed 22 April 2012].

8 Peter Drahos, 'The Universality of Human Rights: Origins and Development', text of presentation at World Intellectual Property Organisation (1998), www.wipo.int/tk/en/hr/paneldiscussion/papers/pdf/drahos.pdf [accessed 22 April 2012].

9 Cohen-Kohler, 'The Morally Uncomfortable Global Drug Gap', 610–14.

TRIPS ensured that criteria for IPRs set out in the agreement would be the minimum for all member states of the WTO, with the lowest income countries being granted a period of up to ten years to implement the required changes.[10]

Before the TRIPS agreement, IPRs depended on individual governments and varied massively across the globe, with countries like India having much looser IPR regimes than countries like the United States.[11] Critics of TRIPS argue that as the primary purpose of granting IPRs has historically been to incentivize innovation, countries should be free to choose if they want to prioritize universal access to current knowledge and technology at the expense of innovation.[12] After noting that patents work by restricting access to knowledge, Graham Dutfield states:[13]

> *society needs to strike a balance between private control over the use of information and its diffusion. Where the line should be drawn is very difficult to determine, but its ideal location is likely to vary widely from one country to another.*

Whether a country wants to prioritize access over innovation may broadly, if a little simplistically, be said to differ depending on whether a country is high-income or industrializing. For instance, in the case of medicines, the former group could be said to have more of an interest in incentivizing innovation, as their populations generally do not face access barriers to medicines that are already available, whereas the latter group may be keener to establish basic access to medicines that are already available. However, access problems are not always confined to LMICs; the recent licensing of the drug amifampridine, which was only a slight modification of the unlicenced 3,4-diaminopyridine, but 50–70 times more expensive, caused neurologists in the United Kingdom to voice their concern.[14] Furthermore, lack of research into NDs shows that lack of access is not the only major barrier to healthcare in LMICs. Fourteen million people die of NDs every year and 90 per cent of these deaths occur in LMICs.[15]

While both opponents and proponents of globalizing IPRs agree that there is a lack of research into NDs, they disagree on why this is the case. Proponents argue that loose IPR regimes in LMICs is a factor deterring research into NDs and that lack of IPRs in those countries makes tropical disease research uneconomical. Their view is that the globalization of IPRs provides incentives

10 Ibid.
11 Murphy Halliburton, 'Drug Resistance, Patent Resistance: Indian Pharmaceuticals and the Impact of a New Patent Regime', *Global Public Health* 4 (2009), 515–27.
12 Drahos, 'The Universality of Human Rights: Origins and Development'.
13 Dutfield, 'Delivering Drugs to the Poor: Will the Trips Amendment Help?', 107–24.
14 Nigel Hawks and Deborah Cohen, 'What Makes an Orphan Drug?', *British Medical Journal* 341 (2010), 1076–8.
15 Mrazek and Mossialos, 'Stimulating Pharmaceutical Research and Development for Neglected Diseases', 75–88.

for research into NDs.[16] Opponents believe stricter IPRs will do little to incentivize research into NDs, also termed 'diseases of the poor', because of differences in the ability of people from HICs and LMICs to pay for drugs. They contend that research will continue to focus on developing drugs for those who are able to pay more, and point to the billions poured into 'lifestyle' drugs for the rich, which can be defined as 'drugs used for non-health problems or for conditions that lie at the boundary between a health need and a lifestyle wish'[17] to justify their view.[18] In their opinion, globalizing IPRs will do little to redress the 10/90 gap, whereby 90 per cent of the disease burden in the world only gets 10 per cent of research funding, while the increased prices of drugs and damage to generic drug industries (such as those found in India) will deprive many of life-saving drugs.[19]

The linking of trade and IPRs is particularly interesting if we see the debates as being between the interests of high-income countries versus those of low- and middle-income ones. For instance, let us consider again the fact that all member states of WTO have to sign the TRIPS agreement, which requires minimum IPR standards. Paul Collier in his book 'The Bottom Billion' states:[20]

> The essence of the World Trade Organisation is that the reduction in our trade restrictions is something that we concede only in return for others doing likewise. . . . [Countries at the bottom billion] have virtually no role in an organisation that is designed for bargaining. The countries at the bottom have no markets of any interest to the rest of the world, and so their high trade restrictions are also of no interest.

Applying Collier's argument to TRIPS, HICs are able through the WTO to impose their own priorities of an environment conducive to innovation over the access priorities of LMICs because of their economic dominance. As LMICs have more to lose if HICs impose sanctions upon them than vice versa, LMICs accept the public health losses caused by strict IPRs in favour of being part of a global trade network such as the WTO.[21]

16 Ibid. See also Patrice Trouiller, Els Torreele, Piero Olliaro, Nick White, Susan Foster, Dyann Wirth and Bernard Pécoul, 'Drugs for Neglected Diseases: A Failure of the Market and a Public Health Failure?', *Tropical Medicine and International Health* 6 (2001), 945–51.

17 David Gilbert, T. Walley and B. New, 'Lifestyle Medicines,' *British Medical Journal* 321 (2000), 1341–4.

18 Rajashree Chandra, 'Intellectual Property Rights and the Right to Health', in *Knowledge as Property* (New Delhi: Oxford University Press, 2010), 192.

19 Trouiller, Torreele, Olliaro, White, Foster, Wirth and Pécoul, 'Drugs for Neglected Diseases: A Failure of the Market and a Public Health Failure?', 945–51.

20 Paul Collier, 'Trade Policy for Reversing Marginalisation', in *The Bottom Billion* (Oxford: Oxford University Press, 2008), 161.

21 T. N. Srinivasan, *The Trips Agreement: A Comment Inspired by Frederick Abbott's Presentation*, (2000), www.econ.yale.edu/~srinivas/TRIPS.pdf [accessed 30 November 2010].

Emphasizing safeguards in TRIPS: The Doha Declaration

Recognizing that TRIPS compromised access to medicines in LMICs, the international community adopted the Doha Declaration in 2001, which 'affirmed the right of member states of the WTO to interpret and implement TRIPS in a manner supporting the protection of public health, and, in particular, access to medicines'.[22] The Doha Declaration thus clarified the safeguards in the TRIPS agreement so that LMICs were able to use compulsory licensing and parallel importing provisions in the interest of public health. Through compulsory licensing, 'the practice of authorizing a third party to make, use, or sell a patented invention without the patentee's consent',[23] countries can allow generic manufacture of cheap versions of patented drugs for use within the country. Countries without manufacturing capacity are able to issue compulsory licences to a pharmaceutical company in another country and subsequently import the drug for use in the domestic market, through parallel importing provisions. Middle-income LMICs such as India and Brazil, which have generic pharmaceutical companies, have thus produced cheap anti-retrovirals and exported them to countries that do not have sufficient resources to manufacture generic drugs.[24]

Undermining TRIPS safeguards

Writing for the Lancet in 2009, Mongkol Na Songkhla, former minister of Public Health in Thailand, reports of political pressure pharmaceuticals and governments of more well-off nations placed on Thailand when it employed TRIPS flexibilities and issued compulsory licences for generic versions of the drug 'efavirenz' and the 'lopinavir–ritonavir' combination.[25] While he reports that compulsory licensing caused the number of people on efavirenz to increase from 5,000 to 20,000 and that of lopinavir–ritonavir combination to increase from 300 to 3,000, he voices concerns that in the aftermath of the use of TRIPS safeguards by Thailand and the political pressure put upon it, other LMIC nations may be discouraged from issuing compulsory licensing in the interest of public health. Other academics have noted how the US government questioned the validity of the licence and pressed Thailand to withdraw the decision to issue a compulsory licence for efavirenz and negotiate with the

22   Vanessa Bradford Kerry and Kelley Lee, 'Trips, the Doha Declaration and Paragraph 6 Decision: What Are the Remaining Steps for Protecting Access to Medicines?', *Globalisation and Health* 3 (2007).

23   Colleen Chien, 'Cheap Drugs at What Price to Innovation: Does the Compulsory Licensing of Pharmaceuticals Hurt Innovation?', *Berkeley Technology Law Journal* (2003).

24   Kerry and Lee, 'Trips, the Doha Declaration and Paragraph 6 Decision: What Are the Remaining Steps for Protecting Access to Medicines?'

25   Mongkol Na Songkhla, 'Health before Profits? Learning from Thailand's Experience', *Lancet* 373 (2009), 441–2.

company that held the patent.[26] They believe LMICs are reluctant to exploit TRIPS safeguards and see the American and pharmaceutical industry reaction to the Thai case as being representative of the pressure on LMICs not to make use of TRIPS safeguards, asserting 'maintaining one's standing as a trading partner committed to IPRs has so far taken precedence over access to medicines'.[27]

These TRIPS safeguards are further undermined through TRIPS-plus agreements in bilateral Free Trade Agreements (FTAs) that often require stricter IPR standards. The standards put forward by the United States work either by introducing new measures that are absent from TRIPS, or by requiring countries to forego TRIPS safeguards. A summary of these measures is provided in Table 8.1.

Carsten Fink and Patrick Reichenmiller, in a Trade Note by the World Bank Group, note that the preferential access to US markets that may be given in return for stricter IPRs are time-bound and liable to be taken away in future FTAs, whereas IPR regimes, once implemented, are unlikely to change. They also note that policies, including IPR policies, are evaluated from time to time, but that trade agreements with specific IPR criteria compromise the ability of countries to change course, concluding, 'the benefits and costs associated with protecting pharmaceutical patents vary from country to country . . . insufficient flexibility in over-riding patents can have a detrimental impact on the protection of public health'.[28]

Considering the effort the international community seems to have taken to strengthen TRIPS safeguards in the Doha Declaration, it seems odd that LMICs should sacrifice these provisions so readily in bilateral FTAs. In Krikorian's opinion, due to attempts to reinforce IPR standards in the world for the past 30 years, the United States has advance knowledge of what it wants to obtain from trade negotiations, in contrast to LMICs, which frequently do not have IPRs on the agenda or 'have the vaguest, if any, notion of what is at stake'. In addition to these factors, Krikorian cites the United States' economic dominance and disparities in access to expert knowledge as reasons for why LMICs sign up to the United States' stringent IPR standards.[29]

Krikorian's representation of LMICs as not knowing the implications of IPRs is not wholly convincing, especially in light of her claim in the same chapter that the 2001 Doha discussions led ministries of health and commerce to acquire 'an unparalleled sense of the public health implications of IP protection'. Nevertheless, her analysis of how the choice for LMICs is often between losing the United States as a trading partner and sacrificing access to

---

26 Kerry and Lee, 'Trips, the Doha Declaration and Paragraph 6 Decision: What Are the Remaining Steps for Protecting Access to Medicines?'
27 Ibid.
28 Carsten Fink and Patrick Reichenmiller, *Tightening Trips: The Intellectual Property Provisions of Recent Us Free Trade Agreements* (2005), http://siteresources.worldbank.org/ INTRANETTRADE/Resources/Pubs/TradeNote20.pdf [accessed 30 November 2010].
29 Krikorian, 'New Trends in IP Protection and Health Issues', 52–77.

medicines has been echoed by various other academics.[30] While I have only used examples of American FTAs, it must be noted that the European Union is currently in the process of negotiating TRIPS-plus measures with India, with greatly adverse implications for the world's generic drug market.[31]

Alternatives to IPRs for incentivizing innovation

There appears to be a conflict between the IPRs and the availability of medical care, at least in LMICs, because the former can restrict access to medicines. However, if it is true that IPRs incentivize research and development of healthcare products to a great degree, it is possible that IPRs are, on balance, conducive to greater health. By incentivizing innovation, IPRs bring newer and better drugs into the market, which must be an improvement on lack of new medicines.[32] The latter argument rests on two presumptions: that IPRs incentivize innovation and that they are justified in so far as the effects they have on innovation outweigh the public health compromises made in reduced access. However, a key message of the report of the WHO Commission on Intellectual Property Rights, Innovation and Health is 'because the market demand for diagnostics, vaccines and medicines needed to address health problems affecting LMICs is small and uncertain, the incentive effect of intellectual property rights may be limited or non-existent'.[33] According to the evidence, IPRs are not only restricting access to medicines, but also not providing incentives for research into the diseases that afflict the majority of the world. In light of the failings of the current system to provide adequate healthcare products for many people in LMICs, several initiatives have been proposed.

Public–private partnerships

The various public–private partnerships (PPPs) devoted to research of NDs exemplify the progress being made to tackle the global burden of disease.[34]

30   Carlos Maria Correa, 'Implications of Bilateral Free Trade Agreements on Access to Medicines', *Bulletin of the World Health Organisation* 84 (2006), 399–404. Kerry and Lee, 'Trips, the Doha Declaration and Paragraph 6 Decision: What Are the Remaining Steps for Protecting Access to Medicines?'

31   'Europe! Hands off Our Medicine', in *Medecins Sans Frontieres* (2010), www.msfaccess. org/sites/default/files/MSF_assets/Access/Docs/ACCESS_briefing_HandsOffCampaign_FTA_ ENG_2010.pdf [accessed 22 April 2012].

32   Linda R. Cohen and Roger G. Noll, 'Intellectual Property, Antitrust and the New Economy', *University of Pittsburgh Law Review* 62 (2000), 453–73.

33   Tomris Türmen and Charles Clift, '"Public Health, Innovation and Intellectual Property Rights: Unfinished Business', *Bulletin of the World Health Organisation* 84 (2006), 338.

34   Mrazek and Mossialos, 'Stimulating Pharmaceutical Research and Development for Neglected Diseases', 75–88.

Table 8.1 TRIPS-plus measures

Measure	Explanation	Implications
Patent-term extension	Extension of patents to compensate for delays in examining patent applications and granting marketing approval. It appears that delays in other countries also have to be taken into account, as has happened in the case of Bahrain.	Extension of patents will directly affect the time period after which generics can enter the market.
Test data exclusivity	TRIPS requires WTO member states to protect undisclosed test data against commercial use, but there is no mention of granting exclusive rights over the data. The bilateral FTAs put forward by the United States, in contrast, require states to grant exclusive rights for a minimum period of five years after approval of the data, regardless of whether or not the data are classed as being 'undisclosed'.	Data exclusivity will delay generic competition, as generic manufactures will not be able to use the data for five years to obtain marketing approval. This greatly undermines the provision of compulsory licensing, as generic manufactures would have to compile their own data, which could be expensive and time-consuming.
Linkage	Linkage requires the registration of drugs to be linked to patent protection, which means that health authorities are not able to grant marketing approval to a generic drug if a patented version is available. Like data exclusivity, linkage is a characteristic of American FTAs, and is not present in TRIPS.	As drugs cannot be brought to the market without the approval of the patent holder, the compulsory licensing provision in TRIPS is yet again undermined.

Grounds for issuing compulsory licences	While TRIPS allows WTO member states to determine the grounds upon which to issue compulsory licences, the US–Vietnam, US–Australia, US–Jordan and US–Singapore FTAs limit the use of compulsory licences to cases of national emergency or non-commercial use.	Specifying the grounds for use of compulsory licensing undermines the ability of states to make decisions on important public health matters.
Limitations on parallel importing	The US–Australia, US–Morocco and US–Singapore FTAs give the patent holder the right to prevent parallel imports, undermining this TRIPS safeguard.	The neighbours of Australia, Morocco and Singapore, who lack manufacturing capacity will not be able to issue compulsory licences and subsequently import generics from these nations, even the event of a national emergency.
Institutional flexibility undermined	Provisions under TRIPS recognize limitations in LMICs in enforcing laws and thus do not create specific obligations to enforce IPRs over enforcing other laws. US agreements with several countries make it clear that resource limitations cannot be used as an excuse for not adhering to intellectual property regimes.	Having to enforce IPRs could direct resources away from important programmes in countries with limited resources.
Fines	In the event of IPR infringement, TRIPS requires fines to be paid in compensation for monetary losses of patent holders. By contrast, all the US FTAs require fines to be paid, whether or not the patent holders are financially affected by the infringement.	Fines that have to be paid even when there has been no financial gain are likely to be detrimental to actors in LMICs.

Source: Correa (2006), Kerry and Lee (2007), Fink and Reichenmiller, (2005).

While many PPPs funnel resources into much-needed research for NDs, some also show an awareness of problems with access and thus incorporate provisions that make access to medical treatment (once the research has delivered a product) a priority. The International Aids Vaccine Initiative is one such PPP, where the possession of IPRs by the private partner is subject to the production of vaccines for LMICs at affordable prices.[35] Another PPP, Medicines for Malaria Venture, retains the IPRs in LMICs, while the private partner possesses the rights in HICs.[36] The Global Fund to Fight AIDS, Tuberculosis and Malaria aims to coordinate the effort of donors and provide incentives for research into NDs.[37]

Health Impact Fund

Recognizing that the patent system was put in place to incentivize innovation, and also noting its shortcomings, namely that 'this system does not encourage development of drugs for diseases that mainly affect poor people', Thomas Pogge and colleagues have proposed the Health Impact Fund (HIF) as an alternative system to incentivize innovation.[38] HIF requires drug developers to register their product, which would entitle them to a share of a 'reward pool' of US$6 billion for ten years. Their share of the reward would depend on the relative impact of their drug compared to other registered drugs in tackling the global burden of disease. The impact would be re-evaluated on a regular basis. Registration to HIF would require drug developers to produce and distribute medicines at the lowest feasible cost of production and distribution for ten years, and then to freely give out licences to generic manufacturers. HIF aims to provide incentives for research into drugs for NDs as well as for more common diseases such as HIV and coronary heart disease, but not into 'lifestyle' drugs. The proposers of HIF hope that the money for the reward pool, although large, would result in savings even for rich-world citizens because the cost of patents would no longer be included in the price of drugs.[39]

Although prize funds are not a new concept, they have never been implemented on the scale that proponents of HIF would do. However, this is hardly a point against HIF, since a larger prize fund must attract more innovation, not less. As the system has broadly worked on a smaller scale, for

---

35 Ibid. See also *International Aids Vaccine Initiative*, www.iavi.org/Pages/home.aspx [accessed 22 April 2012].

36 *Medicines for Malaria Venture*, www.mmv.org [accessed 22 April 2012].

37 Mrazek and Mossialos, 'Stimulating Pharmaceutical Research and Development for Neglected Diseases'. See also *The Global Fund*, www.theglobalfund.org/en/ [accessed 22 April 2012].

38 Amitava Banerjee, Thomas Pogge and Aidan Hollis, 'The Health Impact Fund: Incentives for Improving Access to Medicines', *Lancet* 375 (2010), 166–9.

instance through the Gates Foundation, the concept is at least known to be broadly sound.[40]

As drug manufacturers would have to voluntarily register their product into the HIF, and in doing so forego the absolute monopoly they would otherwise have due to their patented product, their share of the prize fund reward would have to be sufficiently lucrative for them to follow this route. The incentivizing effect of HIF depends on the reward pool that governments agree to support and in the number of products that can simultaneously be registered with the fund. The larger the reward pool and the fewer the number of registrants, the more incentivizing the effect of HIF would be.

The current system of incentives rewards drug manufacturers on the basis of sales of their products only. The manufacturers have every incentive to advertise their product and to lobby doctors to use it. This might not be effective in healthcare systems in many HICs where decisions about the cost-effectiveness and efficacy of drugs are made by independent bodies. However, in LMICs, health-care expenses are usually met out of pocket, and consumers are thus open to exploitation; counterfeits have a big market in many LMICs.[41] If markets are not deemed to be worth advertising in, they are ignored altogether, as firms have no incentive to get their drugs out to those who cannot afford them. The HIF, by altering the reward given to companies and basing it on health impact, has the potential to tackle the 'last mile problem', where consumers in need of medication do not acquire them due to lack of incentives for manufacturers to get medications out to those who are unable to afford them.

As the emphasis of the HIF is on health impact, it should, in theory, be an equitable scheme. However, as high income countries (HICs) will be contributing more to the fund than low- and middle-income countries (LMICs), it is possible that political interests get in the way of implementing such a scheme. It is also probable that those nations that contribute more to the fund will have more voting power and, in the absence of rigorous independent boards to assess the global burden of disease and health impact of a particular drug, it is possible that the fund will not be as equitable as its proponents hope. However, by placing the emphasis on health impact, the HIF could achieve equity both in innovation of new drugs and medical technologies and their subsequent distribution.

39 Ibid.
40 Bill and Melinda Gates Foundation, 'Foundation and U.S. Government Give $2.5 Million Prize for Transforming Banking Sector in Haiti', www.gatesfoundation.org/press-releases/Pages/mobile-money-in-haiti-110110.aspx [accessed 22 April 2012].
41 Shubham Chaudhuri, Pinelopi K Goldberg and Panle Gia, 'Estimating the Effects of Global Patent Protection in Pharmaceuticals: A Case Study of Quinolones in India', *The American Economic Review* 96 (2006), 1477–514. J. Stiglitz, 'Scrooge and Intellectual Property Rights', *British Medical Journal* 333 (2006), 1279–80.

Medical Research and Development Treaty (MRDT)

The MRDT aims to break the link between the cost of production and the cost of research and development, and thus proposes an alternative to the patent system for funding medical research. Countries – high income and low and middle income – would agree to contribute a certain percentage to a research fund, with the contributions increasing according to levels of gross domestic product (GDP) or per capita income.[42]

Priorities of medical research would be identified through a Committee on Priority Medical Research and Development (CPMRD), which would meet once a year. Emphasis would be placed on improving access to knowledge, increasing technology transfer and research into priority medical research and development.[43]

As research will be funded directly, MRDT will no doubt incentivize basic medical research. Whether MRDT will provide sufficient incentives for researchers to translate their research into effective products is much less certain. Nicoletta Dentico and Nathan Ford, in their essay 'The Courage to Change the Rules: A Proposal for an Essential Health R&D Treaty', cite the model used for the Human Genome Project, which was public-sector funded, as an example of the sufficiently incentivizing effect of basic research funding.[44] However, in the absence of clear aims, such as those of the Human Genome Project, and in the face of competition for funding from different researchers with varying research agendas, it is unclear whether the 'public-goods model' that worked for the Human Genome Project would necessarily work as well when implemented on a broader scale.

It is possible, however, that if the MRDT was subject to good governance, research funds would flow between countries, research efforts would not be duplicated and the research base of LMICs would be strengthened, thus contributing to their growth, and aiding research into diseases that primarily afflict populations of these countries, namely the communicable tropical diseases. Taking into consideration the various and sometimes opposing political commitments of the parties that will make up the governing body of the MRDT, this may be an unrealistic prospect.

The concerns about the distribution of benefits of research raised by the current IPR system are no doubt a major contributing factor to the open-access model purported by the MRDT. However, just as there may be a lack of incentives for researchers to translate basic research into usable goods, there may also be a lack of incentive in ensuring physicians and consumers of

---

42   Medical Research and Development Treaty (MRDT): Discussion Draft 4 (2005), www.cptech.org/workingdrafts/rndtreaty4.pdf [accessed 22 April 2012].

43   Ibid.

44   Nicoletta Dentico and Nathan Ford, 'The Courage to Change the Rules: A Proposal for an Essential Health R&D Treaty', *PLoS Medicine* 2 (2005), 96–9.

products are knowledgeable about new products.[45] Even if the goodwill of the actors in question was deemed to be sufficient motivation, it is not clear how such diffusion schemes would be funded. This is in contrast to the HIF where, as inventors are rewarded on the basis of health impact, they are incentivized to ensure that the distribution networks that would maximize the impact of their products are working properly.[46]

A particular strength of the MRDT is its international nature; by signing up, countries would be jointly invested in important health research. Furthermore, coordination has the potential to minimise duplication of research efforts. A solution that draws on the strengths of both the HIC and the MRDT could take the shape of a global R&D treaty, the funds from which would then be used as the 'reward pool' of a HIF-style scheme.

Conclusion

The merits and drawbacks of intellectual property rights (IPRs) have been debated for as long as IPRs have been in place. In recent decades, the impact of IPRs on the health outcomes, particularly of those in LMICs, has been noted. In light of the significant drawbacks of the current system, and the potential merits of alternatives that have been proposed, a rethink of the model of incentivizing innovation is in order.

---

45   Joseph DiMasi and Henry Grabowski, 'Patents and R&D Incentives: Comments on the Hubbard and Love Trade Framework for Financing Pharmaceutical R&D', Submission for WHO Commission on Intellectual Property Rights, Innovation and Public Health (2004), www.who.int/intellectualproperty/news/en/Submission3.pdf [accessed 22 April 2012].
46   Selgelid, 'A Full-Pull Program for the Provision of Pharmaceuticals: Practical Issues', *Public Health Ethics* 1 (2008), 134–45.

9

Drug Resistance, Patents and Justice: Who Owns the Effectiveness of Antibiotics?

James Wilson

Introduction

The wide availability of penicillin from 1945 onwards, and the subsequent rapid progress in discovering new antibiotics revolutionized medicine.[1] Salk's polio vaccine, and the success of the campaign to eradicate smallpox further contributed to a widespread optimism that infectious disease had been conquered.[2]

This has proved a vain hope. Communicable diseases still account for 15 million deaths per year. Communicable diseases still account for 13 million deaths per year. This is 25 per cent of the global burden of disease.[3] The slow progress on the burden of communicable disease is due most obviously to a collective failure to secure the basic prerequisites of healthy life for more than a billion of the world's poorest people: clean water, access to improved sanitation, adequate nutrition, shelter, air quality and health facilities.[4]

---

1 For an accessible introduction to these changes, see James Le Fanu, *The Rise and Fall of Modern Medicine* (London: Little, Brown and Company, 1999).
2 A widely-quoted, but possibly apocryphal, statement by the US Surgeon General, William Stewart has come to emblematize this mood of optimism: 'The time has come to close the book on infectious diseases. We have basically wiped out infection in the United States.' This statement is said to have been made around 1970, though as Battin et al. relate, it is difficult to find an original source for it: see Margaret P. Battin, Leslie P. Francis, Jay A. Jacobson and Charles B. Smith, *The Patient as Victim and Vector: Ethics and Infectious Disease* (Oxford: Oxford University Press, 2008), 3.
3 Rafael Lozano, Mohsen Naghavi, Kyle Foreman et al. 'Global and regional mortality from 235 causes of death for 20 age groups in 1990 and 2010: a systematic analysis for the Global Burden of Disease Study 2010', *The Lancet*, 2012, 380(9859): 2095–128.
4 See Yvonne Rydin, Ana Bleahu, Michael Davies, Julio D. Davila, Sharon Friel, Giovanni De Grandis, Nora Groce, Pedro Hallal, Ian Hamilton, Philippa Howden-Chapman, Ka Man Lai, C. J. Lim, Juliana Martins, David Osrin, Ian Ridley, Ian Scott, Myfanwy Taylor, Paul Wilkinson and James Wilson, 'Shaping Cities for Health: The Complexity of Planning Urban Environments in the 21st Century', *The Lancet*, 2012, 379(9831): 2079–108, available at http://press.thelancet.com/healthycities.pdf.

It is also becoming increasingly apparent that the microbes which cause communicable diseases provide an even sterner long-term challenge to earlier optimistic predictions. This is the challenge of drug resistance. The burden of disease from drug-resistant pathogens is already considerable, and is expected to continue to rise. Multi-drug-resistant tuberculosis alone now accounts over 15,000 deaths per year.[5] Even in the European Union, multi-drug-resistant bacteria account for over 25,000 deaths per year.[6]

This chapter examines how we should think about intellectual property in antibiotics, given the fact of drug resistance. I argue that even when a company is granted a patent on the manufacture of antibiotics, the resource of antibiotic effectiveness that is depleted when those drugs are used remains the common property of humanity. As we shall see, this result has important implications for how antibiotics may legitimately be used, and who should profit from them.

The nature of antibiotic resistance

Antibiotics are drugs that aim to cure disease by interfering with some aspect of the life processes of pathogens such as microbes and viruses.[7] In order to be useful as drugs, antibiotics need to be selective in their action: they need to be able to interfere with the life processes of pathogens, without interfering too much with the life processes of the human body. We can distinguish between narrow and wide spectrum antibiotics: narrow spectrum antibiotics are highly specific in the pathogens that they target, while wide spectrum antibiotics are effective against a broader range.

Pathogens are said to develop *antibiotic resistance* when specific antibiotics lose their ability to kill or inhibit the pathogen's growth. Given the variety of pathogens, antibiotics and possible dosing regimes, a more precise definition of antibiotic resistance would be 'the capability of a *particular* pathogen population to grow in the presence of a *given* antibiotic when the antibiotic is used according to a *specific* regimen'.[8]

5 World Health Organisation, *Fact Sheet 194: Antimicrobial Resistance* (Geneva: World Health Organisation, 2011), www.who.int/mediacentre/factsheets/fs194/en/.
6 European Medicines Agency and European Centre for Disease Prevention and Control, *Joint Technical Report: The Bacterial Challenge – Time to React*, 2009, http://ecdc.europa.eu/en/publications/Publications/0909_TER_The_Bacterial_Challenge_Time_to_React.pdf.
7 Karl Drlica and David S. Perlin, *Antibiotic Resistance: Understanding and Responding to an Emerging Crisis* (New Jersey: FT Press, 2011), 31. In non-technical usage, antibiotics are often treated as synonymous with antibacterials, as, for example, when it is argued that doctors should not prescribe antibiotics for a viral infection. As it is the phenomenon of resistance we are interested in here, and the problem of drug-resistant pathogens goes broader than drug-resistant bacteria, I use antibiotic in this broader sense in this chapter.
8 Drlica and Perlin, *Antibiotic Resistance*, 8.

Antibiotic resistance is ancient.[9] Bacteria and other pathogens have existed as part of a Darwinian struggle for life for over three billion years. Those that have survived this far have already faced selection pressures in which the ability to resist naturally occurring antibiotics has increased reproductive fitness. For example, some bacteria have developed efflux pumps – and so can automatically pump antibiotics out of their cells before the antibiotics have a chance to kill them. Antibiotic resistance which predates the introduction of a given antibiotic is known as inherent resistance.

Other antibiotic resistance is acquired: this occurs when pathogens that were previously susceptible to antibiotics become resistant to them as a result of genetic mutations: for example, by modifications of the target site or metabolic pathway that the antibiotic had previously made use of. The greater the number of pathogen cells that come into contact with a given antibiotic, the greater the likelihood of mutations which confer antibiotic resistance developing. Although mutations which increase antibiotic resistance are rare, the number of pathogen cells exposed to antibiotics is so large that such mutations occur frequently.[10]

Antibiotic stewardship

There are three main strategies for controlling the spread of antibiotic resistance, which must be used together in a coordinated fashion. Given that antibiotics by their nature create selection pressures for new resistant strains, the first plank of responsible antibiotic stewardship is to limit the use of antibiotics. Antibiotic use can be limited in the first instance by ensuring (where time and resources allow) that antibiotics are appropriately targeted to pathogens. Ruling out prescribing antibacterials for viral infections and banning worldwide the addition of antibiotics to feed for healthy farm animals would greatly help.[11] Second, and more controversially, even where the specific pathogen is

9   Vanessa D'Costa, Christine King, Lindsay Kalan, Mariya Morar, Wilson Sung, Carsten Schwartz, Duance Froese, Grant Zazula, et al., 'Antibiotic Resistance Is Ancient', *Nature*, 2011, 477 (7365): 457–61.

10 Drlica and Perlin relate that the number of antibiotic prescriptions in the United States is 100 million per year, and that the number of pathogen cells in an infection is usually over 1 million. This would imply that somewhere in the region of 10^{14} pathogen cells are subjected to antibiotics per year in the United States alone (*Antibiotic Resistance*, 76)

11 Over 50 percent of the antibiotics used in the United States are used in agriculture. See M. Lipsitch, R. S. Singer, B. R. Levin, 'Antibiotics in Agriculture: When Is It Time to Close the Barn Door?', *Proc Natl Acad Sci USA*, 2002, 99: 5752–4. Examples of increased antibiotic resistance in humans from agriculture include the rise of quinolone-resistant enteritis after the introduction of fluoroquinolones in poultry feed. See K. E. Smith, J. M. Besser, C. W. Hedberg, F. T. Leano, J. B. Bender, J. H. Wicklund, B. P. Johnson, K. A. Moore and M. T. Osterholm, 'Q'uinolone-Resistant Campylobacter Jejuni Infections in Minnesota, 1992–1998', *The New England Journal of Medicine*, 1999, 340 (20):1525.

susceptible we can appeal to the opportunity cost of prescribing antibiotics for relatively trivial ailments.[12] Any proposed use must be of sufficiently high value that it is worth the opportunity cost of later persons suffering a greater risk that their treatment will be ineffective.[13]

The second plank is to ensure that where antibiotics *are* used, they are used in a way that will minimize the risk of resistant strains developing and spreading. The best treatment regimen to do this will vary from pathogen to pathogen, depending among other factors on the number mutations that are necessary for a wild-type strain to undergo before it gains resistance to a given antibiotic, the frequency of such mutations, and what costs these mutations place on reproductive fitness.[14] The emerging picture of research is that appropriate regimens can help us to eke out the effectiveness of antibiotics, but cannot prevent its inexorable rise.[15]

The third plank is to ensure that new antibiotics are discovered and brought onto the market, to replace those that are becoming ineffective. Currently new antibiotics are being brought to market much more slowly than already existing antibiotics are losing their effectiveness.[16]

12 K. R. Foster and H. Grundmann, 'Do We Need to Put Society First? The Potential for Tragedy in Antimicrobial Resistance', *PLoS Med*, 2006, 3: e29.

13 I discuss inter temporal opportunity costs and healthcare resource allocation in James Wilson, 'Paying for Patented Drugs is Hard to Justify: An Argument about Time Discounting and Medical Need', *Journal of Applied Philosophy*, 2012, 29(3): 186–99.

14 It has often been assumed that the best model is aggressive drug treatment which is continued until the end of the prescribed course, even if the patient feels better much before this. However, recent work on mathematical models of drug resistance has shown that there can be cases (e.g. in malaria treatment) where aggressive treatment may be less effective at limiting drug resistance. See Andrew F. Read, Troy Day and Silvie Huijben, 'The Evolution of Drug Resistance and the Curious Orthodoxy of Aggressive Chemotherapy', *Proceedings of the National Academy of Sciences*, 2011, forthcoming, doi:10.1073/pnas.110029910. See also L. B. Rice, 'The Maxwell Finland Lecture: For the Duration – Rational Antibiotic Administration in an Era of Antimicrobial Resistance and Clostridium Difficile', *Clinical Infectious Diseases*, 2008, 46(4): 491–6.

15 It was initially thought that the effectiveness of antibiotics could be maintained by employing them in scientifically determined rotation. The assumption was that maintaining resistance to a particular antibiotic would have some cost in fitness to the bacterium in an environment where this antibiotic was not present, and so we should expect drug-resistant strains to die out if we allowed particular antibiotics to lie fallow for a period of time. However, evidence of the effectiveness of antibiotic cycling is weak, and in addition there are a number of theoretical reasons for thinking that it could at best somewhat retard, but not stop, the growth of antibiotic resistance. For a review of the empirical evidence, see E. M. Brown and D. Nathanwi, 'Antibiotic Cycling or Rotation: A Systematic Review of the Evidence of Efficacy', *Journal of Antimicrobial Chemotherapy*, 2005, 55: 6–9. At a more theoretical level, the problem is that there need only be a very small number of resistant bacteria in the environment for resistance to be a problem: as soon as the antibiotic that has been lying fallow is brought back, we then select in favour of the resistant bacteria, and soon see a sharp rise in their numbers. Second, the assumption that resistance to antibiotics inevitably has a high cost for the bacterium is not true: bacteria can and do mutate in such a way as to reduce the survival cost of antibiotic resistance.

16 Cantal M. Morel and Elias Mossialos, 'Stoking the Antibiotic Pipeline', *BMJ*, 2010, 340, bmj.c2115.

Each of these three strategies only underscores the starting point of my argument, which is that the effectiveness of each particular antibiotic is a limited resource. The correct analogy for any particular antibiotic is not something like the stocks of a particular fish which can be prudently managed so that they replenish themselves over time, but rather a limited resource like oil or coal. We can steward antibiotics more or less responsibly, but whenever we use any particular antibiotic we contribute to the conditions in which it becomes ineffective.

Three levels of ownership in antibiotics

We can distinguish between three different levels at which the resources required to deliver effective antimicrobial treatments can be owned. Our interest is in the relationship between the second and the third.

1   *Ownership of physical stocks of antibiotics.* Stocks of antibiotics are physical goods. Ownership of physical stocks of antibiotics raises ethical issues where there is either a scarcity in the supply of the tablets in question, or if people who need access to the tablets to prevent them suffering serious harm are denied access to the tablets.

2   *Ownership of the intellectual property on a particular antibiotic compound.* Patents grant ownership and control rights over *types* of objects rather than concrete particulars.[17] Rights are granted over the use of an antibiotic compound for a particular purpose. An antibiotic patent does not give ownership over physical stocks of the compound, but it does give the monopoly right to control the manufacture and use of the compound for the period of the patent claim.

3   *Ownership of the effectiveness of each particular antibiotic.* We have seen that the effectiveness of each particular antibiotic is a limited resource. We cannot distribute and use antibiotics without depleting this resource.

The key question concerns the relationship between the second and the third types of ownership: does ownership of a patent for a given antibiotic bring with it the private ownership of the underlying resource of antibiotic effectiveness during the period of the patent? Or should we think of antibiotic effectiveness as an unowned resource that can be fairly appropriated by anyone? Or should we think of antibiotic effectiveness as a resource that belongs to humanity in common?

---

17   I write about the ethical implications of this fact at much greater length in James Wilson, 'Ontology and the Regulation of Intellectual Property', *The Monist*, 2010, 93(3): 453–66.

Patents do not usually give the patent holder a temporary monopoly on extracting the value from a limited resource that has significant implications for human well-being, and so the question of the relationship between the second and the third types of ownership has so far gone unexamined. Compare granting a patent on a new type of vacuum cleaner to a patent on a new antibiotic. When authorities grant a patent on a new type of vacuum cleaner it is not the case that each time one of these vacuum cleaners is used, it increases the likelihood of the development of mutant hoover-resistant superdust. Nor is it the case that the decision to use vacuum cleaners for relatively trivial things like cleaning out the inside of a car will prevent people in the future from being able to them for more lofty purposes like capturing dust from inside their houses.

Inventions are by nature public goods: that is, they are non-rival and non-excludable. Standard economic theory tells us that unless we do something to incentivize their production we should expect an underproduction of public goods. It will tend to be irrational (in self-interested terms) to expend your own time and money creating a public good, given that everyone else will be able to benefit from the public good as much as you will. It is easier to allow someone else to do the hard work, and then take a free ride on their efforts. But of course, it will tend to be irrational (in self-interested terms) for anyone else to put the effort in either; and so there is a severe risk of under-creation of such goods. Even where such goods are produced, it will usually be rational (in self-interested terms) for the inventor to try to keep the underlying processes and ideas secret, so that she can reap an advantage for her work.[18]

The patent system is usually justified on the grounds that it provides the best solution to this public goods problem. Patents aim to solve the problem of under-provision by making patented inventions *excludable* and *public*. Provision to exclude others from the good is hypothesized to act as an incentive to do the necessary research and development to create useful new inventions: it will become rational to put the necessary effort in if you know that you will be able to recoup your costs (and return a profit) by charging others for access to the good. Patents attempt to solve the problem of secrecy by requiring that patentors disclose the basis of the patented item in such a way that anyone skilled in the art would be able to reconstruct it from the description. In order to gain a patent, the patent holder has to share the underlying knowledge of how the process or product can be made with everyone.

Thus, patent legislation is usually thought to have its justification in a quid pro quo; the inventor receives a temporary monopoly in order that the space of

---

18   In the past there have been some quite significant cases of the withholding of medical information. Most famously, the Chamberlen family kept the discovery of the obstetrics forceps secret for more than 100 years, in order to protect their midwifery business. (See Wendy Moore, 'Keeping Mum', *BMJ*, 2007, 334(7595): 698).

ideas which are available to all for effective use is expanded once the monopoly expires.[19] Patents on antibiotics are difficult to reconcile with this model. While formulae for making antibiotics are public goods – and hence we will be able to make any amount of antibiotic tablets with a particular formula – the effectiveness of antibiotics is not. The knowledge about how to make an antibiotic that is brought into the public domain by the corresponding patent will typically be much reduced in usefulness, once resistant pathogens develop.

So a better mental model for thinking about the way current patents on antibiotics work would be granting a company an exclusive right to exploit a particular oil reserve for a limited period of time, with the stipulation that after the exclusive license period, anyone is permitted to exploit the oil in the reserve. In providing such a licence, we would be allowing the company the exclusive license to extract as much oil as they are able to from the oilfield during this period. We would usually think that this would be a rather unwise way of proceeding if our interest was in maximizing public benefit from the oil once the company's monopoly had expired.

Who owns the effectiveness of antibiotics?

The central moral question that this raises is who owns these resources of antibiotic effectiveness in the first place. There seem to be three basic answers:

1 *Finders Keepers.* On this view, the resource of the effectiveness of a particular antibiotic is owned by whoever discovers it: he or she has created something which did not previously exist (or used their art to refine something which previously did). The inventor has put the effort to turn a (potentially) naturally existing substance into a *drug* with the right pharmacodynamic and pharmacokinetic properties to be a saleable commodity. On this view, the inventor has a property right over this resource; he is within his rights to use up this resource in any way he sees fit, and no one else is able to make use of the resource without his permission.

2 *First come, first served.* On this view, the resource of the effectiveness of a particular antibiotic is initially unowned. Everyone has a liberty right

---

19 The US Constitution explicitly posits this link: the stated purpose of the copyright and patent statutes is to 'promote the Progress of Science and useful Arts, by securing for limited Times to Authors and Inventors the exclusive Right to their respective Writings and Discoveries'. (Article I, Section 8, Clause 8) On this general point, and what it should mean for the future of intellectual property regulation, see for example James Boyle, *The Public Domain: Enclosing the Commons of the Mind* (New Haven: Yale University Press, 2008).

to use this resource in whatever way he or she sees fit: the inventor is permitted to use the resource up, but so is everyone else.

3   *Common ownership.* On this view, the antimicrobial resources are commonly owned by humanity as a whole. There are certain duties of stewardship that make it wrong to use up resources which are held in common.

Let us start by considering a resource allocation case that is familiar from the literature. We can call this *Ordinary Pill Shortage.*

Ordinary Pill Shortage

There is a new deadly disease in our country. The only treatment that is effective against it is a new pill, and there are only 100 of these pills. Each one will be effective in curing the disease for one person. Once these pills are gone, we will not be able to get any more.

In resource allocation cases of this kind, it is standard to begin with two questions. First, who has a claim to be considered for the allocation of these pills? Second, among those who should be considered, how do we decide who should be of higher priority and who of lower priority? Compare this to a second case, which we can call *Super-resistant bacteria.*

Super-resistant Bacteria

There is a new deadly disease wreaking havoc. Knowledge of how to make a pill that will cure the disease is in the public domain, and there are a number of different factories in the world that could cheaply make large numbers of these pills. However, due to the super-resistance of the bacteria, after the hundredth person has taken their pill, the pills will no longer be effective against the disease.

How should we decide who should be allowed to take the 100 pills in this case? One important difference between the cases is that ownership of physical stock of pills plausibly matters in *Ordinary Pill Shortage,* whereas it is of much less relevance in *Super-resistant Bacteria.* In *Super-resistant Bacteria,* lots of different actors have the ability to make more than 100 pills. While ownership of 100 pills gives any actor the *power* to decide how the limited resource of this antibiotic's effectiveness will be used up, the fact that many others also have the same power should make us question whether this power is sufficient to provide the *authority* to decide how the limited resource should be used up.

Let us stipulate that in *Super-resistant Bacteria* no one is responsible for uncovering the knowledge of how to make the pill. (We shall shortly consider a case in which someone has a strong claim to have invented the drug). This leaves us with two possibilities: *First Come, First Served,* or *Common*

Ownership. The pills in *Super-resistant Bacteria* have two morally relevant important properties. First, no one can claim to have a privileged relationship to them in virtue of having invented them, second, many (perhaps all) people need them. If we take for granted the widely shared view of the equal moral status of human beings, then the salient moral question is how a group of moral equals should distribute a scarce and important resource to which none has a privileged claim.[20] If we start from this analysis, then the most important thing is to ensure that the way we distribute such a resource is in line with treating each person as an equal.

First Come, First Served, amounts to the claim that it is fair for those who get to the pills first to take them, and thus exclude others from the benefit. This seems like an implausible account of allocation of scarce resources among equals, as we can readily imagine scenarios in which the 100 doses of the drug go to people who do not really need them, and do not really benefit from them. Is 'I took the drug first' an adequate justification to give to those who are thereby deprived of the drug – especially those who are sickest, or would have benefited most from it?

Common Ownership provides a more plausible answer. On *Common Ownership*, the fairest response would be to view the case as similar to a version of the *Ordinary Pill Shortage* problem in which we stipulate that all human beings count equally as potential claimants of the resource, and we then work out who should be highest priority, and assign the pills to the people who have the strongest claim. It seems unlikely that merely being there first would count as a morally relevant consideration in this context. A common ownership approach may include delaying giving out the pills, if there are people in the world who will have stronger claims in the future than those people have now.[21]

Let us now examine a third scenario. We can call this *Super-resistant Bacteria with patent.*

Super-resistant Bacteria with patent

There is another new deadly disease wreaking havoc. Professor Smith designs and patents a molecule that has never existed in nature before and which can cure the disease. He takes out a patent on it. Knowledge of how to make this drug is again widespread, and there are a number of different factories in the world that could cheaply make large numbers of these pills. Due to the

20 The framing of this argument is taken from Mathias Risse's writings on the common ownership of the world. See for example, Mathias Risse, 'Common Ownership of the Earth as a Non-Parochial Standpoint: A Contingent Derivation of Human Rights,' *European Journal of Philosophy,* 2009, 17(2), 277–304.
21 I discuss time and resource allocation at length in James Wilson, 'Paying for Patented Drugs is Hard to Justify: An Argument about Time Discounting and Medical Need', *Journal of Applied Philosophy,* 2012, 29(3): 186–99.

super-resistance of the bacteria, after the hundredth person has taken their pill, the pills will no longer be effective against the disease.

Does Professor Smith have the right to auction off all the effective doses of the drug while he holds the relevant patent? Of course, if Professor Smith does this, it is unlikely that the doses will get into the hands of those who would get them under the principles that a group of moral equals would institute in common ownership cases. The key question is whether – even if we think that he should have ownership of the intellectual property in the ideas and processes for a limited period of time – this should give Professor Smith the right to use up or sell the entire world's effective doses of this drug?

It is important to clarify what the argument might be for thinking that Smith's invention of the drug gives him the right to appropriate privately the limited resource of the underlying antibiotic effectiveness. The standard view is that the justification of patents is to act as *incentives* to get inventors to act in certain ways, rather than to protect pre-existing moral claims to ownership that arise from invention. In Thomas Jefferson's words, 'Inventions then cannot, in nature, be a subject of property. Society may give an exclusive right to the profits arising from them, as an encouragement to men to pursue ideas which may produce utility, but this may or may not be done, according to the will and convenience of the society, without claim or complaint from anybody.'[22] Standard theories of the role of patents thus do not provide support for the claim that invention brings with it moral entitlements, let alone moral entitlements over scarce and previously unowned resources that would be depleted by the industrial use of the invention.

What would be required would be an argument to establish a moral right not only to exclusively appropriate the fruits of one's intellectual labours, but also whatever other resources are necessary to profit from one's intellectual labours. I have argued at length elsewhere that there can be no moral right to exclusively appropriate the fruits of one's intellectual labours.[23] Hence I am even more sceptical that Smith could have a right to exclusively appropriate the scarce good of antibiotic effectiveness in virtue of having intellectual property rights over the drug compound.

It might be possible to argue that Smith has a claim to ownership of the effectiveness of the antibiotic that derives from somewhere else than his ownership of the intellectual property. Perhaps it could be argued that the case is similar to the case where someone mixes labour with a resource that was otherwise unowned – in this case, by turning what was otherwise merely

---

22   Thomas Jefferson, *Letter to Isaac McPherson*, 13 August 1813, in Writings 13: 333–5. Available online at http://press-pubs.uchicago.edu/founders/documents/a1_8_8s12.html.

23   James Wilson, 'Could There Be a Right to Own Intellectual Property?', *Law and Philosophy*, 2009, 28(4): 393–427.

a molecule into a *drug* with the right pharmacodynamic and pharmacokinetic properties to be a saleable commodity.

However, there are two difficulties for making good on this analogy. First, even though the resource of antibiotic effectiveness is scarce, it is not by nature excludable (any more than other ideas are), and so it is unclear what would give the inventor the right to compel others to desist from making use of this resource. It is particularly unclear why it would be fair for Smith to exclude those who separately discovered the same resource of antibiotic effectiveness from making use of it. Second, even if someone were tempted by such an analogy, it would seem to commit us to a problematically strong view of the rights of pharmaceutical inventors. If someone had a claim to exclusive use of the effectiveness of a particular antibiotic that was separate to any claim in intellectual property, then we would not expect that claim to lapse at the point where the patent lapsed. Absent any further argument – we would expect it to be perpetual – as natural rights to physical property would be.

In view of these difficulties, I am inclined to think that the fact that Smith has invented or discovered the drug is not relevant to the question of the ownership of the resource of the drug's effectiveness. Just as in the case where no one is responsible for our knowledge of how to make the drug, we should adopt a common ownership view of the limited resource of the effectiveness of the drug.

Conclusion and policy implications

Antibiotics present us with a worldwide collective action problem. They are cheap to manufacture (especially when out of patent). Their low price brings with it a standing temptation to use them profligately, thus reducing their effectiveness for future generations. Assuming that a human life in the future is worth the same as one now, then our current use of antibiotics is deeply problematic.

The rise of drug resistance can be slowed by the appropriate use of antibiotics, but it is unrealistic to suppose that it will be halted. Even if we are careful to use antibiotics only in cases where they are medically indicated, then we will still see drug resistance rising over time.[24] The key question is how best to steward the limited resource of antibiotic effectiveness. The main purpose of this chapter has been to argue that antibiotic effectiveness remains the common property of humanity, regardless of who holds the patent on the relevant molecules. Owning a patent on an antibiotic does not bring with it a moral entitlement to deplete the underlying resource of antibiotic effectiveness.

24   Michael R. Millar, 'Can Antibiotic Use Be Both Just and Sustainable . . . or Only More or Less So?', *Journal of Medical Ethics*, 2011, 37: 153–7.

This conclusion should influence how we think about how to fund antibiotic research, and the pricing structure for antibiotics. I have argued that the resource of antibiotic effectiveness should not be thought of as belonging to the patent holder. This provides some, but not complete, support for the claim that we should think of antibiotic research as a public endeavour to be publicly funded for public benefit.[25] It also follows that we should be sceptical about attempts – such as those put forward by Kades – to argue that massively extending patent terms for antibiotics would be a plausible approach to antibiotic stewardship.[26] On this view, by awarding a longer monopoly period on the drugs, the patent holder – through their attempt to maximize profits – will keep the price of the antibiotic high, thus discouraging their use for trivial conditions. Kades even floats the idea that governments should auction expired patent-rights of antibiotics to the highest bidder, to prevent prices falling too low.

While such price signals would undoubtedly reduce the use of antibiotics in some low value areas, by massively extending patents on antibiotics, we would be giving the patent-owner a license to make an enormous economic rent over a period of time which would be unconnected to the length of time necessary to make a profit on their research and development investment. Insofar as we use prices as a signalling mechanism here, there seems little reason to return the excess costs that we want to impose to discourage inappropriate antibiotic use to the patent holder as profits. The resources being exploited and depleted are common, and so (absent some compelling argument to the contrary) should the benefit be. Moreover, there is something decidedly inegalitarian about controlling the usage of a common resource by charging high prices for it; in so doing, we prevent the poor from accessing it. If our aim is to combat the rise of drug resistance, it is important that any strategy also addresses under utilization of antibiotics.

To the extent we use pricing mechanisms to discourage inappropriate antibiotic usage, the tax or levies paid should be agreed at a national and international level by the WHO, and should be imposed as a tax onto healthcare systems when antibiotics are prescribed. This money could then be used for a fund to (a) provide antibiotics in a way that will be maximally effective and least likely to fuel drug resistance in poorer countries, (b) fund further research into antibiotics. Given that generic drugs make the same contribution to antibiotic resistance as branded drugs do, such a tax, if adopted, should be applied not just to makers of branded antibiotics, but to all makers of antibiotics.

---

25 For discussion of the funding of antibiotic research, see Michael Selgelid, 'Ethics and Drug Resistance', 2007, *Bioethics* 21(4): 218–29; Jonny Anomaly, 'Combating Resistance: The Case for a Global Antibiotics Treaty', *Public Health Ethics*, 2010, 3(1), 13–22.

26 Eric Kades, 'Preserving a Precious Resource: Rationalising the Use of Antibiotics', *Northwestern Law Review*, 2005, 99(2): 611–75.

Funding

James Wilson's research was funded by the UCL/UCLH NIHR Biomedical Research Centre. Thanks especially to Jasper Littmann for extensive discussion of the various issues in this chapter, and also to the audience at the Manchester conference at which this chapter was originally presented.

10

Health in the International Governance of Biotechnology – The Real, the Ideal and the Achievable

Catherine Rhodes

Introduction

Biotechnology has great potential to fulfil health needs worldwide. Governance of biotechnology in the health area can help shape its ability to fulfil this potential. By examining the ability of current international governance efforts to promote benefits, identify, assess and manage risks, minimize negative impacts and promote capacity building for health (the ideal), this chapter highlights problems, flaws and weaknesses in the current situation (the real) and points to ways in which it can be improved, given the realities of the international system (the achievable).

Health and biotechnology

Health is one of the main areas in which modern biotechnology is applied and in which it has great potential. New knowledge and techniques enhance understanding of disease processes and susceptibilities and can be applied to assist diagnosis, treatment and prevention of disease and surveillance of infectious disease outbreaks. Biotechnologies also pose potential hazards to health. Concern has, for example, been expressed about: nutritional and other health implications of genetically modified foods; side-effects of gene therapies; and release of genetically modified pathogens into the environment. There is also potential for the new knowledge and technologies to be misused – the production of novel biological warfare agents would be a significant negative impact.

Health is an area of great inequalities within and between nations in regard to research and development (R&D), healthcare systems and infrastructure and availability of and access to treatments. Application of biotechnologies thus raises concerns about the likelihood that the concentration of research and development activities in developed countries[1] will mean that their interests will dominate and benefits will fail to reach those who need them most:

> Fears that the unequal distribution of the potential medical benefits which may be generated by genomics research could exacerbate current inequalities in the provision of healthcare among nations are well founded. Although some progress is being made towards improving the situation, many problems remain, particularly in the areas of infrastructure, biotechnological development, patenting DNA, benefit-sharing, and the commercial implications of large population data collections.[2]

This produces a substantial need for capacity-building and highlights a significant negative impact that could result from advances in biotechnology – that rather than meeting their potential they will simply serve to further entrench existing inequalities.

Taken in isolation of other rules and fully and appropriately implemented, the health rules would contribute significantly to promoting benefits by advancing scientific, health and regulatory capacities. Governance of biotechnology within the health area is adequate for dealing with many of the risks associated with accidental or deliberate disease outbreaks. However, scant attention is given to a major negative impact associated with advances in biotechnology – that of entrenching inequalities between developed and developing countries in regard to knowledge and expertise, scientific and technological capacities, research and development capabilities and supporting infrastructures. This is despite high-level recognition of the problems this situation will cause. There is room for improvement then – but how far this can go towards achieving what is desirable in governance of biotechnology is questionable.

An additional issue is that the health area has substantial interactions with other regulatory areas – both generally and within the governance of biotechnology. While some of these connections are supportive others impede the effective and intended operation of the health rules.

Use of terms

Biotechnology

Biotechnology can refer to any application of the biosciences, however, most references relate to use of modern tools and techniques, for example in genetic

---

1 The United Nations Educational, Scientific and Cultural Organisation (UNESCO) provides figures on global research and development expenditure (GERD), the most recent figures (2008) indicate that science and R&D activities remain overwhelmingly concentrated in developed countries – which account for less than 20 per cent of the global population, but 76 per cent of GERD and 75 per cent of scientific publications. UNESCO, *UNESCO Science Report 2010: The Current Status of Science in the World* (Paris: UNESCO, 2010), http://unesdoc.unesco.org/images/0018/001899/189958e.pdf.

2 WHO, *Genomics and World Health* (Geneva: WHO, 2002), 146.

engineering and genomics. Modern biotechnologies have applications across a range of sectors including healthcare, agriculture, environmental remediation and related industries.

International governance

Global governance refers to rules, mechanisms, procedures and other arrangements which, in the absence of an overarching supranational authority, govern relations between actors in the international system. International governance refers to a subset of these that occurs between states. Finkelstein describes global governance as: 'Any purposeful activity intended to 'control' or influence someone else that either occurs in the arena occupied by nations or, occurring at other levels, projects influence into that arena.'[3]

International regulation

These are rules agreed between states to govern their relations and actions. The term is used to cover both the 'hard' and 'soft' elements of international law – that is legally binding treaties and voluntary standards, guidelines and codes – because both influence state behaviour. It refers here only to those rules that are potentially universal – that is open to any state to subscribe to.

International organizations

Often associated with particular rules, these are organizations of states that serve to facilitate cooperation, provide forums for discussion and negotiation and oversee and support implementation of rules. Again, the term refers to those which are open to all states, having potentially universal membership.

The need to govern biotechnology

As in the area of health – where it has potential to bring great benefits, carries risks, will give rise to negative impacts (some of which may be severe and irreversible), and can impact inequalities – biotechnology has similar implications for a range of other areas, including conservation of biodiversity, food security and agricultural production. These outcomes are not inherent to the technology but result from how it is applied, under which conditions and in

---

3   Lawrence S. Finkelstein, 'What is Global Governance?', *Global Governance*, 1995, 1(3): 363–72.

which context. This can be shaped by governance measures such as regulation. The dimensions of benefits, risks, negative impacts and inequity produce four key roles for governance of biotechnology:

1 Promotion of benefits

2 Identification, assessment and management of risks

3 Minimization or avoidance of negative impacts

4 Promotion of capacity-building[4]

As an illustration – regulation of a genetically modified food could fulfil these roles by: promoting the benefit of enhanced nutritional value; requiring the identification and assessment of any risks to human health resulting from the changes made to the food and their management, for example by setting a recommended daily intake; banning types of changes that produce too high a risk to human health, for example insertion of genetic material from known allergenic sources; and promoting capacity-building in the conduct of effective risk assessment.[5] This fits quite closely the current international regulatory approach to such foods.[6]

In the context of this chapter governance that fulfils these four roles will be viewed as the 'ideal'.

International governance of biotechnology

The applications and impacts of biotechnology are not limited by national boundaries. Knowledge, technology material resources and people are highly mobile and the governance mechanisms of a single state can easily be

4 Catherine Rhodes, *International Governance of Biotechnology: Needs, Problems and Potential* (London: Bloomsbury Academic, 2010), 49.

5 Ibid., 50.

6 See, Codex Alimentarius Commission, *Codex Principles for the Risk Analysis of Foods Derived from Modern Biotechnology* (2003a). Accessed 31 October 2011 through http://codexalimentarius.org/standards/list-of-standards/en/; Codex Alimentarius Commission, *Guideline for the Conduct of Food Safety Assessment of Foods Derived from Recombinant-DNA Plants* (2003b). Accessed 31 October 2011 through www. codexalimentarius.org/standards/list-of-standards/en/. Codex Alimentarius Commission, Guideline *for the Conduct of Food Safety Assessment of Foods Produced Using Recombinant-DNA Microorganisms* (2003c). Accessed 31 October 2011 through www.codexalimentarius.org/standards/list-of-standards/en/. Codex Alimentarius Commission, *Guideline for the Conduct of Food Safety Assessment of Foods Derived from Recombinant-DNA Animals* (2008). Accessed 31 October 2011 through www. codexalimentarius.org/standards/list-of-standards/en/.

circumvented by locating activities elsewhere. Murphy makes this point in relation to xenotransplantation:[7]

> national regulations may be developed in some states to prevent animal viruses from spreading to humans. However, if comparable regulations do not exist in other states, leading to the risk of such viruses originating elsewhere and then travelling to the highly regulated states, then the national regulations will be undermined.

The impacts of biotechnology are shaped by the global context in which it is being applied. As previously mentioned, this is a context of great inequalities. It is also one of deep interdependence between states which provokes a need for cooperative action on issues of common concern.

International governance efforts have 'greater potential than those at other levels to contribute to a more even distribution of benefits and to establish measures to ameliorate negative impacts', they can 'play a role in introducing accountability and responsibility for transnational risks; help balance the varying needs and interests of different countries; and to promote transfer of technology, financial assistance, information and skills for capacity-building'.[8]

In any area in which there is a high degree of international interdependence – where separate actions by individual states will be insufficient to address issues of common concern – there is a need for rules and other governance mechanisms in order to coordinate state action. In coordinating state action, international regulation and other forms of governance fulfil several core functions such as: establishing and shaping expectations; defining rights and obligations; simplifying and facilitating transactions; reducing uncertainty; authorizing or prohibiting certain actions; guiding policy-making; reducing the costs of individual actions; and channelling conflict and providing mechanisms for its resolution.[9]

Biotechnology has significant applications and impacts in several areas in which international interdependence is high, these include:

- Arms control

Biotechnology has the potential for misuse in production of novel warfare agents and can also be applied to biodefence research. In the arms control area there are rules which prohibit non-peaceful uses of biology and that promote scientific and medical research for peaceful purposes.

---

7   Sean D. Murphy, 'Biotechnology and International Law', *Harvard International Law Journal*, 2001, 42(1): 47–139, 60.
8   Rhodes, *International Governance of Biotechnology*, 51.
9   Ibid., 57–8.

- Development

Biotechnology – in the way it is applied and the uses to which it is put – has significant implications for several aspects of development. Rather than there being separate regulations relevant to the development implications of biotechnology, there are development-related clauses within about half of the other regulations. These include, for example, clauses on provision of scientific and technical advice, financial resources and training, and various forms of capacity-building, for example in infrastructure and administration.

- Drugs control

This includes control of the illicit international drugs trade and prohibitions on the use of doping in sport. In both cases biotechnology could be applied to produce novel drugs that may be misused; it can also assist in producing sufficient supplies of (e.g. pain relieving) drugs for medical and scientific purposes – something that is promoted by rules in this area.

- Environmental protection

Biotechnologies could have both protective and damaging effects on the environment, with a particular area of international concern being their impacts on biodiversity. This concern is most strongly raised in relation to planting of genetically engineered crops which may reinforce monocultural agricultural practices, push out wild relatives and result in gene transfer to other crops and weeds.[10]

- Health

As mentioned earlier, biotechnology has many applications and impacts of relevance to health. Relevant international governance efforts include those on disease control (for plant, animal and human health), food safety, and laboratory biosafety and biosecurity.

- Social impacts of human genetics

There are four international declarations which deal with the human rights and other social implications of human genetics research and its applications.

- Trade

---

10   See, for example, John Madeley, *Yours for Food: Plant Genetic Resources and Food Security* (London: Christian Aid, 1996); David Zilberman, Holly Ameden and Matin Qaim, 'The Impact of Agricultural Biotechnology on Yields, Risks and Biodiversity in Low Income Countries', *Journal of Development Studies Special Issue – Transgenics and the Poor: Biotechnology in Development Studies*, 2007, 43(1): 63–78.

The products of biotechnology and their constituent parts are traded internationally. Relevant rules include those on free trade, intellectual property rights and access to genetic resources.

There are currently 37 regulations relevant to biotechnology within these areas and 15 international organizations directly associated with these rules. These are listed in Table 10.1 at the end of this chapter. Most of the rules were not developed with the specific aim of addressing the applications and impacts of biotechnology, but do so as part of a wider purpose. They developed largely in separation from one another, at different times (ranging from 1925–2010) and for different purposes. It is not surprising, therefore, to find that these regulations lack coherence – a point which has implications for the effective operation of the health rules.

Health in the International Governance of Biotechnology (The 'Real')

There are three strands of health regulations that have particular relevance to the governance of biotechnology – those on disease control, on laboratory biosafety and biosecurity, and on food safety.

Disease control rules have been created in the domains of human, animal and plant health. These rules aim to limit the spread of disease through international travel and trade links. Biotechnology is particularly relevant to these rules because it can assist in the detection, identification, surveillance, tracking and response to disease outbreaks. The key rules and their associated organizations are:

- The International Health Regulations – World Health Organisation (WHO).

- The Terrestrial Animal Health Code, Aquatic Animal Health Code, Manual of Diagnostic Tests and Vaccines for Terrestrial Animals and Manual of Diagnostic Tests for Aquatic Animals – World Animal Health Organisation (OIE).

- The International Plant Protection Convention – Food and Agriculture Organisation (FAO).

These rules will also be relevant to the control of any disease outbreaks caused by accidental or deliberate release of pathogens that have been genetically modified or otherwise used within biotechnological processes. This is not a remote possibility – the 2007 Foot-and-Mouth disease outbreak in the United

Table 10.1 International regulations relevant to biotechnology and their associated international organizations

Regulation	Associated organization
Arms Control	
1925 Geneva Protocol for the Prohibition of the Use in War of Asphyxiating, Poisonous or Other Gases and of Bacteriological Methods of Warfare	
Biological Weapons Convention	
Chemical Weapons Convention	Organisation for the Prohibition of Chemical Weapons
Convention on the Prohibition of Military or Any Other Hostile Use of Environmental Modification Techniques	
Drugs Control	
Single Convention on Narcotic Drugs	United Nations (UN) Office on Drugs and Crime; International Narcotics Control Board; Commission on Narcotic Drugs
Convention on Psychotropic Substances	UN Office on Drugs and Crime; International Narcotics Control Board; Commission on Narcotic Drugs
Convention against the Illicit Traffic in Narcotic Drugs and Psychotropic Substances	UN Office on Drugs and Crime; International Narcotics Control Board; Commission on Narcotic Drugs
World Anti-Doping Code	World Anti-Doping Association
International Convention against Doping in Sport	UN Educational, Scientific and Cultural Organisation
Environmental Protection	
Convention on Biodiversity	Convention on Biodiversity Secretariat
Cartagena Protocol on Biosafety	Convention on Biodiversity Secretariat
Health	
International Health Regulations	World Health Organisation
Terrestrial Animal Health Code	World Animal Health Organisation
Aquatic Animal Health Code	World Animal Health Organisation
International Plant Protection Convention	Food and Agriculture Organisation
Manual of Diagnostic Tests and Vaccines for Terrestrial Animals	World Animal Health Organisation

Manual of Diagnostic Tests for Aquatic Animals	World Animal Health Organisation
Laboratory Biosafety Manual	World Health Organisation
Laboratory Biosecurity Guidance	World Health Organisation
Guidance on Regulations for the Safe Transport of Infectious Substances	World Health Organisation
Codex Principles for Risk Analysis of Foods Derived from Modern Biotechnology	Codex Alimentarius Commission
Codex Guideline for Safety Assessment of Foods Derived from Recombinant-DNA Plants	Codex Alimentarius Commission
Codex Guideline for Safety Assessment of Foods Produced Using Recombinant-DNA Microorganisms	Codex Alimentarius Commission
Codex Guideline for Safety Assessment of Foods Derived from Recombinant-DNA Animals	Codex Alimentarius Commission

Social Impacts of Human Genetics

Universal Declaration on the Human Genome and Human Rights	UN Educational, Scientific and Cultural Organisation
International Declaration on Human Genetic Data	UN Educational, Scientific and Cultural Organisation
Universal Declaration on Bioethics and Human Rights	UN Educational, Scientific and Cultural Organisation
United Nations Declaration on Human Cloning	UN General Assembly

Trade

Agreement on the Application of Sanitary and Phytosanitary Measures	World Trade Organisation
Agreement on Technical Barriers to Trade	World Trade Organisation
Agreement on Trade Related Aspects of Intellectual Property Rights	World Trade Organisation
Patent Law Treaty	World Intellectual Property Organisation
Patent Cooperation Treaty	World Intellectual Property Organisation
Budapest Treaty on the Deposit of Microorganisms for the Purpose of Patent Procedure	World Intellectual Property Organisation
Convention on the Protection of New Varieties of Plants	Union for the Protection of New Varieties of Plants
International Treaty on Plant Genetic Resources	Food and Agriculture Organisation
Nagoya Protocol on Access to Genetic Resources and the Fair and Equitable Sharing of Benefits Arising Out of their Utilisation	Convention on Biodiversity Secretariat

Kingdom was almost certainly caused by the release of a virus strain used in the production of vaccines in a laboratory facility.[11]

These long-standing rules[12] are based on the need to protect life and health from infectious disease with minimal interference in travel and trade.

> The purpose and scope of these Regulations are to prevent, protect against, control and provide a public health response to the international spread of disease in ways that are commensurate with and restricted to public health risks, and which avoid unnecessary interference with trade.[13]

> Safety of international trade in animals and animal products depends on a combination of factors which should be taken into account to ensure unimpeded trade, without incurring unacceptable risks to human and animal health.[14]

They prescribe mechanisms for surveillance, communication, reporting and import and travel controls. The importance of capacity-building is acknowledged in the IHR, particularly in relation to surveillance, reporting, risk analysis and regulation.[15] The International Plant Protection Convention (IPPC) asks its contracting parties to provide technical assistance to developing countries to assist their implementation of the Convention.[16]

Laboratory biosafety and biosecurity rules aim to protect the health and safety of workers involved in the transport, handling and use of infectious substances and to protect human and animal health and the environment from disease outbreaks that might originate from laboratory facilities. The following extract from the WHO Laboratory Biosafety Manual[17] explains the distinction between biosafety and biosecurity in this context:

> 'Laboratory biosafety' is the term used to describe the containment principles, technologies and practices that are implemented to prevent unintentional exposure to pathogens and toxins, or their accidental release. 'Laboratory biosecurity' refers

11 Brian G. Spratt, *Independent (Spratt) Review of the Safety of UK Facilities Handling Foot-and-Mouth Disease Virus* (Defra: UK, 2007), http://archive.defra.gov.uk/foodfarm/farmanimal/diseases/atoz/fmd/documents/spratt_final.pdf.
12 The first version of the International Health Regulations was adopted in 1951, the first version of the Terrestrial Animal Health Code in 1968 and the first version of the International Plant Protection Convention in 1952.
13 World Health Organisation, *International Health Regulations (2005)* (Geneva: WHO, 2008), Article 2, http://whqlibdoc.who.int/publications/2008/9789241580410_Eng.pdf.
14 Office International des Epizooties, *Terrestrial Animal Health Code* (20th edn) (Paris: OIE, May 2011), Article 5.1.1., www.oie.int/international-standard-setting/terrestrial-code/access-online/.
15 World Health Organisation, *International Health Regulations (2005)*, para 5.
16 Food and Agriculture Organisation, *International Plant Protection Convention* (Rome: FAO, 1997), Article XX, www.ippc.int/file_uploaded//publications/13742.New_Revised_Text_of_the_International_Plant_Protectio.pdf.
17 World Health Organisation, *Laboratory Biosafety Manual* (Geneva: WHO, 2004), 47, www.who.int/csr/resources/publications/biosafety/Biosafety7.pdf.

to institutional and personal security measures designed to prevent the loss, theft, misuse, diversion or intentional release of pathogens and toxins.

The Laboratory Biosecurity Guidance broadens this to cover 'the safekeeping of all valuable biological materials (VBM), including not only pathogens and toxins, but also scientifically, historically and economically important biological materials'.[18] This was done to highlight the fact that there are many reasons to secure these materials, not just prevention of misuse.

The World Health Organisation has a biosafety programme which includes three key publications: the Laboratory Biosafety Manual; Biorisk Management: Laboratory Biosecurity Guidance; and Guidance on Regulations for the Safe Transport of Infectious Substances. The Laboratory Biosecurity Guidance and Laboratory Biosafety Manual both have specific guidance relating to genetically modified organisms (Chapter 16 of the Manual and p. 17 of the Guidance) as well as applying more generally to all laboratory work.

Laboratory biosafety is also covered in a section of the Terrestrial Animal Health Code (Chapter 5.8) and is addressed in more detail in Chapter 1.1.2 – Biosafety and Biosecurity in the Veterinary Microbiology Laboratory and Animal Facilities – of the Manual of Diagnostic Tests and Vaccines for Terrestrial Animals.

The WHO and OIE guidance take a very similar approach, advising on risk analysis and assignment of pathogens to one of four risk groups. Particular containment and handling requirements apply to four biosafety levels to which different pathogens are assigned (these levels 'relate' but don't 'equate' to the risk groups[19] because local conditions, e.g. levels of immunity in the population and availability of treatments also have to be taken into account).

In 1963 the WHO and FAO formed a joint body to take forward their work developing standards and guidelines for safety in the international food trade – known as the Codex Alimentarius Commission (CAC). The CAC has since produced more 300 standards and set nearly 3000 maximum residue limits for pesticides and around 440 maximum residue limits for veterinary drugs in food (see[20] and www.codexalimentarius.org).

In 2003, the Commission adopted a set of Principles for Risk Analysis of Foods Derived from Modern Biotechnology. These were viewed as a necessary supplement to its standard risk analysis principles because these did not deal with assessment of whole foods. At the same time, CAC adopted the two sets of guidelines on assessment of foods derived from recombinant-DNA plants

18 World Health Organisation, *Biorisk Management: Laboratory Biosecurity Guidance* (Geneva: WHO, 2006), 5, www.who.int/csr/resources/publications/biosafety/WHO_CDS_EPR_2006_6.pdf.

19 World Health Organisation, *Laboratory Biosafety Manual*, 1.

20 FAO/WHO, *Understanding the Codex Alimentarius*, (Rome: FAO, 2006), ftp://ftp.fao.org/codex/Publications/understanding/Understanding_EN.pdf.

and produced using recombinant-DNA microorganisms. In 2008, guidelines for assessment of foods derived from recombinant-DNA animals were added.

The Principles present a reasoned modification of and supplement to the CAC's standard risk analysis approach and aim to 'provide a framework for undertaking risk analysis on the safety and nutritional aspects of foods derived from modern biotechnology'.[21] They cover the steps of risk assessment (relative to a 'conventional counterpart'), risk management and risk communication. The three guidelines give more specific recommendations on the structure and content of food safety assessments. The assessments are intended to identify any new or altered hazards. If such hazards are determined to be a risk to human health, this should then be dealt with under the risk management considerations outlined in the Principles.[22] The Principles outline a need for capacity-building in capabilities to assess and manage risks:

> Efforts should be made to improve the capability of regulatory authorities, particularly those of developing countries, to assess, manage and communicate risks, including enforcement, associated with foods derived from modern biotechnology or to interpret assessments undertaken by other authorities or recognised expert bodies, including access to analytical technology.[23]

The above health rules, taken in isolation and implemented as intended, could serve the four roles quite well, promoting benefits while using science-based risk assessment and management processes, and supporting effective and rapid response to any disease outbreaks. They also have some capacity-building clauses, which, if fully implemented, could make a significant contribution.

The health rules do not operate in isolation of other rules. There are significant interactions with other rules in the governance of biotechnology – some of these are complementary and supportive but some (and in fact often the same) rules can also conflict and/or impede the effective operation of the health rules. Not all of these interactions are outlined here, instead examples from the areas of trade and arms control are provided.

Trade

There are three types of trade rule relevant to the governance of biotechnology – those on reduction of barriers to trade, on protection of intellectual property rights and on access to and benefit-sharing from the use of genetic resources – all three have implications for the operation of the health rules.

---

21 Codex Alimentarius Commission, *Codex Principles for the Risk Analysis of Foods Derived from Modern Biotechnology*, point 7.

22 See, Codex Alimentarius Commission, *Guideline for the Conduct of Food Safety Assessment of Foods Derived from Recombinant-DNA Plants*, point 5.

23 Codex Alimentarius Commission, *Codex Principles for the Risk Analysis of Foods Derived from Modern Biotechnology*, point 27.

The World Trade Organisation's Agreement on the Application of Sanitary and Phytosanitary Measures (SPS Agreement) aims to limit trade measures put in place for health reasons to those that are scientifically justified. Health-based trade restrictions must also not be applied in a discriminatory manner. The Agreement promotes harmonization of international standards and use of those standards as the basis for health-related trade rules.

> Members shall ensure that any sanitary or phytosanitary measure is applied only to the extent necessary to protect human, animal or plant life or health, is based on scientific principles and is not maintained without sufficient scientific evidence.[24]

> Sanitary or phytosanitary measures which conform to international standards, guidelines or recommendations shall be deemed necessary to protect human, animal or plant life or health, and presumed to be consistent with the relevant provisions of this Agreement.[25]

It refers specifically to standards associated with the World Animal Health Organisation, Codex Alimentarius Commission and International Plant Protection Convention as acceptable sources of international standards. The SPS Agreement also promotes capacity building in relation to the application of health measures.[26]

Rules on protection of intellectual property rights influence the operation of health rules in various ways. For example, they have implications for access to medicines and for benefit-sharing from research on viral genetic resources. Relevant rules include: the WTO's Agreement on Trade Related Aspects of Intellectual Property Rights (TRIPS Agreement), the Patent Cooperation Treaty and Patent Law Treaty of the World Intellectual Property Organisation (WIPO) and the Convention for the Protection of New Varieties of Plants. It is the TRIPS Agreement that has had the most notable impacts through its provisions requiring harmonized minimum standards for patenting, which must extend to pharmaceutical products. This is because it requires that patents 'be available for any inventions, whether products or processes, in all fields of technology'.[27]

This has undermined generic production in developing countries and made many medicines unaffordable to their populations. It should be noted that the Agreement itself contains flexibilities intended to avoid such problems, for example allowing compulsory licensing subject to certain conditions in Article 31.

There has also been subsequent work by WTO member states to promote use of these flexibilities and interpretation of the Agreement in ways supportive of the

24 World Trade Organisation, *Agreement on the Application of Sanitary and Phytosanitary Measures* (Geneva: WTO, 1995a), Article 2, www.wto.org/english/tratop_E/sps_E/spsagr_E. htm.
25 Ibid., Article 3.2.
26 Ibid., Article 9.1.
27 World Trade Organisation, *Agreement on Trade Related Aspects of Intellectual Property Rights* (Geneva: WTO, 1995b), Article 27.1, www.wto.org/english/docs_E/legal_E/27-trips. pdf.

right to health, including the 2001 Doha Declaration on the TRIPS Agreement and Public Health, which emphasized that the Agreement should be applied in ways supportive of public health and access to medicines and that states are free to 'determine the grounds' under which they grant compulsory licenses.[28] Paragraph 6 of the Declaration instructed the Council for TRIPS (a body within WTO) to find a solution to the problem that 'members with insufficient or no manufacturing capacities in the pharmaceutical sector could face difficulties in making effective use of compulsory licensing'.[29] This led to a 2003 Decision on the Implementation of Paragraph 6 of the Doha Declaration on the TRIPS Agreement and Public Health which created the 'paragraph six mechanism', allowing import of generic medicines manufactured under compulsory licensing, where the importing country lacks domestic manufacturing capability.[30] The provisions of this decision were incorporated in an amendment to the TRIPS Agreement adopted by the WTO General Council in December 2005.[31] This will take effect once two-thirds of WTO's members have accepted it.

There are also two international rules on access to genetic resources that have relevance to health. Both focus on plant genetic resources, some of which have potential uses in medicine, but the main link to health is their connection to food security. International exchange of plant genetic resources assists in maintaining their diversity, which in turn provides greater resilience to disease and changing environmental conditions. There are very strong connections between health and nutrition. Research involving plant genetic resources that, for example, increases yields of key food crops, or enhances their micronutrient value, could help to reduce incidence of calorie and micronutrient deficient malnutrition. The Food and Agriculture Organisation's most recent estimates are that over 925 million people worldwide are undernourished;[32] more than twice this number suffer from micronutrient deficiencies.[33]

28 World Trade Organisation, *Declaration on the TRIPS Agreement and Public Health* (Geneva: WTO, November 2001a), para 4, www.wto.org/english/thewto_E/minist_E/min01_E/mindecl_trips_E.htm.

29 Ibid., para 6.

30 World Trade Organisation, *Decision on Implementation of Paragraph 6 of the Doha Declaration on the TRIPS Agreement and Public Health* (Geneva: WTO, 2003), www.wto.org/english/tratop_E/trips_E/implem_para6_E.htm.

31 World Trade Organisation, *Amendment of the TRIPS Agreement* (Geneva: WTO, 2005), www.wto.org/english/tratop_E/trips_E/wtl641_E.htm.

32 Food and Agriculture Organisation, Press Release 'World Hunger Report 2011: High, Volatile Prices Set to Continue' (Rome: FAO, 10 October 2011), www.fao.org/news/story/en/item/92495/icode/.

33 World Health Organisation, *Worldwide Prevalence of Anaemia Report 1993–2005* (Geneva: WHO, 2008), www.who.int/vmnis/anaemia/prevalence/en/; World Health Organisation, *Micronutrient Deficiencies: Vitamin A Deficiency* (Geneva: WHO, no date a), www.who.int/nutrition/topics/vad/en/index.html; Food and Agriculture Organisation, *The Scourge of 'Hidden Hunger': Global Dimensions of Micronutrient Deficiencies* (Rome: FAO, 2003), ftp://ftp.fao.org/docrep/fao/005/y8346my8346m01.pdf.

The International Treaty on Plant Genetic Resources was adopted by the FAO in 2001, to promote 'the conservation and sustainable use of plant genetic resources for food and agriculture and the fair and equitable sharing of the benefits arising out of their use'.[34] It covers a core set of plant genetic resources that are considered to be important to food security and created a 'multilateral system of access and benefit-sharing' through which they can be exchanged.

The Nagoya Protocol on Access to Genetic Resources and the Fair and Equitable Sharing of the Benefits Arising out of their Utilisation was adopted by the states parties to the Convention on Biodiversity in 2010.[35] It sets out a system for prior informed consent of countries of origin (and also local and indigenous groups) to use of their genetic resources. Its coverage is limited to those genetic resources that fit within Article 15 of the Convention on Biodiversity – those being accessed for 'environmentally sound purposes'.

There is a strong connection between the rules on intellectual property rights and on access and benefit-sharing. Article 27.3b of the TRIPS Agreement (a clause which has been controversial since its drafting) states that:

Members may also exclude from patentability: . . .

(b) plants and animals other than microorganisms, and essentially biological processes for the production of plants and animals other than non-biological and microbiological processes.[36]

Whether and how this applies to genetic resources (and of which types) is somewhat ambiguous, and there are large controversies over the patenting of genetic material, particularly that which is related to disease.

The relationship between intellectual property rights and access and benefit-sharing has been raised within the World Health Organisation in relation to viral genetic resources. The WHO first became concerned about this issue in 2003 during the SARS (severe acute respiratory syndrome) outbreak and faced significant problems during an avian influenza outbreak in 2007 when Indonesia stopped sharing viral samples with its collaborating research centres due to concerns that private companies were patenting products based on the research conducted on these resources and would price them at a level

---

34   Food and Agriculture Organisation, *International Treaty on Plant Genetic Resources for Food and Agriculture* (Rome: FAO, 2001), Article 1, ftp://ftp.fao.org/docrep/fao/011/i0510e/i0510e.pdf.

35   Convention on Biodiversity Secretariat, *Nagoya Protocol on Access to Genetic Resources and the Fair and Equitable Sharing of the Benefits Arising Out of their Utilisation* (Montreal: CBD Secretariat, 2010), www.cbd.int/abs/doc/protocol/nagoya-protocol-en.pdf.

36   World Trade Organisation, *Agreement on Trade Related Aspects of Intellectual Property Rights*, Article 27.3b.

unaffordable to its population.[37] WHO stated that 'there has been a breakdown in trust in this essential system of the international collaboration and collective action' relating to 'sharing of viruses and specimens, the development and production of preventive and curative measures such as vaccines and antivirals' and that 'the current system does not deliver the desired level of fairness, transparency and equity'.[38] Its member states have developed various mechanisms and guidance on sharing viruses including adoption of a Pandemic Influenza Preparedness Framework: Sharing of Influenza Viruses and Access to Vaccines and Other Benefits in May 2011 (WHA64.5).[39] However, the issue of intellectual property rights has been largely excluded from these outputs and it remains to be seen whether the problem will re-occur in future.

The SPS Agreement seems largely supportive of the health rules; TRIPS – in the way it is currently implemented – poses various problems for their effective operation; and rules on access- and benefit-sharing may generally be supportive of health, but also have significant omissions in relation to human, viral and other disease-related genetic resources.

Arms control

Many of the health rules are supportive of the Biological Weapons Convention. Effective implementation of laboratory biosafety and biosecurity measures will close one route to accessing dangerous pathogens. The Laboratory Biosecurity Guidance also recommends that laboratories' risk management culture involve consideration of bioethics; ethics education has been recommended as part of national implementation measures for the Biological Weapons Convention. The surveillance and monitoring capacities promoted in the disease control rules will also be useful in the event of any deliberate disease outbreaks. The International Health Regulations, for example, cover any disease 'irrespective of origin or source, that presents or could present significant harm to humans' (Article 1). The connection is recognized by the World Health Organisation – for example in its work on preparedness for deliberate epidemics[40] and within

37   World Health Organisation, *Patent Applications for SARS Virus and Genes* (Geneva: WHO, 2003), www.who.int/ehtics/topics/sars_patents/en/print.html; World Health Organisation, Press Release 'Indonesia to resume sharing H5N1 avian influenza virus samples following a WHO meeting in Jakarta' (Geneva: WHO, 27 March 2007), www.who.int/mediacentre/news/releases/2007/pr09/en/index.html.

38   World Health Organisation, *Interim Statement of the Intergovernmental Meeting on Pandemic Influenza Preparedness: Sharing of Influenza Viruses and Access to Vaccines and Other Benefits* (Geneva: WHO, 23 November 2011), www.who.int/gb/pip/pdf_files/IGM_PIP_Int_Statement_En.pdf.

39   World Health Assembly, *WHA65.4. Pandemic Influenza Preparedness Framework: Sharing of Influenza Viruses and Access to Vaccines and Other Benefits* (Geneva: WHO, May 2011), http://apps.who.int/gb/ebwha/pdf_files/WHA64/A64_8-en.pdf.

40   World Health Organisation, *Preparedness for Deliberate Epidemics* (Geneva: WHO, no date b), www.who.int/csr/resources/publications/preparedness/en/.

the Laboratory Biosecurity Guidance – the Food and Agriculture Organisation and the World Animal Health Organisation (OIE) and by states parties to the Biological Weapons Convention. The three organizations have given presentations and participated as observers in recent meetings of states parties to the Biological Weapons Convention.[41]

The problem of deliberate misuse is addressed within some of the health rules which support provisions of the Biological Weapons Convention, both at the stage of prevention (the rules on laboratory biosafety and biosecurity) and in the event of any use (through provisions for tracking and containing disease outbreaks in the disease control rules). There are concerns about the robustness of the current biological weapons control regime, but these are not due to weaknesses in the health rules.

Assessment against the ideal (four roles)

In relation to the 'ideal' of fulfilling the four roles, these examples suggest that:

The health rules do not specifically promote benefits of biotechnology but they have the potential to facilitate benefits by providing for products of biotechnology to be researched, handled, traded and consumed safely. All of the health rules incorporate processes for risk assessment and management approaches, as does the Sanitary and Phytosanitary Agreement. There is, however, a lack of reflection on the risks that arise due to the inequitable context in which biotechnology is being applied.

The negative impact of entrenched inequalities is not adequately addressed. A need for capacity-building is recognized in some of the rules and by their associated organizations but action remains small-scale and provisions are not fully implemented by states. The adequacy of the provisions on capacity-building is questionable. There is high demand for capacity-building activities and finance, but effective support and enforcement mechanisms are lacking. Other

41   See, for example, World Health Organisation, *WHO's response in the case of an alleged use of a biological agent* (Geneva: BWC Implementation Support Unit, 2010), www.unog. ch/80256EDD006B8954/(httpAssets)/CA61BD8F4B4AA1B7C125778B0046A0DF/$file/1_ WHO.pdf; Office International des Epizooties, *Statement for the Biological and Toxin Weapons Convention Meeting of States Parties* (Geneva: BWC Implementation Support Unit, 2010), www.unog.ch/80256EDD006B8954/(httpAssets)/89A67AFC0499190BC12577F2003 9690B/$file/BWC_MSP_2010-OIE-101206.pdf; Food and Agriculture Organisation, *Current FAO Mechanisms for Dealing with the Deliberate Release of Detrimental Biological Agents – Biological Weapons Convention (BWC) Meeting of States* (Geneva: BWC Implementation Support Unit, 2007), www.unog.ch/80256EDD006B8954/(httpAssets)/56FF617B870F4D12 C12573AF0051BF53/$file/BWC_MSP_2007_Statement-FAO-071210AM.pdf.

negative health impacts, for example the introduction and spread of infectious diseases are addressed adequately by the rules.

The achievable – signs of progress

There are some initiatives and activities that indicate improvements in some of the deficient areas are likely. Examples include:

- Collaboration among international organizations

For example, the World Intellectual Property Organisation has, on request, been sharing information with the WHO on patent landscapes for avian influenza which has supported its work on access and benefit-sharing for viral genetic resources.[42]

- Development agendas

The WTO's member states adopted a development agenda in the Doha Ministerial Declaration of 2001 providing a work programme for the organization in which developing countries' needs and interests are to be central.[43] The World Intellectual Property Organisation's member states adopted a development agenda in 2007 to promote consideration of development issues across the organization's activities and established a Committee on Development and Intellectual Property.

- Capacity-building funds/programmes

These include the Standards and Trade Development Facility which provides project grant funding to support capacity-building for the implementation of sanitary and phytosanitary standards. It is a partnership of the FAO, OIE, World Bank, WHO and WTO. Three of the organizations have also established journal access initiatives providing free online access to many journals for developing countries including: Hinari (Access to Research in Health Programme) linked to

---

42 World Intellectual Property Organisation, *Patent Issues Related to Influenza Viruses and their Genes* (Geneva: WIPO, 19 October 2007), www.who.int/csr/disease/avian_influenza/WIPO_IP_%20paper19_10_2007.pdf; World Intellectual Property Organisation, *Patent Landscape for the H5 Virus: Interim Report* (Geneva: WIPO, November 2007), www.who.int/csr/disease/influenza/avian_flu_landscape.pdf.

43 World Trade Organisation. *Doha Ministerial Declaration* WT/MIN(01)/DEC/1 (Geneva: WTO, November 2001b), www.wto.org/english/thewto_E/minist_E/min01_E/mindecl_E.htm.

the WHO;[44] Agora (Access to Global Online Research in Agriculture) linked to FAO;[45] and aRDI (Access to Research for Development and Innovation) linked to WIPO.[46] WIPO has also recently launched 'Re:Search' in partnership with WHO, major pharmaceutical companies, the US National Institutes of Health and non-profit research organizations. This initiative has been set up to 'share valuable intellectual property (IP) and expertise with the global health research community to promote development of new drugs, vaccines, and diagnostics to treat neglected tropical diseases, malaria and tuberculosis'.[47]

The achievable – obstacles remaining

Various obstacles to progress remain. The biggest problems are in the area of capacity-building for science and technology, health research and development, effective regulation, technology and risk assessment and related infrastructure. States still generally perceive their national interest in narrow terms largely related to economic competitiveness and short-term gain rather than cooperative action in pursuit of long-term welfare improvements. As Dresner explains:

> In a world of competing states, each has an incentive to go for the maximum growth and become dominant. The societies that fail to grow . . . end up losing their influence to those who do grow. So each state has an incentive to follow the path of modernity in the short to medium term, even if it is likely to lead to global disaster in the long term.[48]

Combined with power relations this means that the short-term interests of developed states continue to dominate international relations and 'there are still considerable doubts about the will of governments of developed countries to help solve problems which do not appear directly germane to their own populations'.[49] With the result that, for example: cooperative activities between international organizations are curtailed; issues are dropped from negotiating agendas even when their value is fully recognized; and flexibilities provided

44 World Health Organisation, Health Internetwork Access to Research Initiative, www.who. int/hinari/en.
45 Food and Agriculture Organisation, Access to Global Online Research in Agriculture, www. aginternetwork.org/en.
46 World Intellectual Property Organisation, Access to Research for Development and Innovation, www.wipo.int/ardi/.
47 World Intellectual Property Organisation, Press Release PR/2011/699. 'Leading Pharmaceutical Companies and Research Institutions Offer IP and Expertise for use in Treating Neglected Tropical Diseases as Part of WIPO Re:Search' (Geneva: WIPO, October 2011), www.wipo.int/pressroom/en/article_0026.html.
48 Simon Dresner, *The Principles of Sustainability* (London: Earthscan, 2002), 170.
49 World Health Organisation, Genomics and World Health, 105.

in trade agreements are circumvented by the application of bilateral pressures (the paragraph 6 mechanism has, for example, only been used once since its creation). Funding commitments are also under-fulfilled. For example, although the Standards and Trade Development Facility has a relatively small annual budget of $5 million, donations between 2007 and 2010 contributed only an average of 86 per cent of this target.[50]

Power relations are unlikely to change significantly in the near future, but can be balanced to an extent by developing countries working together – indeed without such efforts the development agendas of the WTO and WIPO are unlikely to have been created.

Lessons

The design and implementation of health rules needs to take into account the impacts of rules in other areas that might support or hinder their operation. Likewise, the design and implementation of rules in other areas of biotechnology governance ought to take into account the impact they might have on the operation of health rules. The global context needs to be adequately taken into account with far more effort being made to ensure that inequalities are not entrenched by scientific advances being concentrated in developed countries and that biotechnologies can fulfil their beneficial potential for those with greatest need.

50 Standards and Trade Development Facility, *Donor Support* (no date), www.standardsfacility. org/en/AUDonorSupport.htm.

11

Awareness of and Education about the Biological and Toxin Weapons Convention (BTWC): Why this is Needed by All Life Scientists and How it Might be Achieved

Malcolm Dando

Introduction

The threat to global health comes from natural disease, accidental disease and the deliberate causation of disease by use of biological and chemical agents.[1] We strive to deal with natural disease by improving measures of public health and we use biosafety measures to reduce the chance of accidental disease. Deliberately caused disease, in the form of bioterrorism and State offensive biological weapons programmes[2] is less well known outside of security circles, but we attempt to minimize such malign misuse of the modern life sciences through an integrated web of preventive policies[3] to support the international prohibition norm embodied in the Biological and Toxin Weapons Convention (BTWC) and the Chemical Weapons Convention (CWC). This is important because it is clear, particularly from the offensive biological weapons programmes of major states in the last century, that in the right conditions very-large-scale casualties and deaths could be caused to humans, animals and plants. Furthermore, ongoing advances in the life and associated sciences could make it easier for states, sub-state terrorist groups or even deranged individuals to carry out such attacks. This chapter considers the problem of deliberate disease, but it should be understood that there is an overlap in the impact of policies concerned with dealing with disease. Thus good laboratory biosecurity will also assist in

---

1   Geoffrey L. Smith and Neil Davison, 'Assessing the Spectrum of Biological Risks', *Bulletin of the Atomic Scientists*, 2010, January/February: 1–11.
2   Mark Wheelis, Lajos Rosza and Malcolm R. Dando, *Deadly Cultures: Biological Weapons Since 1945* (Cambridge, MA: Harvard University Press, 2006).
3   Board of Science and Education, *Biotechnology, Weapons and Humanity II* (London: British Medical Association, 2004).

preventing accidental disease, and good public health measures will assist in dealing with any disease outbreak – natural, accidental or deliberate.

The biological and toxin weapons convention

Article I of the BTWC states that:

> Each State Party to this Convention undertakes never in any circumstances to develop, produce, stockpile or otherwise acquire or retain:
>
> 1. Microbial or other biological agents, or toxins whatever their origin or method of production, of types and in quantities that have no justification for prophylactic, protective or other peaceful purposes . . .

So any peaceful purpose is allowed but there is a sweeping prohibition of other uses embodied in the Convention. Moreover, in order to ensure that the prohibition is effective, Article IV states:

> Each State Party to this Convention shall, in accordance with its constitutional processes, take any necessary measure to *prohibit and prevent* the development, production, stockpiling, acquisition or retention of the agents, toxins . . . specified in Article I of the Convention . . . (emphasis added)

So measures such as national laws are required to prohibit what is banned by Article I, but there is an additional need to take measures to prevent malign misuse of the agents and toxins.

The Convention is assessed at a special Review Conference every five years and a consensus Final Declaration shows the agreed understandings of States Parties in regard to each Article. Thus they agreed at the Second Review Conference in 1986 under Article IV that:

> The Conference notes the importance of. . . .
>
> – inclusion in textbooks and in medical, scientific and military educational programmes of information dealing with the prohibition of microbial or other biological agents or toxins and the provisions of the Geneva Protocol [of 1925, which bans use of such agents] . . .[4]

States Parties also agreed that such measures would strengthen the Convention, and they have made similar statements at subsequent Review Conferences. Thus it is clear that in-depth implementation of the Convention requires a

---

4   United Nations, *Final Declaration,* Second Review Conference of the Parties to the Convention on the Prohibition of the Development, Production and Stockpiling of Bacteriological (Biological) and Toxin Weapons and on Their Destruction. (1986) BWC/CONF.II/4, 18 August, Geneva: United Nations.

high level of awareness and education of life scientists. How else could they contribute to the development and maintenance of any necessary oversight systems of potentially dangerous research that others might misuse (dual-use research) or codes of conduct, let alone know what activities might contravene the Convention?

The awareness and education of life scientists

Unfortunately, when States Parties met in the 2005 Inter-Sessional Process between the Fifth and Sixth Five Year Review Conferences, Australia reported that:

> Amongst the Australian scientific community, there is a low level of awareness of the risk of the misuse of the biological sciences to assist in the development of biological or chemical weapons. Many scientists working in 'dual-use' areas simply do not consider the possibility that their work could inadvertently assist in a biological or chemical weapons programme.

Australia is far from unique in this respect. At the same meeting I reported work with Brian Rappert in which we used his interactive seminar to assess the views of practising life scientists in the United Kingdom about the Convention. We concluded that:

There is little evidence from our seminars that participants:

a regarded bioterrorism or bioweapons as a substantial threat;

b considered that developments in life sciences research contributed to biothreats;

c were aware of the current debates and concerns about dual-use research; or

d were familiar with the BTWC.

In the following year we reported further seminars in the United Kingdom and in Finland, Germany, the Netherlands, South Africa and the United States that produced very similar results[5] and subsequently we found much the same in Argentina, Australia, India, Israel, Japan, Kenya, Sweden, Switzerland, Uganda and the Ukraine. It is very difficult to avoid the conclusion that ignorance of the BTWC and the dangers of deliberate disease are widespread among practising life scientists around the world.

---

5   Malcolm R. Dando and Brian Rappert, *In-depth Implementation of the BTWC: Education and Outreach*, Review Conference Paper No. 18, November (Bradford: University of Bradford, 2006).

There could, of course, be many reasons for these findings. For example, in the fast-moving revolution in the life sciences, there is a vast amount of new information and many new technologies to be mastered by practising life scientists before they get down to the tough task of carrying out their own work. There may thus be little time to consider the potential misuse of the materials, technologies and information they are generating day by day. Yet we reasoned that if the essential material required for understanding the importance of the BTWC was incorporated into their university education at undergraduate and postgraduate levels it would be most unlikely that the widespread ignorance we encountered would have been possible.

We therefore began to examine what was being taught in university Life Sciences departments in different countries and regions of the world. The results again were very clear. In co-operation with Italian colleagues we first carried out a survey of courses in Europe. Using a sample of 142 courses from 57 universities in 29 countries, a search was made for evidence of biosecurity modules, bioethics modules and biosafety modules. These were the results:

> This research suggested that only 3 out of the universities identified in the survey currently offered some form of specific biosecurity module and in all cases this was optional for students.[6]

We felt reasonably sure that this was a correct assessment of the situation because if more such modules existed they would likely have been discovered in larger numbers as the survey also found that nearly half of the degree courses surveyed had a bioethics module and a fifth had a biosafety module. Efforts to dig deeper into the material being taught by searching even for references to issues such as the BTWC brought equally bleak results. Similar findings resulted from a survey in Japan[7] and subsequently in Israel and the Asia-Pacific region. In short, it is clear that there is a major gap in the current education of life scientists at university level around the world. It is very unlikely that they are receiving the education that States Parties to the BTWC considered important in strengthening the Convention two-and-a-half decades ago.

Correcting the education and awareness deficiency

When we followed up our surveys by asking lecturers why they did not cover the absent material, some said that they did not see the relevance of the problem.

---

6   Guilio Mancini and James Revill, *Fostering the Biosecurity Norm: Biosecurity Education for the Next Generation of Life Scientists* (Landau Network and University of Bradford, 2008), available at www.dual-use bioethics.net.
7   Masamichi Minehata and Nariyoshi Shinomiya, *Biosecurity Education: Enhancing Ethics, Securing Life and Promoting Science* (Japan, National Defence Medical College, and Bradford: University of Bradford, 2009), available at www.dual-use bioethics.net.

Others, however, did see that there was an important gap, but said that they lacked the knowledge, resources and space on the timetable to deal with it. We thus came to the conclusion that one way, among a number, in which we could help was to provide a wide-ranging internet-based 'open-source' Education Module Resource (EMR) that could easily be used by lecturers to add material, as they saw fit, to their ongoing courses.[8]

The question then was what material should go into our EMR? In deciding, we were guided by the States Parties to the BTWC giving more detailed consideration to the problem of education and the outcome of the BTWC Inter-Sessional Process meeting in December 2008,[9] which concluded in part that:

> State Parties noted that formal requirements for seminars, modules or courses, including possible mandatory components, in relevant scientific and engineering training programmes and continuing professional education could assist in raising awareness and in implementing the Convention.

The States Parties then went on to agree on the value of such programmes including:

a Explaining the risks associated with the potential misuse of the biological sciences and biotechnology;

b Covering the moral and ethical obligations incumbent on those using the biological sciences;

c Providing guidance on the types of activities which could be contrary to the aims of the Convention and relevant national laws and regulations and international law; and

d Being supported by accessible teaching materials, train-the-trainer programmes, seminars, workshops, publications and audio-visual materials . . .

In order to meet such objectives we decided, with our colleagues at the National Defence Medical College (NDMC) in Japan, that the EMR should have three main sections together with an introductory overview and a concluding look forward.

Thus the 21 lectures of the EMR are designed as follows:

A Introduction and Overview (Lecture 1).

B The Threat of Biological Warfare and Terrorism and the International Prohibition Regime (Lectures 2–10).

---

8   James Revill, *Developing Metrics and Measures for Dual-Use Education* (Bradford: University of Bradford, 2010), available at www.dual-use bioethics.net.
9   United Nations, *Report of the Meeting of States Parties*, BWC/MSP/2008/5, 12 December, Geneva: United Nations, 2008.

C   The Dual-Use Dilemma and the Responsibilities of Scientists (Lectures 11–18).

D   National Implementation of the BTWC (Lectures 19–20).

E   Building an Effective Web of Prevention (Lecture 21).

To assist with the use of the EMR, each of the lectures consists of 20 powerpoint slides in a standard format. Additionally, notes are provided for the lecturers and direct links on the Internet are made to the references used for the slides. There are also some background papers on issues that life scientists are less likely to know about and sets of questions for students related to each lecture.

The first major section (B) of the EMR therefore has the following series of lectures:

2   Biological weapons from Antiquity to World War I

3   Biological weapons from WWI to WWII

4   Biological weapons during the Cold War

5   The impact of biological weapons agents

6   Assimilation of biological weapons in State Programmes

7   International legal agreements

8   Strengthening the BTWC 1980–2008

9   The 2003–2005 Inter-Sessional Process

10 The 2007–2010 Inter-Sessional Process.

However, this unfamiliar material for life scientists was made 'user-friendly' by introducing modern accounts of the traditional biological agents and toxins such as anthrax, smallpox and botulinum toxin in the historical accounts of the twentieth-century offensive biological weapons programmes in major states such as the United Kingdom, United States, Union of Soviet Socialist Republics, France, Germany and so on.

Section C of the EMR then introduces the recent concerns about dual-use research and publications as follows:

11 Bioethics methodology

12 Obligations derived from the BTWC

13 The growth of dual-use bioethics

14 Dual-use: The US National Academy of Sciences Fink Report

15 Dual-use examples

16 The US National Academy of Sciences Lemon-Relman Report

17 Weapons targeted at the nervous system

18 Regulation of the life sciences.

Because life scientists have little knowledge of the BTWC, again an effort has been made to ensure that the module is user-friendly by suggesting that the problem of dual-use is best seen as an ethical problem since life scientists are often taught about ethical issues such as those, for example, surrounding GMOs and stem cell research. More specifically, we use the original outlining of the problem of dual-use in the US National Academy of Sciences Fink Committee Report and the expansion of concern across the life sciences in the Lemon-Relman Report to clearly demonstrate high-level scientific concerns about this issue.

The following section (D) sets the regulation of dual-use within the wider context of international efforts to regulate the biotechnology revolution as a whole and the national implementation of the BTWC:

19 International regulation of biotechnology

20 National implementing legislation.

Finally, the last lecture – number 21 – looks forward to examine how all elements of the overall web of preventive policies may be improved. Currently, the EMR is available in English, Japanese, French and Russian, and other translations are in progress. We have also tested out the use of parts of the module in Italy and Japan with our colleagues and reported the successful outcomes to BTWC meetings in Geneva. However, the question now is – how can this successful project, or other such projects, be used to inform the majority of practising life scientists?

Effective education?

There are obviously problems in converting small-scale projects of the kind illustrated by the development of the EMR into large-scale programmes of education. A basic difficulty is the way in which the problem of biosecurity has been formulated for scientists. Following the terrorist attacks in the United States in 2001 and the subsequent mailing of anthrax-contaminated letters, the most prominent concern has focused on terrorism and the dangers that could arise from the later misuse of dual-use experiments or publications. This approach is epitomized by the Fink Committee's designation of seven classes of experiment of concern that require, in their opinion, a form of oversight in a pre-project review. Such reviews would weigh the benefits of the research against the potential future risks. Unfortunately, as Brian Rappert and I were often told in our seminars with life scientists, it will be very difficult to achieve a consensus that the biosecurity risks of almost any experiment will outweigh the benefits. The fact that the benefits of reconstructing the deadly Spanish influenza virus (and publication of the details) were seen to outweigh the risks is surely a good illustration, as is the vanishingly small number of publications that have been withheld on the grounds of biosecurity risk.

As Catriona McLeish has argued, there are a number of different ways in which the concept of dual-use can be understood.[10] From the perspective of the BTWC the problem is not just about individual experiments and publications but with the probability that the scope and pace of change in the biotechnology revolution could facilitate both old and new means of biowarfare and bioterrorism. Yet the last thing we want to do is to prohibit beneficial science and technology. So, properly formulated, the problem is how to prevent malign misuse without, in trying to prevent the most exceptionally dangerous research and publication, preventing beneficial work.

Put simply, it would appear that we have formulated the problem incorrectly. The problem is not (or very rarely) concerned with the benignly intended work of individual scientists but with the protection of all such work from misuse. In such circumstances it seems difficult for bioethicists to offer much help to the scientist about what to do and that may partly explain the limited forays of bioethicists to date into the field of dual-use.[11] My own guess is that Aquinas' Doctrine of Double Effect might help.[12] The original argument is that if I inadvertently kill an attacker in defending myself then I can hardly be called to account. However, if I am reckless in my defence, that may not hold. So if I carry on with my life science research and publication but take part in efforts to prevent misuse, I have a defensible case if my work is misused, but if I recklessly ignore the possibility of misuse, that may not hold. And maybe, also, other ethical principles can be used to help scientists decide what to do.

Even if a satisfactory bioethical approach to dual-use is developed there will clearly be a problem in transmitting it effectively to life scientists. As Jane Johnson explained:

> Analysing the relatively limited literature regarding teaching philosophy to science students reveals that at the broadest level student difficulties stem from a difference in culture and norms of the humanities and sciences . . .

10   Caitriona McLeish, 'Reflecting on the Problem of Dual-Use', in Brian Rappert and Caitriona McLeish McLeish (eds), *A Web of Prevention* (London: Earthscan, 2007).
11   Michael Selgelid, 'Ethics Engagement of the Dual-Use Dilemma: Progress and Potential', in Brian Rappert (ed.), *Education and Ethics in the Life Sciences*, (Canberra: ANU E Press, 2010).
12   Stanford Encyclopedia of Philosophy, *Doctrine of Double Effect*, (2011), available at plato. stanford.edu/entries/double effect.

She detailed the problems that arise from this difference as follows:

> ... science students frequently not having the requisite skills in writing, reading, and so on, to perform well in philosophy subjects generally ... in their not knowing, understanding or being comfortable with the culture and expectations of philosophy ...

Indeed:

> ... in their possibly having a hostile orientation towards a discipline which they may perceive as either challenging or inferior to their chosen career path in science ...[13]

There may, of course, be imaginative teachers who can overcome what I suspect are widespread characteristics among science students, but it will surely not be easy to make a lasting impact with a measurable effect.[14]

It is for such reasons, I suspect, that a more popular approach with scientists is to aim to develop responsible conduct of research in a much more straightforward manner with little recourse to overt philosophical (ethical) arguments. Yet for those interested in dealing with the dual-use/biosecurity problem, even this approach can present difficulties, as is easily seen by an analysis of the widely used US National Academies book, *On Being a Scientist: A Guide to Responsible Conduct of Research*.[15] This book has 12 substantive chapters following the introduction which cover issues such as advising and monitoring, the treatment of data, research misconduct and so on (see Table 11.1). The issue of dual-use is covered in the final chapter (13), which is titled 'The Researcher in Society'. This chapter takes a wide-ranging view of the researcher's responsibilities, stating:

> The standards of science extend beyond responsibilities that are internal to the scientific community. Researchers also have a responsibility to reflect on how their work and the knowledge they are generating might be used in the broader society.

It goes on to mention different roles that scientists might play in the wider society such as providing expert advice to government or lobbying policy-makers on topics in which they specialize but, interestingly, the 'Historic Case Study' for the chapter concerns a dual-use issue and is titled 'Ending the Use of Agent Orange'. This historic study recounts how, in the 1940s, Arthur Galston

---

13   Jane Johnson, 'Teaching Ethics to Science tudents: Challenges and a Strategy', in Rappert (ed.), *Education and Ethics in the Life Sciences*.
14   National Academies, *Ethics Education and Scientific and Engineering Research: What's Been Learned? What Should Be Done?* (Washington DC: National Academies Press, 2009).
15   Committee on Science, Engineering and Public Policy, *On Being a Scientist: A Guide to Responsible Conduct in Research* (3rd edn) (Washington DC: National Academies Press, 2009).

Table 11.1 Chapters and Case Studies*

Chapter	Case Studies	Advice	Historic Case Study	Appendix
1**	-	-	-	-
2	y***	y	-	y
3	y	-	-	y
4	y	-	y	y
5	yy	-	y	yy
6	y	-	y	y
7	yy	-	-	yy
8****	-	-	-	-
9	y	y	y	y
10	y	-	y	y
11	y	-	-	y
12	y	y	-	y
13	-	-	y	-

*From Committee on Science, Engineering and Public Policy (2009), on Being a Scientist: A Guide to Responsible Conduct in Research, 3rd edn (Washington DC: National Academies Press).
**Introduction.
*** Symbol 'y' indicates presence.
****Biosafety chapter with checklist.

discovered plant bioregulators that could hasten the flowering of plants. This allowed particular plants to be grown in colder climates because it shortened the growing season required. However, in larger concentrations these synthetic chemicals could be used as herbicides to defoliate and kill the plants. When Galston discovered that the US military were using thousands of tons of the chemicals (mainly Agent Orange) as defoliants in the Vietnam War in the 1960s he actively opposed this abuse of his work. The historic case study ends by quoting Galston:

> I used to think that one could avoid involvement in the anti-social consequences of science simply by not working on any project that might be turned to evil or destructive ends. I have learned that things are not that simple … The only recourse is for a scientist to remain involved with it to the end.

However, no further advice is offered to the scientist about how to do this.

As Table 11.1 illustrates, this is in stark contrast to the other substantive chapters of the book. Some have historic case studies and a few also have advice sections, but all have one or more hypothetical case studies backed up by additional analyses and answers to some of the questions raised by these case studies in an appendix. So what this text on responsible conduct of research lacks is precisely what the scientist needs to be responsible about biosecurity: information on dual-use and biosecurity and the BTWC.

Yet I think this approach of developing a wider sense of the responsible conduct of research can be of use in regard to dealing with the wider social responsibilities of scientists under the Convention. For example, a straightforward list of practical questions such as the following would alert the scientist to what he or she needed to find out.

A In regard to work in their scientific field:

Would you be able to spot an experiment of real dual-use concern?

B In regard to their workplace:

Is there a mechanism in place where you could raise concerns about a dual-use experiment of concern with your superiors?

C In regard to their scientific associations:

Are dual-use and biosecurity policy developments (nationally and internationally) being carefully followed and are you being kept informed so that you can contribute your expertise to finding solutions?

D In regard to national implementation of biosecurity policies:

Are you well informed about the national laws and regulations that could affect your country's obligations under the Biological Weapons Convention?

E In regard to the Biological Weapons Convention:

Are you aware of the key provisions of the Convention and of how efforts are being made to keep it up-to-date with ongoing scientific advances?

It seems possible that a new version of *On Being a Scientist* could include a case study, advice and answers to some such questions in a new section of the appendix.

Yet even if that were done and other non-governmental initiatives were undertaken it does not seem possible that a large-scale change in the culture of the life sciences towards the problem of dual-use and biosecurity could take place without government action at the national level. Some of what that might involve was set out in a US National Science Advisory Board for Biosecurity (NSABB) report on a *Strategic Plan for Outreach and Education on Dual-Use Research Issues* in 2008. According to this report:

First and foremost, the target audience must be identified and assessed as to their level of understanding of the issues since this will guide the educational strategies.

Then:

Messages should be tailored to specific target audiences. Key points must be identified and specifically crafted to effectively convey the nature and importance of the information while simultaneously addressing the unique concerns of different stakeholder groups.

And finally:

> ... it is important to select those methods that will most effectively reach the intended audiences.[16]

Even more daunting, when all of that theoretical analysis is completed for diverse stakeholder groups, an implementation plan still has to be devised, carried out and monitored to completion.

What needs to be done?

In the face of such a set of difficulties it might seem that it is an almost impossible task for the international community to deal with this gap in the web of preventive policies and to enlist the help of an aware and well-educated scientific community in the protection of their work from malign misuse. I do not agree with that assessment.[17] It will be recalled that in 2008 State Parties to the BTWC agreed a set of sensible means by which the level of awareness and education of life scientists could be improved in order to strengthen the Convention.

Of course, given the different circumstances in each country there will be no 'one size fits all' solution. Each State would have to take what actions it felt would be most appropriate to achieve the desired end and then report back to the hopefully reinvigorated system of annual meetings[18] in order that 'Best Practice' could more rapidly evolve. Most importantly, I think it is necessary to understand that some massive, cumbersome, top-down system is just what is *not* required. Instead, a series of low cost, imaginative, practical projects could be initiated that would help to develop and demonstrate what needs to be done. Properly reported in the scientific and educational literature, these projects would, I think, certainly then be taken up by other life scientists and the idea and implementation of the new culture could be expected to spread nationally and internationally.

For example, State-level Research Councils could deliberately advertise grants that would be available for groups to develop and implement new dual-use and biosecurity educational material and make it available 'open-source' on the internet. National and private funders could also make grants available for the

---

16   National Science Advisory Board for Biosecurity, *Strategic Plan for Outreach and Education on Dual-use Research Issues* (Washington DC: NSABB, 2008).

17   Simon Whitby and Malcolm R. Dando, *Effective Implementation of the BTWC: The Key Role of Awareness Raising and Education*, Review Conference Paper No. 26, November (Bradford: University of Bradford, 2010).

18   Nicholas A. Sims, *An Annual Meeting for the BTWC*, Review Conference Paper No. 22, June (Bradford: University of Bradford, 2010).

development and implementation of Train-the-Trainer programmes[19] to help with the teaching of the new material or with short courses specifically designed for particular stakeholders (e.g. industry) within the country. Furthermore, grants could be made available for networks of interested lecturers to be organized, course material to be developed into textbooks and for professional associations to help develop international competency standards in biosecurity. So there are many low-cost, efficient and effective actions that could be taken by State Parties if it is decided to act upon the agreement made in 2008 (see Table 11.2).

None of that kind of funding would incur large-scale costs and could, in any event, be distributed over a number of government agencies and private sources. Moreover, it can surely be expected that as awareness and education levels improve, the scientific community will give consideration to appropriate codes of conduct and oversight systems as they appear necessary.

Conclusion

There is undoubtedly a serious gap in the overall web of preventive policies designed to minimize the possibility that the modern life sciences will be used for hostile purposes. Most practising life scientists still are unaware that there is a problem and we are certainly only in the early stages of working out how to close this dangerous gap – a gap that will certainly grow more dangerous as the biotechnology revolution continues to advance and spread.

Yet despite the difficulties in changing the culture of the life sciences – some of which, as noted here, are indeed formidable – it seems that effective action at relatively low cost could build a self-sustaining process by which the life sciences community will carry out the necessary actions itself. All that is required now is for the Seventh Review Conference of the BTWC to take the decision to act on awareness-raising and education in December 2011 and for State Parties to ensure funding for small-scale, imaginative practical projects which, when well reported, can be the model for many others to follow. In short, there is the possibility of a huge gearing up of projects by life scientists because the last thing they want to see is their benignly intended work being misused for hostile purposes.

However, the danger is that with so many possible issues to deal with and so little time at the Review Conference itself, awareness-raising and education (and, by implication, codes of conduct and oversight systems) will just get lost among what are perceived to be more important or pressing issues.[20] Yet a successful

19   Whitby and Dando, *Effective Implementation of the BTWC*.
20   Graham S. Pearson, *Preparing for the BTWC Seventh Review Conference in 2011*, Review Conference Paper No. 21, May (Bradford: University of Bradford, 2010).

Table 11.2 Actions that could be taken to implement the 2008 agreements on education

i. Explaining the risks associated with the potential misuse of the biological sciences and biotechnology;

Action	The government could send a message to all Universities setting out the risks and asking that this information be circulated to all heads of departments in life and associated sciences with a view to actions being taken in regard to the education of students.
Objective	The aim would be to rapidly raise awareness of the risks among those with professional expertise and to engage them in considering what should be done about the education of their students.

ii. Covering the moral and ethical obligations incumbent on those using the biological sciences;

Action	The government could send a letter to all Universities requesting that the information given in the letter described in section (i) above be circulated to all philosophy departments with a view to action being taken to develop an ethical approach to questions of dual-use, biosecurity and the BTWC.
Objective	To assist life and associated scientists to add this material on their moral and ethical obligations under the Convention to the material being taught on bioethics and medical ethics.

iii. Providing guidance on the types of activities which could be contrary to the aims of the Convention and relevant national laws and regulations and international law;

Action	The government could issue a short statement setting out the national laws and international laws in brief and why they are needed to minimize the risk of biowarfare and bioterrorism.
Objective	To provide a coherent context and rationale for the development of new educational courses and materials.

iv. Being supported by accessible teaching materials, train-the-trainer programmes, seminars, workshops, publications and audio-visual materials;

Action	Funding Agencies (government and non-governmental) could be asked to provide small grants, for example to assist in the development of new courses on dual-use bioethics and biosecurity that could then be made available 'open source' on the web or for seminar series and network building.
Objective	To develop and spread best practice effectively and efficiently.

v. Addressing leading scientists and those with responsibility for oversight of research or for evaluation of projects or publications at a senior level, as well as future generations of scientists, with the aim of building a culture of responsibility;

Action	The government could convene a meeting of representatives of all the relevant professional associations and industry associations to consider how they could assist in the promotion of a culture of responsibility and ownership in relation to the Convention, for example through the development of appropriate elements of continuing professional development.
Objective	To engage leading scientists in the process of developing this element of the web of prevention.

vi. Being integrated into existing efforts at the international, regional and national levels;

Action	The government could set up an interdepartmental committee to monitor and integrate these efforts at awareness raising and education and to report what is being done to the relevant meetings of the BTWC and other international meetings.
Objective	To make the overall national effort as effective as possible and to assist others in such developments.

outcome should not be seen as farfetched, indeed it may eventually be seen as mainstream when, for example, the US Presidential Commission for the Study of Bioethical Issues, in its 2010 report *New Directions: Ethics of Synthetic Biology and Emerging Technologies*, stated in its Recommendation 9:

> Because synthetic biology and related research cross traditional disciplinary boundaries, ethics education similar or superior to the training required today in the medical and chemical research communities should be developed and required for all researchers and student investigators outside of the medical setting, including in engineering and material science . . .

The Recommendation continued, in part:

> . . . the Executive Office of the President . . . should convene a panel to consider appropriate and meaningful training and models. This review should be completed within 18 months and the results made public.[21]

Just in case there is any misunderstanding, it should be noted that the recommendation is introduced in the Executive Summary by a paragraph that suggests that *'Creating a culture of responsibility in the synthetic biology community could do more to promote responsible stewardship in synthetic biology than any other single strategy'* (emphasis added).

Encouraging signs in regard to action on education and awareness-raising also became clear at the meeting of G8 Foreign Ministers in March 2011 in the lead-up to the April meeting of the Preparatory Committee for the Seventh Review Conference. In Paragraph 9 of their concluding *Statement* the Foreign Ministers argued that:

> The involvement of civil society, particularly the academic and industrial sectors, is essential to the effective implementation of the Convention. We will therefore step up such engagement to fully take account of scientific and technical developments in the biological area . . .

They continued, significantly:

> . . . We will likewise work on better awareness raising among those involved in the development of life sciences in order to limit the possibilities of misuse of technical developments, including supporting dual-use education programs on bioethics.[22]

This forward-looking stance was repeated by the United States Ambassador in her opening *Statement* at the Preparatory Committee. In the view of the United

21   Presidential Commission for the Study of Bioethical Issues, *New Directions: The Ethics of Synthetic Biology and Emerging Technologies* (Washington DC: Presidential Commission, 2010).
22   Meeting of G8 Foreign Ministers, *Statement on the Seventh Review Conference for the Biological and Toxin Weapons Convention*, 14–15 March 2011.

States,[23] one of the priority topics for the inter-sessional work between the Seventh and Eighth Review Conference (of 2016) should be:

> Strengthening and promoting outreach, education, and awareness to and of those engaged in the life sciences to reinforce strong norms of responsible, ethical and safety- and security-conscious behaviour.

Finally, at the Preparatory Committee meeting an important Information Paper was produced by Australia, Japan and Switzerland on behalf of the JACKSNNZ group of States, and Sweden.[24] This Paper recounted the efforts that the countries had made to improve education and awareness-raising, supported the view that consideration should be given to awareness-raising and education at the Review Conference and made a number of suggestions as to what might be done by State Parties. Crucially, the Paper pointed out that State Parties could report on what they had done under the Annual Confidence Building Measure 'E' on the *Declaration of legislation, regulations and other measures* as measures that they had taken to strengthen the implementation of the Convention and then noted that:

> ... With the publication of this material, inter alia in CBM returns, those State Parties which are at a more advanced stage in the implementation of their dual-use awareness-raising and education activities would be able to identify, and offer appropriate cooperation to State Parties at a less advanced stage in such activities.

In short, a positive feedback system could rapidly accelerate the generation and implementation of best practice and thus lead quickly to a strengthening of the Convention and the prohibition it embodies.

---

23   Ambassador Laura Kennedy, *Statement of the US Special Representative for the Biological and Toxin Weapons Convention Issues at the Preparatory Committee for the BWC Review Conference*, 14 April (Geneva: United Nations, 2011).
24   Australia, Japan and Switzerland on behalf of 'JACKSNNZ', and Sweden, *Possible Approaches to Education and Awareness-Raising among Life Scientists* BWC/CONF. VII/ PC/INF.4, 15 April, (Geneva: United Nations, 2011).

PART THREE

Political and Regulatory Responses in Global Health

12

The Human Right to Health: Whose Obligation?

Doris Schroeder

Introduction

The highest attainable standard of health is a fundamental human right,[1] which has been part of international law since 1948. The preamble to the Universal Declaration of Human Rights states that: '*every individual and every organ of society* ... shall strive ... by progressive measures, national and international, to secure their [human rights] universal and effective recognition and observance'.[2]

This chapter analyses and compares obligations vis-à-vis the human right to health of the following groups: governments, affluent individuals, non-governmental organizations (NGOs) and pharmaceutical companies. To focus the discussion, the case of access to life-saving medicines is considered. As the authors of the Millennium Development Goals Gap Task Force have noted, access to medicines is a vital component of realizing the human right to health.[3]

Nearly 30 per cent of the world population do not have access to life-saving medicines, as Anand Grover reported to the United Nations in 2009. According to him, 'improving access to medicines could save 10 million lives a year'.[4] Implied in this mortality figure is immense human suffering. Parents lose their children, children their carer, husbands their wives. And a mortality figure does not even capture the additional suffering associated with avoidable ill health and morbidity.

Who are the individuals and organs of society, who must strive to secure the universal and effective recognition of human rights, in particular the human

---

1 Henceforth, 'Human Right to Health'.
2 Universal Declaration of Human Rights 1948: Preamble, emphasis added; available at www.un.org/en/documents/udhr/index.shtml#a25
3 United Nations MDG Gap Task Force, *Delivering on the Global Partnership for Achieving the Millennium Development Goals* (New York: United Nations, 2008), 42.
4 Anand Grover, *Promotion and Protection of All Human Rights, Civil, Political, Economic, Social and Cultural Rights, Including the Right to Development, a Report of the Special Rapporteur on the Right of Everyone to the Enjoyment of the Highest Attainable Standard of Physical and Mental Health*, U.N. Doc. A/HRC/11/12 (New York: United Nations, 2009), 6, 7, 28.

right to health and its sub-goal, the human right to access life-saving drugs? Figure 12.1 captures the essence of the question, which will occupy us for the remainder of this chapter.

Governmental obligations

The one entity from our set of potential duty holders that undisputedly carries obligations towards the human right to health are governments. Governments or states have legal obligations to respect, protect and fulfil the right to health, which includes assuring access to life-saving medicines for all and – for developed countries – providing international assistance. The relevant legal instruments which enshrine the above obligations are listed in Table 12.1.

With reference to access to life-saving medicines, Anand Grover makes it clear that these fall squarely within state obligations. He writes:

> States have an obligation under the right to health to ensure that medicines are available, financially affordable, and physically accessible on a basis of non-discrimination to everyone within their jurisdiction. Developed States also have a responsibility to take steps towards the full realization of the right to health through international assistance and cooperation.[5]

The reason state obligations are stringent is that they are contractual. States have committed themselves to abiding by these obligations through binding legislation such as the International Covenant on Economic, Social and

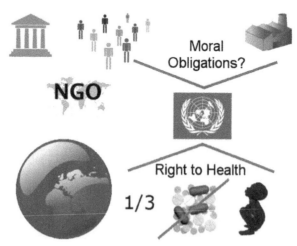

Figure 12.1 The human right to health – whose obligation?

5 Ibid.

Table 12.1 The human right to health – relevant legal instruments

Government obligations towards their own citizens	Government obligations for international assistance
O Universal Declaration of Human Rights, Art.25(1)[a] O International Covenant on Economic, Social and Cultural Rights, Art.12[b] O Convention on the Elimination of All Forms of Discrimination against Women, Art.12[c] O Convention on the Rights of the Child, Art.24(1–3)[d]	O Declaration of Alma-Ata, Art.II[e] O UN Committee on Economic, Social and Cultural Rights E/C.12/2000/4, General Comment No.14.[f] O Millennium Development Goals 4, 5 and 6[g] Convention on the Rights of the Child, Art.24(4)[h]

a   www.un.org/en/documents/udhr/.
b   www2.ohchr.org/english/law/cescr.htm.
c   www.un.org/womenwatch/daw/cedaw/text/econvention.htm.
d   www2.ohchr.org/english/law/crc.htm.
e   www.who.int/hpr/NPH/docs/declaration_almaata.pdf.
f   www.unhchr.ch/tbs/doc.nsf/(symbol)/E.C.12.2000.4.En.
g   www.un.org/millenniumgoals/bkgd.shtml.
h   www2.ohchr.org/english/law/crc.htm.

Cultural Rights. However, it is noteworthy that the United States of America, South Africa and Cuba have not ratified the Covenant.[6] Hence, there are some exceptions. Likewise, the United States and Somalia have not ratified the Convention on the Rights of the Child. But with the exception of the United States, the duties towards one's own and other countries' citizens that derive from the above legal instruments are widely accepted, if judged on accession and ratification. However, a more detailed comparison of ratification with human rights commitment is not encouraging.

In 2009 the Lancet published a study which assessed whether the ratification of human rights treaties was linked to improved health indicators. The study analysed

> data for health (including HIV prevalence, and maternal, infant, and child [<5 years] mortalities) and social indicators (child labour, human development index, sex gap, and corruption index), gathered from 170 countries. [The results] showed no consistent associations between ratification of human-rights treaties and health or social outcomes.[7]

6   See: http://treaties.un.org/Pages/ViewDetails.aspx?src=TREATY&mtdsg_no=IV-3&chapter=4&lang=en.
7   Alexis Palmer, Jocelyn Tomkinson, Charlene Phung, Nathan Ford, Michel Joffres, Kimberly A. Fernandes, et al., 'Does ratification of human-rights treaties have effects on population health?', *The Lancet*, 2009, 373(9679): 1987–92.

Thus, pinpointing who has a stringent obligation to secure the human right to health for all does not by itself mobilize sufficient resources or willingness. However, recent developments in international 'soft law', that is non-binding law, may help expand the group of agents who have stringent obligations and may therefore be mobilized alongside governments.

Affluent individuals' obligations

In general, human beings value life and want to enjoy its full length from childhood to adulthood to seniority. In recognition of this human *joie de vivre*, heroic life-saving acts occur all over the world. For instance, in New York, Wesley Autrey jumped onto a subway track to help a fallen teenager when a train was approaching. Unable to hoist the unresponsive teenager onto the platform, he decided to cover him with his body and lie still in the drainage trough while the train passed. Both men survived. Autrey later commented: 'I don't feel like I did something spectacular; I just saw someone who needed help. I did what I felt was right.'[8]

Yet, while a heroically courageous man feels that rescuing a complete stranger is simply the right thing to do, the essence of such an act rarely translates into rescuing the lives of *distant* strangers. 'We can reasonably believe that the cost of saving a life through ... [specified] charities is somewhere between $200 and $2000.'[9] This aligns roughly with the costs of providing patent-protected drugs to AIDS patients. In 2008, the yearly cost of providing second-line[10] anti-retrovirals was $US 1,105 per patient in low-income countries.[11] This means that affluent individuals could regularly save other people's lives without major restrictions on their own.

> The question how much the relatively well off are obligated to do for the needy is one of the most interesting areas ... in moral theory ... We frequently wonder whether we are doing what morality requires of us in terms of helping others. And it is far from obvious that any familiar moral theory has an intuitively acceptable line on this matter.[12]

Brad Hooker, the author of the above excerpt, is right. Intuitively acceptable answers on this matter are not easily available. Table 12.2 therefore simplifies some relevant answers.

---

8   See: www.msnbc.msn.com/id/16444249/.
9   Peter Singer, *The Life You Can Save* (Melbourne: Text Publishing, 2009), 111.
10 Second-line drugs are used when the standard therapy fails, and are often much more expensive than the first drug of choice.
11 Avert, *Aids, Drug Prices and Generic Drugs*.
12 Brad Hooker, *Ideal Code, Real World* (Oxford: Clarendon Press, 2000), 159.

Table 12.2 Why promote distant strangers' human right to health?

Author	Principle	The case of life-saving medicines
Peter Singer	'If it is in our power to prevent something bad from happening, without thereby sacrificing anything of comparable moral importance, then we ought, morally, to do it.'[a]	The death of 10 million people p.a. from lack of access to medicines is a typical case for the application of Singer's utilitarian principle. Affluent individuals can prevent something bad from happening without sacrificing anything of comparable moral importance by, for instance, donating to charity.
Immanuel Kant	'Act only according to that maxim whereby you can, at the same time, will that it should become a universal law.'[b]	One cannot universalize a maxim that lets 10 million people die every year unnecessarily because the affluent refuse to assist the poor. No reasonable person would want to live in this world.
Aristotle	'. . . happiness is an activity of soul in accordance with perfect virtue.' (1102a)[c]	Generosity is a virtue situated between wastefulness and meanness. In order to achieve happiness through perfect virtue, it is important not to be mean; more important than not to be wasteful. Hence, one should err on the side of giving too much to benefit others.

[a] Singer, Peter (2009) The Life You Can Save, Melbourne: Text Publishing.
[b] Kant, Immanuel (1965, 1785) Grundlegung zur Metaphysik der Sitten, Hamburg: Felix Meiner Verlag, 42 (421).
[c] Aristotle (1985) Nikomachische Ethik, Hamburg: Felix Meiner Verlag, 22 (1102a).

As Table 12.2 shows, Singer, Kant and Aristotle provide good philosophical reasons for requiring affluent individuals to take action on securing the human right to health for the global poor. However, while some philosophers believe that our duties towards distant strangers are nowhere near this pressing,[13] there

13   See, for instance, Warwick Fox who argues that we only have one duty towards distant others, namely not to harm them. When it comes to providing assistance, Fox distinguishes between strong duties of benevolence one has towards one's partner, children and close relatives ('supersignificant others') from weaker duties towards one's friends, close colleagues or mentors ('significant others'). To distant others, we have no duties of benevolence, he argues (*A Theory of General Ethics: Human Relationships, Nature, and the Built Environment* (Cambridge, MA: MIT Press, 2007)).

is an even more obvious reason why affluent individuals have no stringent[14] obligation to help secure the human right to health for others. Benevolence and charity, as requested by all three of the above philosophers, leave considerable space for individual decision-making. If an affluent individual decides to spend her resources on improving food security for the global poor to the neglect of their health-care needs, she still fully complies with her moral obligations. Hence, there is no philosophical justification for requiring any particular affluent individual to help secure universal and effective recognition and observance of the human right to health per se. As long as the individual does *something* to relieve the burden of suffering from the poor, relative to her means, all is well, morally speaking.

Contrary to the above, Thomas Pogge offers a justification for a stringent obligation on why affluent individuals *must* assist the global poor in their right to access to life-saving medicines. We are not faced here with a question of beneficence, that is of how philanthropy ought to set in to rescue a distant stranger. As Pogge puts it: 'we are not bystanders who find ourselves confronted with foreign deprivations whose origins are wholly unconnected to ourselves.'[15] We are benefactors of an intellectual property rights framework that systematically favours our interests and the interests of the pharmaceutical industry over those of 'desperately poor people, often stunted from infancy, illiterate and heavily preoccupied with the struggle to survive, [who] can do little by way of either resisting or rewarding their local and national rulers, who are therefore likely to rule them oppressively while catering to the interests of other (often foreign) agents'.[16]

It is important here to consider Anand Grover's judgement on the causes for 10 million deaths per year. He noted that:

> the inability of populations to access medicines is partly due to high costs[17] [. . . as] TRIPS and FTAs [Free Trade Agreements] have had an adverse impact on prices and availability of medicines, making it difficult for countries to comply with their obligations to respect, protect, and fulfil the right to health.[18]

It is therefore clear that the current intellectual property rights system, which Pogge singles out as one reason for imposing a duty on affluent individuals, does indeed contribute to these 10 million deaths each year.

To sum up this section, while traditional philosophical theories on beneficence cannot justify a stringent obligation that affluent individuals must

---

14   By stringent, I mean an obligation that cannot be avoided without failing in one's duties as a moral agent. One could also use the Kantian term 'perfect duty'. Immanuel Kant, *Grundlegung zur Metaphysik der Sitten* (Hamburg: Felix Meiner Verlag, 1965, [1785]), 43 (421).

15   Thomas Pogge, 'Priorities of Global Justice', in Thomas Pogge (ed.), *Global Justice* (Oxford: Blackwell Publishers, 2001), 14.

16   Ibid., 8.

17   Grover, *Promotion and Protection of All Human Rights*, 7, point 14.

18   Ibid., 28, point 94.

assist in securing the human right to access to life-saving medicines, Pogge's philosophical insight and Grover's confirmation of the detrimental effects of the international intellectual property rights system lead to a different conclusion. As benefactors of a system that tailors medicines to diseases of the affluent who can afford monopoly prices, while foreseeably harming the poor,[19] we do have a specific duty to help the poor access life-saving medicines. It is a duty that stems from a combination of benefits received with harm foreseeably done rather than our obligations of beneficence. I shall return to this topic when discussing the obligations of pharmaceutical companies.

NGO obligations

The term non-governmental organization (NGO) is used in many different settings for a wide range of bodies. Yet, some features are common to all. An NGO must:

- be independent from direct government control;

- not constitute a political party;

- be non-profit-making; and

- be non-violent.

The above characteristics are required for recognition by the United Nations. An NGO can therefore be understood as:

> an independent voluntary association of people acting together on a continuous basis, for some common purpose, other than achieving government office, making money or illegal activities.[20]

At first hand, it may seem obvious that some NGOs have obligations to help the 10 million who currently die from lack of access to life-saving medicines. They would then be one of the organs of society, which are meant to strive to secure the human right to health for all. Organizations such as *Médecins Sans Frontières*, the Clinton Foundation, the Medicines for Malaria Venture, or the Foundation for Innovative New Diagnostics are already working towards this aim highly successfully. However, voluntary organizations can by their very nature not have any *stringent* or to use Kant's term *perfect* obligations to secure a particular common good.

19   Aidan Hollis and Thomas Pogge, *The Health Impact Fund: Making New Medicines Accessible for All* (Incentives for Global Health, 2008).
20   Peter Willetts, *What is a Non-Governmental Organization?* (UNESCO Encyclopaedia of Life Support Systems, 2002) Section 1: www.staff.city.ac.uk/p.willetts/CS-NTWKS/ NGO-ART.HTM#Part1.

The above-named NGOs may have relevant mission statements. For instance, the Medicines for Malaria Venture envisions 'a world in which ... innovative medicines will cure and protect the vulnerable and under-served populations at risk of malaria, and help to ultimately eradicate this terrible disease'.[21] But their efforts are truly voluntary and charity-based. That they have chosen to collaborate on ventures to secure the human right to health is supererogatory rather than obligation-based. They fall under the precept that was discussed above for affluent individuals, namely that we may all have duties of beneficence but how we discharge them is up to us. No affluent individual and no NGO can be forced, morally, to undertake charitable efforts in a particular area.[22] At the same time, the Poggean argument of benefitting from a system that imposes foreseeable harm on the poor cannot be made with regard to NGOs. Hence, there is no stringent obligation upon NGOs to help secure the human right to health.

Pharmaceutical industry obligations

The main role of a pharmaceutical company is to develop and produce innovative drugs and services that improve the quality of life of patients. No other societal actor assumes this responsibility as their main task. Paul Hunt, Anand Grover's predecessor as UN Special Rapporteur on the right to health formulates it thus:

> A pharmaceutical company that develops a life-saving medicine has performed a vitally important medical, public health and right-to-health function. By saving lives, reducing suffering and improving public health, it has not only enhanced the quality of life of individuals, but also contributed to the prosperity of individuals, families and communities. The company, and its employees, has made a major contribution to the realisation of the rights to life and the highest attainable standard of health.[23]

Yet beyond this traditional role, increasing demands are made on pharmaceutical companies to recognize and fulfil further obligations in relation to the right to health. This development became most obvious with the adoption of the Millennium Development Goals (MDGs). MDG 8 Target E requires that governments 'in cooperation with *pharmaceutical companies*, provide access to

---

21 See: www.mmv.org/about-us.
22 Of course, if an NGO has already announced its mission and collected relevant donations, it may be bound to particular efforts, but I am here talking about formulating mission statements in the first place.
23 Paul Hunt, *Report of the Special Rapporteur on the right of everyone to the enjoyment of the highest attainable standard of health: Annex – Mission to Glaxosmithkline* (New York: United Nations, 2009), 11: 35.

affordable essential drugs in developing countries'.[24] While the private sector in general is mentioned elsewhere (e.g. MDG 8F), no other industrial sector is named explicitly. Likewise a Lancet editorial assigns responsibilities to the pharmaceutical sector:

> Almost 2 billion people worldwide lack access to essential medicines. The human rights responsibility to improve access lies mainly with the state. However, non-state actors, such as the pharmaceutical industry, share that responsibility too.[25]

Additional pressure comes from NGOs. In *Investing for Life – Meeting poor people's needs for access to medicines through responsible business practices,* Oxfam states:

> there are major shortcomings in the pharmaceutical industry's current initiatives to ensure that poor people have access to medicines . . . The time is ripe for a bold new approach. The industry must put access to medicines at the heart of its decision-making and practices . . . The industry's failure to comprehend access to medicines as a fundamental human right enshrined in international law, and to recognise that pharmaceutical companies have responsibilities in this context, has prevented the adoption of appropriate strategies.[26]

The remainder of this section examines whether and if so how the above demands could be philosophically justified. Does the pharmaceutical sector have a co-responsibility, together with governments, to fulfil the human right to health?[27]

The starting point for an investigation of the above question has to be the international intellectual property rights system, and more particularly patents. Patents bar entry to the market for products copied from the original for a specified interval so that innovators can recoup research and development costs through charging monopoly prices.[28] Among those who benefit from intellectual property rights protection, the pharmaceutical industry is the

---

24 See: www.un.org/millenniumgoals/global.shtml.

25 Editorial, 'Right-To-Health Responsibilities of Pharmaceutical Companies,' *The Lancet*, 2009, 373: 1998.

26 Oxfam. *Investing for Life – Meeting Poor People's Needs for Access to Medicines through Responsible Business Practices* (Oxfam Briefing Paper 109, 2007), 1: www.oxfam.org/sites/ www.oxfam.org/files/bp109-investing-for-life-0711.pdf.

27 I shall take it for granted that pharmaceutical companies *respect* the human right to health and, for instance, do not harm their employees in unsafe working conditions or undertake trials on human participants with an unjustifiable harm–benefit ratio; This section is based on: Doris Schroeder, 'Does the Pharmaceutical Sector have a Co-Responsibility to Secure the Human Right to Health?', *Cambridge Quarterly of Healthcare Ethics*, 2011, 20(2): 298–308.

28 P. M. Danzon and A Towse, 'Differential Pricing for Pharmaceuticals: Reconciling Access, R&D and Patents', *International Journal of Health Care Finance and Economics*, 2003, 3: 183–205, 185.

only industry that trades in goods that are required to satisfy basic human needs.[29]

Films, software, books, designs, circuit layouts, computer programs, etc. – none of these satisfy basic human needs. The only exception is the seeds industry, which does benefit from intellectual property rights protection while providing for basic human needs. However, considerable farmers' rights against multinational corporations have been established under the International Treaty on Plant Genetic Resources for Food and Agriculture (ITPGR). This treaty exempts a number of basic food and seed crops from patenting and makes them accessible to all member states through a facilitated system.[30] There are no such exemptions for the pharmaceutical industry, and countries face serious difficulties when they invoke the compulsory licensing exemption[31] of the Trade-Related Aspects of Intellectual Property Rights (TRIPS) agreement.[32] Hence, the pharmaceutical sector is unique in benefiting from monopoly pricing powers at the same time as providing for a basic human need. However, the justification for pharmaceutical obligations is more subtle than a benefit granted through patents on the one hand and access to medicines for the poor on the other. The most obvious response would be that innovators have a human right to the protection of their invention, which is of equal standing to the human right to life of the poor. This claim has been discussed elsewhere and it was shown that the right to life trumps when colliding with the natural right to intellectual property protection.[33]

Given Anand Grover's statement that TRIPS 'had an adverse impact on prices and availability of medicines, making it difficult for countries to comply with their obligations to respect, protect, and fulfil the right to health',[34] would one not need to question intellectual property rights in general? In particular, if they cannot be maintained against the right to life of the poor? If 'patents are killing people',[35] should the system not be abandoned rather than maintained to secure profits for the pharmaceutical industry?

---

29   In line with Art. 25(1) of the Declaration of Human Rights I take basic human needs to comprise: food, clothing, housing and medical care.

30   Laurence R. Helfer, *Intellectual Property Rights in Plant Varieties – International Legal Regimes and Policy Options for National Governments*, FAO Legislative Study 85 (Rome: United Nations, 2004), Part IV.

31   With a compulsory license, a government forces a patent holder to allow the manufacture of generic copies of a drug at significantly reduced prices.

32   SciDevNet, Drug Licences All for the Poor, Says Thai Minister: www.scidev.net/en/news/drug-licences-all-for-the-poor-says-thai-minister.html.

33   Doris Schroeder and Peter Singer, 'Access to Life-Saving Medicines and Intellectual Property Rights – An Ethical Assessment', *Cambridge Quarterly of Healthcare Ethics*, 2011, 20(2): 279–89.

34   Grover, *Promotion and Protection of All Human Rights*, 28, point 94.

35   Madeleine Bunting, Profits that Kill, *The Guardian* (2001): www.guardian.co.uk/world/2001/feb/12/wto.aids.

The obvious answer to this question is that profits for the pharmaceutical industry are not the main justification for the patent system. As stated in the preamble of the 1970s Patent Cooperation Treaty, which covers 142 countries,[36] the reason governments support intellectual property rights is because patents 'make a contribution to the progress of science and technology' and 'facilitate and accelerate access by the public to the technical information contained in documents describing new inventions'.

While patents are 'a tortured solution to the problem of providing a public good',[37] it is not yet clear that there is an alternative. Providing a public good in the form of a product that is cheaply and easily copied, yet requires significant investment, is highly difficult, although efforts are being made.[38] This does not mean that the system could not be improved[39] or that the pharmaceutical industry cannot be assigned a special obligation towards the human right to health given their considerable benefits from a system that foreseeably harms the poor. This argument from harm was already discussed in the section on affluent individuals. In the case of the pharmaceutical industry, the argument is even stronger as it has more recently benefitted from a system change (the adoption of TRIPS) that is less relevant to affluent individuals (at least in the North) than it is to industry.

For example, before the adoption of TRIPS, Indian law only allowed patents on processes, not on products. As a result, India had a thriving generic pharmaceuticals industry that supplied copies of patented medicines cheaply throughout the world's poor regions. However, in 1994 India signed up to TRIPS and as a result, was required to introduce patents on products by January 2005. This change to Indian patent rules affects the world's poor in two ways; directly by undercutting the supply of affordable medicines and indirectly by removing the generic competition that reduced the cost of brand-name medicines.[40] These poor populations are now worse off and possibly dying, due to a tightening of the existing intellectual property system. At least some of the 10 million avoidable annual deaths alluded to above can be attributed to current developments in the patent system. Hence, we can speak of a direct, recent harm, which relates to the patent system and which could have been avoided without the adoption of the TRIPS agreement. The

36 World Intellectual Property Organization, Treaties and Contracting Parties: www.wipo.int/ treaties/en/ShowResults.jsp?lang=en&treaty_id=6.

37 Suzanne Scotcher, *Innovation and Incentives* (Cambridge, MA: MIT Press, 2004), 34.

38 Carl Nathan, 'Aligning Pharmaceutical Innovation with Medical Need', *Nature Medicine*, 2007, 13(3): 304–8; Josephine Johnston and Angela A. Wasunna, 'Patents Biomedical Research and Treatments – Examining Concerns, Canvassing Solutions', *A Hastings Centre Special Report*, 2007, 37(1): S1–S36.

39 See for instance, Hollis and Pogge, *The Health Impact Fund: Making New Medicines Accessible for All.*

40 Editorial, 'India's Choice', *New York Times* (2005), www.nytimes.com/2005/01/18/ opinion/18tues2.html.

argument that patents are a tortured solution to providing a social good, but alas necessary, does not work for those poor who may die due to the TRIPS regime. Prior to its adoption, pharmaceutical companies researched, developed and produced medical interventions. It was not necessary to adopt TRIPS to provide incentives for pharmaceutical research. But again, the problem is more subtle than this.

High prices of drugs under patent protection are not the only problem endangering poor people's health. Given that the pharmaceutical industry operates almost exclusively within the profit-making sector in line with its primary obligation in a market system (to develop and produce innovative drugs and services that improve the quality of life of patients), diseases that burden the poor are often not investigated in the first place. One can therefore speak of an accessibility problem (i.e. that existing drugs are priced beyond the reach of the poor) and an availability problem (i.e. that drugs are not being developed to address the needs of the poor).[41] It is assumed that stronger patent protection in countries like India, Brazil and South Africa will lead to the growing interest of pharmaceutical companies in so-called neglected diseases, given that purchasing power in those countries is significantly on the increase. Hence, while TRIPS creates direct harm for those poor people who can no longer access cheap generic copies of patented drugs in, say India today, it contributes (at least potentially) to resolving the neglected diseases issue. Going back to the pre-TRIPS regime is therefore no straightforward solution, morally, if one considered future benefit. At the same time, the pharmaceutical sector benefits from a system that imposes direct harm, for instance on the current severely poor in India who would have had access to generic copies of patented drugs without TRIPS.

Corporate social responsibility is usually discussed within the realm of law, enlightened self-interest or benevolence. Either a duty is instructed by law (e.g. health and safety for workers) or self-interest (e.g. continuing education of staff) or benevolence (e.g. donations) or a mixture of the three. But for one business sector, namely those companies that benefit from patents on goods required to satisfy basic needs, a fourth realm must be added; namely a duty of redress for harm from which one benefits.

What follows from this? The creators of the international intellectual property rights system are policy-makers, pressured by lobbyists, among them the pharmaceutical industry. The strongest duty to reduce any foreseeable harm from the current patent system lies with its creators, who have to fine-tune the system to a degree of maximum benefit and minimum harm. One possibility

41   Michael J. Selgelid and Eline M. Sepers, 'Patents, Profits, and the Price of Pills: Implications for Access and Availability,' in P. Illingworth, U. Schuklenk and J. C. Cohen (eds), *The Power of Pills: Social, Ethical and Legal Issues in Drug Development, Marketing and Pricing Policies* (London: Pluto Press, 2006), 153.

is the Health Impact Fund, a reform plan suggested by a team working with Thomas Pogge,[42] and discussed alongside alternative possibilities in Sadie Regmi's chapter in this volume.

At the same time, the system has not only creators, but also beneficiaries, most notably the pharmaceutical industry and those who are affluent enough to enjoy the fruits of scientific progress. Duties of redress for harm imposed on some which achieves benefits for others, apply to both these groups. It is here that one can most reasonably apply the Kantian 'ought implies can'[43] maxim. Pharmaceutical corporations in affluent countries are better placed than civil society to have a fast impact on the health of the poor. They must therefore discharge their responsibility to reduce the harm generated by a system from which they benefit, that is, this is not a supererogatory act.

Conclusion

Each year, 10 million people die unnecessarily, because they have no access to life-saving drugs. To provide such access is generally regarded as a government obligation. Ignoring the notable exception of the United States, almost all states world-wide have accepted this obligation through ratification of relevant human rights instruments. The Millennium Development Goals have added to these instruments by requiring the pharmaceutical industry to help provide access to affordable essential drugs in developing countries. This imposition of duties on industry can be morally justified, while an equivalent duty on affluent individuals and NGOs cannot. Pharmaceutical innovation is the only research activity protected through patents, which targets basic human need satisfaction. As such it is the only research activity, which benefits from intellectual property rights protection while foreseeably harming the poor. Abolishing patents is not the answer, yet giving the industry a share in fulfilling human rights could be. How far this will improve on governments' track record to fulfil the human right to health remains to be seen. Novartis' long-term commitment to leprosy-elimination could point the way.[44]

---

42 See http://healthimpactfund.com
43 'He must judge that he *can* do what the law imposes on him unconditionally that he *ought* to do.' Kant, Immanuel (1990, [1797]) Metaphysische Anfangsgründe der Tugendlehre, Hamburg: Felix Meiner Verlag, 12 (380), my translation.
44 www.novartisfoundation.org/page/content/index.asp?MenuID=217&ID=493&Menu=3& Item=43.2.

13

Institutionalizing Solidarity for Health

Thomas Gebauer

Health: A global common good

Talking about *global health* is certainly fashionable! All over the globe, politicians, scientists and also representatives from NGOs have started to refer to these two words – with notions, however, that widely differ. Most likely, a German journalist being asked about his concept of *global health* would mention global threats such as AIDS/HIV, avian flu, perhaps also tuberculosis, whereas a WHO official may call for a better coordination in a fragmented global landscape of health actors. But *global health* refers to more than just controlling pandemics or calling for managerial improvements. In the first instance, it refers to the need to re-conceptualize health under the premise of the globalized world. Health is an essential condition for human and social development. Thus, from the human-rights perspective *global health* stands for the internationally shared responsibility for the global common good 'health'.

The ambitious goal *Health for All* is not new. It inspired the establishing of the World Health Organisation (WHO) in 1948. Considering the global wealth that has been generated in today's world, the prospect of *Health for All* must not be an illusion any longer. It could have been achieved long ago. *Health for all* is not an issue of creating more wealth, but of the redistribution of existing wealth and income. The world is awash with money. What is missing is the political will for change and the public pressure to make change happen.

In view of the appalling global health crisis, change is urgently needed. Although average life expectancy of the global population has constantly increased over the past 50 years, in Africa and some countries of the former Eastern world, it is declining. Also the second health indicator, the infant mortality rate (IMR), illustrates the inequalities that exist in today's health. From 1,000 live births in Chad, 124 children die before they reach their first birthday. In Sweden, by contrast, the IMR is two.[1]

In the course of economic globalization the world has progressed, no doubt, but the gap between the rich and the poor has become bigger rather than

---

1 WHO, *World Health Statistics 2011* (Geneva: World Health Organisation, 2011), www.who. int/whosis/whostat/EN_WHS2011_Full.pdf, 45–8.

smaller. The neo-liberal promise that the poor would also benefit from the liberalization of trade in goods and capital has been proven wrong. Instead of a trickle-down effect, we witness an expansion of poverty following a cynical hidden agenda: *Take it from the needy, give it to the greedy*. More than ever it makes a difference whether we are born in one of the prosperous regions of the world, the 'global north', or in the zones of social exclusion, poverty and the denial of future perspectives, the 'global south', which in the meantime has also evolved alongside all European and United States – cities.

The good news is that alternatives to the present health inequalities are possible; at least they do not fail because of a lack of resources. However, as alternatives will not appear from nowhere, they can only be realized by dealing with the prevailing power relations that are responsible for the maintenance of the *status quo*. Change for better health requires amendment to, or abolition of, those structural circumstances that fuel the persisting inequalities; it requires social movements guided by a vision of a different world. Academics can be part of this struggle. They can contribute by providing social movements with proper concepts and strategies for creating health justice.

The two areas of change for better health

It is necessary to recognize two areas of struggle that have to be pursued, both at the same time. Getting rid of health inequalities requires both a response to the so-called *Social Determinants of Health* (SDH) and *Universal Coverage* in health-care protection. The first refers to the creation of a social environment that allows people to develop and activate their own health potentials. Appropriate living conditions include access to income or land, to adequate nutrition, housing, education, full participation in cultural life and so on. By emphasizing the importance of the *Social Determinants of Health*, action for global health has to be connected with the struggle for the protection and recovery of fundamental commons such as land (for nutrition), rivers (for clean water), environmental issues and also knowledge (for access to medicine). Besides the struggle for the Social Determinants of Health there is the need also to make every effort for effective health-care services. Even in a perfect world, in which all the Social Determinants of Health are fully recognized, people will fall ill and will suffer accidents and need medical assistance, for example during pregnancy, in old age and so on. Thus, Universal Coverage is not contradictory to the SDH-approach. Universal Coverage means that everyone must have access to preventive, curative and rehabilitative health care when needed. Universal Coverage implies equality of access and financial risk protection.

In this chapter, I concentrate on Universal Coverage. I am doing that surely not with the intention of diminishing or denying the importance of the Social

Determinants of Health. The world is far from having universally healthy living conditions, *and* there is far from universal access to the highest attainable standard of health care. The statistics are appalling:

Every year 18 million die of diseases, which would be preventable through sufficient nutrition, safe water, etc., or easy to treat with essential medicines, re-hydration salt, etc.[2]

- Developing countries account for 84 per cent of global population and 90 per cent of the global disease burden, but only 12 per cent of global health spending.[3]

- Forty-one low-income countries are too poor to generate sufficient resources required to achieve the Millennium Development Goals by 2015.[4]

- Every year about 100 million people are pushed under the poverty line because they need to pay for health services.[5]

Owing to these scandalous global inequalities, the health of the majority of the world population remains insufficiently protected and promoted. Only a minority enjoys complete financial risk protection. The poorer the country, the larger the private share of health expenditure. In 2007, in 33 mostly low-income countries, more than 50 per cent of health expenses were direct out-of-pocket payments charged when people access doctors or health facilities. Such out-of-pocket payments go along with incalculable financial risks. They are the most inequitable source of health financing.[6]

In 2010, on the occasion of presenting the World Health Report: 'Health Systems Financing' in Berlin WHO Director General Margaret Chan called for the abolition of out-of-pocket payments and particularly 'user fees'. Dr Chan has not had a good word to say for the latter. 'User fees' are punishing the poor, said the DG of the WHO,[7] in the presence of representatives of the World Bank, which in the late 1980s and 1990s, together with the International Monetary Fund, heavily promoted 'user fees' as part of the structural adjustment programmes forced on the developing world. From both a development and a human-rights perspective, the past two decades have to be characterized as lost decades.

2   Thomas Pogge, *Poverty and Human Rights* (Geneva: UN-OHCHR, 2008) www2.ohchr.org/english/issues/poverty/expert/docs/Thomas_Pogge_Summary.pdf.
3   Pablo Enrique Gottret and George Schieber, *Health Financing Revisited – A Practitioner's Guide* (Washington DC: The World Bank Publication, 2006), 2.
4   WHO, *World Health Report: Health Systems Financing – The Path to Universal Coverage* (Geneva: WHO, 2010), xiii.
5   Ibid., 5.
6   Ibid., xiv.
7   Thomas Gebauer, 'Universal Coverage – A Shift in the International Debate in Global Health', *Equinet Newsletter*, 2011, 119: 1.

At least, and this is remarkable too, international politics again recognizes what our ancestors have known for centuries: that poverty fuels sickness, and sickness poverty. Because of the correlation between ill-health and poverty, universal access to health care cannot be achieved by connecting health to individual purchasing power. It is right that health experts again search for ways to break out of the vicious cycle of poverty and sickness. A promising strategy consists of five key actions.

Key actions to enhance universal coverage

First and foremost, it is necessary to challenge the neoliberal paradigm of self-responsibility and entrepreneurship. Second, as a prerequisite for improving state accountability there is the need for a health governance reform. Third, out-of-pocket payments have to be reduced by enhancing financial risk protection. Fourth, pooled funds have to be created, and – last but not least – the principle of solidarity recalled and implemented.

Challenging the neoliberal ideology

The struggle for Universal Coverage starts with challenging the still dominant neoliberal paradigm. It is well known that globalization has widened health inequalities. However, more emphasis should be given to the fact that the transforming of health services into commodities, the linkage of access to health care to individual purchasing power, the dismantling of public health systems, has only been possible in the context of a specific ideology – an ideology that has widely affected those who are suffering its negative consequences, the global poor.

At the core of the neo-liberal ideology is a concept that has replaced social values and institutions such as solidarity and common goods by self-responsibility and individual entrepreneurship. Although there is plenty of evidence that health is primarily determined by the social environment, neo-liberalism has succeeded in pushing the responsibility for health away from public and state institutions to private actors and individuals – individuals seen as business entrepreneurs in a liberalized market. Even those spheres of societies that traditionally do not belong to the field of business, such as health, education and culture have been increasingly penetrated by market values.

In his contribution to the conference that gave rise to this book, Professor Angus Dawson stressed the need to consider other values than just the value of Liberty.[8] That's true: we should remind ourselves that the French

Revolution, which came up with the first comprehensive lists of Human Rights in 1789, called for; Liberty, Equality and Fraternity. 'Fraternity', the revolutionary agenda's third pillar, may be equated with 'solidarity' in today's discourse. It is of tremendous importance in the context of achieving Universal Coverage.

During the last decades the idea of solidarity has been under constant siege. 'There is no such a thing as society', Margret Thatcher said in the early 1980s – paving the way for the cynical credo of neoliberal politics; if everyone takes care of him/herself, then 'all' are taken care of. Millions of people have been excluded from health and social care as a consequence of neglect of the social principles that nurture the cohesion of societies. Only by revitalizing solidarity – both as an ethical principle and in its public institutions – can health inequalities be tackled and *Health for All* achieved. Indeed, there is such a thing as society.

The creation of a social environment favourable to health and health protection cannot be settled by market forces alone. Commercial actors might play a role as service providers. However, since their ultimate goal is to make a profit, they have to be regulated by institutions that are committed to the public interest of promoting health.

Improving state accountability

While talking about the accountability of governments and public institutions we should not disregard the amazing fragmentation that has taken place in the international health landscape during the last two decades. On the one hand the rapid emergence of new actors, such as corporate and private foundations, multinational companies, public–private partnerships, has highlighted health as a priority, but at the same time this has also contributed to the weakening of mandated state institutions at all levels.

Particularly the health ministries of many countries in the South have to navigate a verily maze in today's health governance. It is almost impossible to make a national health ministry accountable if it has to deal with dozens of private and international actors, all pursuing their own interests. Similar problems afflict the WHO at the international level.

It is obvious that the chaotic situation that has emerged with the fragmentation has to be overcome. In order to stop the wasting of resources, to avoid duplications of activities, to support national ownership, publicly mandated institutions have to be strengthened – a giant task indeed. It is encouraging that the debate on governance reform has commenced. The best solution is to bring health ministries and the WHO back into the 'driver's seat'. Only if mandated

8   Professor Dawson's talk is available as a podcast: www.isei.manchester.ac.uk/research/ resources/.

institutions again serve as directing and coordinating authorities can we make them accountable: accountable, for example, for introducing financial risk protection schemes – and that is my third point.

Enhance financial risk protection

Financial risk protection means that the major source of health funding needs to come from prepaid and pooled contributions rather than from fees and payments charged once a person falls ill. Universal Coverage will only be possible if direct payments are progressively replaced by pre-payment plans. The most effective ones are legally binding Social Health Insurance (SHI) schemes that are mandatory for all (partly realized in Germany) and tax-based public health systems (as in the United Kingdom). Sometimes health services in tax-based systems are described as being free of charge. That, of course, is not strictly true. State revenues come from tax-payers, and the paying of taxes is – comparable to premiums to social insurance schemes – a kind of pre-payment that protects against financial risks in case of ill-health.

There is a long-standing debate about the advantages and disadvantages of the two systems. It is obvious that tax-based systems are more adequate for countries with a high part of population that is too poor to pay premiums to SHI. The latter, on the other hand, may be better for wealthier countries since the funds collected through SHI schemes are earmarked for health and cannot be misused for other purposes in case of budget constraints.

Besides tax-based systems and SHI plans there are other options, such as the idea of Health Saving Accounts (HSA) as promoted in the United States. The concept of HSA is to oblige people to build up individual savings to be used when health care is needed. With respect to achieving universal coverage such saving accounts are counterproductive. They are part of a consumer-driven health-care system, opposing the idea of health as a common good. They undermine social cohesion: healthy people with higher incomes will prefer HSA while people with health problems will avoid them. Instead of private savings, effective financing for health require pooled funds, and that is my fourth point.

Setting up pooled funds

Both tax-based health systems and social insurance schemes work on the basis of pooled funds. At its best, a pooled fund comprises all citizens of a country and is therefore large enough to cover the risks of all its members. The smaller the group contributing to a pooled fund, the more unlikely it is that all risks can be met. Only if the number of those contributing is great enough can an expensive treatment of a particular person be covered.

The figure shows the WHO model of pooled funds as presented in the World Health Report 'Health Systems Financing'. It works along three

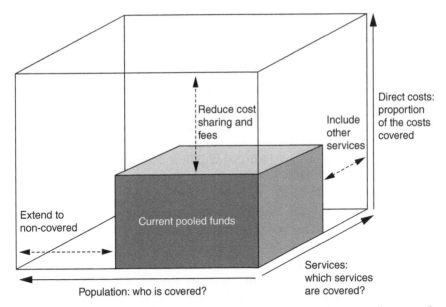

Figure 13.1 **Three dimensions to consider when moving towards universal coverage**[9]

dimensions: expanding the number of people covered; expanding the scope of services; and reducing cost sharing (direct payments such as user fees).

Most remarkably, the WHO model does not speak about just going for some coverage and it also does not advocate for basic protection packages like the ILO does with its concept of a 'Social Protection Floor'.[10] Rather it urges all states to do their utmost to set up pooled funds that provide equal care for everybody. It is a dynamic model that never loses sight of the claim to fully realize the Right to Health. Even if this may not be possible from one day to the next, the duty bearers, the states, are obliged to present strategies and corresponding plans of action describing the way towards the goal to achieve universal coverage. Such an approach opens the space for national adaptations based on democratic decision-making and invites civil society organizations to continuously challenge their governments.

Under ideal conditions all citizens of a country enjoy social health protection, without compromises in the service package and without any extra-payments. Although that sounds utopian it can be achieved – by reiterating solidarity.

The principle of solidarity

Since in every country a part of the population is too poor to contribute to pooled funds, Universal Coverage requires the presence of a permanent and

9 WHO, *World Health Report*, xv.
10 See: www.ilo.org/gimi/gess/ShowTheme.do?tid=1321.

institutionalized system of redistributing wealth. The poor need to be subsidized by those who are in the position to contribute more. Precisely this balancing is established through the principle of solidarity. It is perhaps the most important key to establishing an effective health-care system.

In this context, it does not matter whether a system is tax-financed or based on SHI schemes. Both are socially agreed funding schemes guaranteeing that even members who are not in a position to contribute a single shilling or cent to national budgets or social insurance will receive the same services as all the others members when they need them. While individual contributions (in terms of taxes or insurance premiums) are dependent on financial capacities, the entitlement to and claiming of services is only determined by need. It is the principle of solidarity that disconnects access to health care from individual purchasing power: those who are wealthier support those who are poorer, younger or elderly. Those who are economically active, support children and those who are unemployed or retired.

Thus, the principle of solidarity goes far beyond what is usually meant when solidarity refers to empathy and charity. The principle refers rather to an institutionalized solidarity that organizes a fair burden sharing. It is fundamental to the 'social infrastructure' of societies. Like the hard infrastructure such as transportation, energy, administration, law enforcement, police and so on, the social infrastructure also needs to be publicly regulated and funded. The term social infrastructure stands for an ensemble of common goods, such as effective health-care services, proper education systems, social protection schemes, food security and so on. In other words, it covers social institutions that are essential for the social cohesion of societies and should therefore be accessible to everybody, regardless of any individual's purchasing power.

Sooner or later, societies will collapse if they lack the social institutions that protect healthy relationships among their citizens. Fair burden sharing, however, needs to be based on mandatory contributions. Otherwise the rich will opt out. It is sad but a fact that all over the globe the rich prefer private assurances or seek tax-dodging and tax avoidance. The corporate sector has done a lot to achieve tax exemption.[11] Sufficient funding to cover the needs of the poor requires compulsory contributions from the rich.

Innovative funding for health

Achieving proper health care depends on the availability of adequate financial resources. The existing health inequalities can only be abolished

---

11 For further reading see, for example Trades Union Congress, *The Missing Billions – The UK Tax Gap*, www.tuc.org.uk/touchstone/missingbillions/1missingbillions.pdf.

through increased public spending rather than continuing social cuts. In view of the global poverty that has already affected one third of the world's population, fiscal policy-making has again to focus on the redistribution of wealth. That sounds quite radical, but even the WHO goes along with it. The World Health Report 'Health Systems Financing' (WHO, 2010) invites the WHO Member States to introduce new fiscal measures in order to enhance governmental revenue capacities. Taxation is seen as one of the key policy instruments to widen the fiscal space. As suitable options WHO proposes:

- A special levy on large and profitable companies;
- A levy on currency transactions;
- A financial transaction tax; and
- Taxes on tobacco, unhealthy food, etc.[12]

It is remarkable that the Report does not mention public–private partnerships as a source of new funding opportunities. Resource innovation goes far beyond the attempt to attract private foundations and the corporate sector. The call for tax justice through progressive taxation is back on the political agenda; it provides civil society organizations with a powerful tool to challenge their governments. Governments should not be allowed to remain inactive just given the assertion that there are no or insufficient resources. In order to properly respond to the social needs of their populations, governments are encouraged to widen their fiscal space. Accountability implies financial capacity, and only adequately funded institutions can be made accountable. If the call for health as a common good in collective responsibility is not just dealing with nice words, health needs to be essentially seen in the context of financing for health.

However, some of the poorest countries will not be able to raise sufficient funds to meet all the health needs even if their governments show the political will for change and try to activate the necessary resources. Maybe because the domestic economy is too weak or the negative impact of the global economy too strong they fail to balance needs with capacities. In these countries, governments have limited ability to collect taxes or premiums to SHI schemes because people simply are poor or work in the informal sector.

As mentioned above, only 8 of the 49 low-income countries will be able to finance the required level of services from domestic resources in 2015.

In 2001 the WHO Commission on Macroeconomics and Health estimated that even a very basic set of services for prevention and treatment would cost

---

12 WHO, *World Health Report*, 29.

in excess of US$ 34 per person per year. However, 31 countries spend less than US$ 35 per capita on health.[13]

Of course there is every reason to strive for self-reliance and to resist any kind of economic dependency, but change may take time or may fail because of circumstances that cannot be influenced by single governments, such as the effects of climate change and natural disasters. In these cases, the gaps between the fiscal needs and fiscal capacity of particular countries can only be bridged by financial support from abroad – support that should be based on global solidarity. And that is where the call for an 'International Fund for Health' comes in.

Globalizing the principle of solidarity

At an international conference on 'Strengthening Local Campaigns for National and International Accountability for Health and Health Services', held in Johannesburg, South Africa in March 2011, delegates called for 'the principles of social solidarity that are an accepted part of governance within many nations to be extended to the international level'.[14]

Health-care systems based on the principle of solidarity (still) exist in European countries, where they form part of the foundations of societies. Most likely these systems can only be defended by extending them to the international level. In dealing with the neo-liberalism that is persistently posing threats to societies by dismissing solidarity institutions as a proof of 'devilish socialism', it is crucial to again to struggle for solidarity. This struggle needs to be waged at the national level, but it also includes an international dimension. To bridge the gaps, an international financing mechanism is required that obliges rich countries to contribute also to the health budgets of poorer ones.

The Universal Declaration of Human Rights provides the legal foundation for such obligations. Paragraph 28 states that everyone is entitled to a social *and international* order in which the rights and freedoms that are set forth in this Declaration can be fully realized. 'The existing international institutional order fails this test, it aggravates extreme poverty', says the Yale philosopher Thomas Pogge: 'The rich countries (are) violating human rights when they, in collaboration with Southern elites, impose a global institutional order

---

13 Ke Xu, David B. Evans, Guido Carrin, Ana Mylena Aguilar-Rivera, Philip Musgrove and Timothy Evans, 'Protecting Households from Catastrophic Health Spending – Moving Away from Out-of-Pocket Health Care Payments to Prepayment Mechanisms Is the Key to Reducing Financial Catastrophe', *Health Affairs*, 2007, 26(4): 979.

14 Conference Statement, *Strengthen Local Campaigns for National and International Accountability for Health and Health Services*, Section 27 (2011), www.section27.org.za/wp-content/uploads/2011/04/Johannesburg-Conference-Consensus-and-Resolutions-final.pdf.

under which, foreseeably and avoidably, hundreds of millions cannot attain "a standard of living adequate for the health and well-being of himself and of his family (Paragraph 25 of Universal Declaration of Human Rights)".'[15]

From a human-rights perspective, establishing a global institution that would correct the negative effects of the current global order by redistributing wealth and health-related resources is not a matter of nice-to-have, but an obligation. Such an institution would have to manage two main tasks. It should organize a fair burden sharing between those countries providing the funds. And it should also see to it that these funds are properly used by recipient countries. Such an institution could be seen as 'a method to transpose collective entitlements and duties into individual states' entitlements and duties'.[16]

The managing of an International Fund for Health does not necessarily require the creation of a new big bureaucratic body – another Geneva-based health actor with thousands of staff members centrally designing programmes and vertically dominating recipient countries. Gorik Ooms and Rachel Hammonds propose to transform the existing Global Fund to Fight AIDS/HIV, Tuberculosis and Malaria (GFATM) into a Global Health Fund by expanding GFATM's mandate from a limited vertical disease approach to a horizontal strengthening of national health systems.[17] It would also be possible to create a small new authority that completely refrains from any operational activity and is just in charge of running a horizontal equalization payment scheme.

Such equalization payments exist at national, regional and even international levels. They exist in countries such as Australia, Belgium, Canada and Germany. The German model is of particular interest here. To balance the economic gaps among the 'Bundesländer' (federal states), those with higher fiscal capacity are legally obliged to transfer funds to those lacking fiscal capacity. The German equalization payment works horizontally between the federal states. It is based on highly complex calculations taking into account things such as the tax revenues of the states, their population figures and the population density. In 2010 the volume that has been transferred between the states accounted for almost €7 billion; organized by an institution that does not play a big role in the public's mind because it is just raising the right data, feeding computers and arranging it so that equalization payments can be made.[18]

---

15 Pogge, *Poverty and Human Rights*, 3.
16 Gorik Ooms and Rachel Hammonds, 'Correcting Globalisation in Health: Transnational Entitlements versus the Ethical Imperative of Reducing Aid-Dependency', *Public Health Ethics*, 2008, 1(2): 160.
17 Ibid., 154–170. See also Ooms and Hammonds' chapter in this book.
18 For further reading, see Bundesfinanzministerium (Federal Ministry of Finance) The Federal Financial Equalisation System in Germany, available at www.bundesfinanzministerium.de/ nn_4480/DE/BMF__Startseite/Service/Downloads/Abt__V/The_20Federal_20Financial_20E qualisation_20System_20in_20Germany,templateId=raw,property=publicationFile.pdf.

Comparable schemes exit at regional levels: the European Social Fund, for example, which was established to balance the needs of the European regions in the context of education, services for unemployed and so on, is handling €75 billion at present. And even at the international level there is an example for an equalization payment mechanism. It is part of the Universal Postal Union that was founded in 1874. At that time the national postal authorities agreed on a treaty regulating the financial requirements that arise when a letter, sent, for instance, in Germany is to be delivered in India, Malawi or the United Kingdom. In other words, when a fee charged in Germany has to also cover the expenses of services provided in other countries. Today, hardly anybody knows of the existence of the Universal Postal Union. But its creation was crucial to allowing global communication, and it still works. The Universal Postal Union shows that the best common goods are those that do their work without causing a fuss. If establishing such an international equalization payment scheme was possible in the nineteenth century, why not again today in the context of global governance for health?

International Fund for Health

The lessons learned in the context of the Global Fund to Fight AIDS, Tuberculosis and Malaria (GFATM) show the way to universal coverage. On one side the progress achieved in responding to HIV/AIDS not only demonstrates the effectiveness of international funding instruments, but it also makes clear that an approach focusing on just three diseases is inadequate to address the problems in the longer term. Ad hoc success stories like these cannot last unless effective health systems are built up. Long-term results – and experience with the GFATM demonstrates this – require mandatory rather than voluntary contributions: there must be contractually guaranteed funding.

Therefore an International Fund for Health should be firmly based on a legally binding treaty. Both fair burden sharing among the countries that contribute to the fund as well as the claiming of access should be transparently regulated, based on a human rights approach. An international legal agreement could be arranged either by signing a treaty that just covers the global funding aspect or as an additional protocol to a 'Framework Convention on Global Health' (FCGH), as proposed by Larry Gostin and the 'Joint Action and Learning Initiative' (JALI).[19]

Obviously an International Fund for Health would change the existing paradigm of international co-operation. It would transform Official Development

---

19   Lawrence O. Gostin, Eric A. Friedman, Gorik Ooms, Thomas Gebauer, Narendra Gupta, Devi Sridhar, Wang Chenguang, John-Arne Røttingen and David Sanders, 'The Joint Action and Learning Initiative: Towards a Global Agreement on National and Global Responsibilities for Health', *PLoS Medicine*, 2011, 8(5): e1001031. See also Gostin's chapter in this book.

Assistance (ODA) from a donor–recipient interest-driven type of aid to a system of co-operation that is based on entitlements and joint responsibility. Particularly, because an 'International Fund for Health' will not operate as a global body vertically implementing health programmes, the use of transferred funds has to be legally bound by appropriate guidelines and principles. And these guidelines already exist. First and foremost the International Covenant of Economic, Social and Cultural Rights plus the General Comments, the Primary Health Care Declaration of the WHO, the concept of Universal Coverage claiming equal access for all and other such instruments. Undoubtedly there is sufficient knowledge of how to achieve Health for All. And there are already internationally agreed principles. All that is missing are the institutions to set the knowledge and principles into force.

However, what are the costs? Would it not be much too expensive to run such a fund? Again, it is not the money that is missing. Paying for an International Fund for Health would be feasible. The existing figures provide clarity. The World Health Report mentions an annual amount of US$ 60 per capita to realize access to appropriate health care in today's poor countries. Below the line the total amount required would still be in the range of what is already promised by high-income countries. The costs to significantly improve health-care funding in the least-developed world would not exceed the 15 per cent margin of health out of the 0.7 per cent goal for ODA. But even if we insist on global health equity – and there is no reason not to go for equity – and calculate US$ 500–700 per capita there would be no need to generate new funds. US$ 500–700 would certainly be a good start to enable all citizen of the world to enjoy health-care protection – without exceeding the total of global expenditures for health: in 2007 the world has spent US$ 4.1 trillion for health, which amounts to US$ 639 per person per year.[20]

Taking the principle of solidarity forward internationally is not a matter of finding missing resources. It is rather a matter of the political will to create a new institutional norm ensuring that richer countries with higher fiscal capacity are obliged to transfer funds to poorer countries, as long as these are lacking adequate fiscal capacity. However, this may raise another concern that has to be taken seriously. How can we avoid internationally supplied resources displacing national efforts? In fact, today's international aid quite often brings with it the effect that recipient countries decrease the allocation of domestic resources. However, having a closer look at the facts it becomes obvious that it is precisely the unreliability of today's international aid that prevents countries from allocating more of their own resources.

Setting up a proper health system in poor countries is certainly quite cost-intensive. A government that is trying to do this by using international

20   WHO, *Spending on Health: A Global Overview: Fact sheet No. 319* (Geneva: WHO, 2007), www.who.int/mediacentre/factsheets/fs319/en/index.html.

donations given just for a short period could find itself left behind with unaffordable costs when funding from aboard stops. Under these circumstances countries may prefer not to invest in national health-care systems. Thus, it is rather the long-term reliability of international co-financing that allows and motivates national planning based on a steady increase of internal resources.[21]

To summarize, innovative mechanisms for health systems financing need to be based on the redistribution of wealth, a kind of social transfer that goes beyond charity. Funding for health addresses the entitlements of human beings. People in need should not be seen as objects of good will activities. They are human beings enjoying the legal claim to health. To be able to respond to the entitlements of people, mandatory and predictable funding mechanisms have to be created that regulate a fair burden sharing and ensure the proper use of funds. However, international funding mechanisms, even the proposed International Fund for Health, are only the second best option. As their task would be to balance existing financial gaps, everything has to be done to strengthen national capacities on the front line. The global south needs to regain control over its own resources.

Yes, utopian

An International Fund for Health may be considered as utopian. Yes, there is a kind of utopianism, but change will only be possible if we go beyond pragmatism. Looking to all that is happening in today's world in the name of realism, we see that 'realism' has long proven to be wrong-headed. And there is a window of opportunity for change. Margret Thatcher's dictum: 'There Is No Alternative' – known as the TINA principle – is no longer convincing.

Change can be successful if there is the 'desire for change', actively expressed by an engaged international public: by social movements, community organizations, civil society creating a 'countervailing power'. Precisely this strong public is needed to gain the 'diplomatic space' that allows the negotiation of new norms and the setting up of new institutions.

Globalization has reached a point where, for the first time ever, signs of a world society are emerging. This is good news. The creation of an International Health Fund firmly belongs on the political agenda. For the benefit of all in the globalized world, national solidarity institutions such as a tax-based health system or mandatory social health insurance schemes will only survive if the principle of solidarity itself becomes globalized. That is the level where self-interest meets ethics.

---

21   Gorik Ooms, 'Fiscal Space and the Importance of Long Term Reliability of International Co-Financing', *JALI*-Working paper No. 1 (2011).

14

Reinforcing Global Health Normative Frameworks and Legal Obligations: Can Adaptive Governance Help?

William Onzivu

Introduction

Global health law: A challenge of governance

The world population faces unprecedented transnational public health threats due to increased travel, environmental changes, modern communications and other technological change.[1] The double burden of infectious and non-infectious diseases,[2] including influenza A (H1N1), HIV/AIDS, malaria, tuberculosis, maternal and child diseases and tobacco demonstrate the globalized nature of contemporary public health threats.[3] Globalization in the face of poor domestic health systems[4] has accentuated the spread of disease and harmful products, undermining public health.[5] Public health legislation in most of the developing world is obsolete and in urgent need of reform.[6] Unfortunately, the governance of international health cooperation is not optimized to promote global health. First, global health institutions including the World Health Organization (WHO), face challenges in tackling the underlying determinants of health, such as poverty, which in turn damages global health.[7] Secondly, the inhabitants of international health space now include a multiplicity of States, international

1   Tony McMichael and Robert Beaglehole, 'The Global Context of Public Health', in Robert Begalehole (ed.), *Global Public Health, a New Era* (Oxford: Oxford University Press, 2003).
2   World Health Organization, *World Health Report 1999: Making a Difference*, (WHO, 1999).
3   World Health Organization, Influenza A(H1N1): Frequently Asked Questions: www.who.int/csr/disease/swineflu/frequently_asked_questions/en/.
4   World Health Organization, *World Health Report 2008: Primary Health Care – Now More than Ever* (WHO, 2009).
5   William Onzivu, 'Globalism, Regionalism or Both: Health Policy and Regional Economic Integration in Developing Countries, an Evolution of a Legal Regime?', *Minnesota Journal of International Law*, 2006, 15(1): 117.
6   Commonwealth Secretariat review of public health legislation across the 54 Member States of the Commonwealth Secretariat, report on file with the author, 22 July 2011.
7   Allyn Taylor, 'Global Governance, in International Health Law and WHO: Looking towards the Future', *Bulletin of the World Health Organization*, 2002, 80(12): 975–80.

organizations and other non-state actors.[8] The roles of these actors in shaping global health governance continue to evolve.[9] The multiplicity of actors has also led to challenges of accountability, institutional fragmentation and normative congestion in global health. Thirdly, existing health governance models have not optimized global health despite the pluralistic discourses in biomedicine, economics, human rights, security and neo-liberalism.[10] Therefore, the search for alternative models is critical. In this chapter, I argue that adaptive governance has the potential to reinforce global health governance.

Global health legal and normative frameworks: Definition

The WHO Constitution defines health as a 'state of complete physical, mental and social well-being and not merely the absence of disease or infirmity'. Global health law includes several multilateral treaties, rules, regulations and dispute settlement mechanisms that all contribute to promoting health, addressing global health threats such as infectious diseases, tobacco control and food safety.[11] It also includes resolutions adopted by WHO organs such as its World Health Assembly,[12] and WHO Regional Committees.[13] The emerging field of global health law has expanded the scope of health beyond the domestic to the comparative, regional and global.[14] Gostin defines global health law as the body of substantive, procedural and institutional laws that aim at creating conditions for the highest attainable physical and mental health.[15]

8   Kent Buse and Gill Walt, 'An Unruly Melange? Coordinating External Resources to the Health Sector: A Review', *Social Science & Medicine*, 1997, 45: 449–63; Kelly Lee, Suzanne Fustukian and Kent Buse, 'An Introduction to Global Health Policy', in Kelly Lee, Kent Buse and Suzanne Fustukian (eds), *Health Policy in a Globalising World* (Cambridge: Cambridge University Press, 2002), 3–17; Kelly Lee and Hillary Goodman, 'Global Policy Networks: The Propagation of Healthcare Financing Reform since the 1980s', in Kelly Lee, Kent Buse and Suzanne Fustukian (eds), *Health Policy in a Globalising World* (Cambridge: Cambridge University Press, 2002).

9   Obijior Aginam, 'Health or Trade? A Critique of Contemporary Approaches to Global Health Diplomacy', *Asian Journal of WTO and International Health Law and Policy*, 2010, 5(2): 355–80.

10   Kelly Lee, 'Understanding of Global Health Governance: The Contested Landscape', in Adrian Kay and Owain Williams (eds), *Global Health Governance: Crisis, Institutions and Political Economy* (London: Palgrave, 2009); Ibid.

11   David Fidler, 'International Law and Global Public Health', *Kansas Law Review*, 1999, 48: 1–26.

12   WHO Resolution. WHA61.19: www.who.int/whr/2008/whr08_En.pdf.

13   WHO Regional Office for Africa, *The Work of WHO in the African Region 2008: Annual Report of the Regional Director* (Reg'l Comm. Res. AFR/RC59/2, 2009), 26.

14   Michel Belanger, *Global Health Law, an Introduction* (Cambridge: Cambridge Scientific Publishers & Editions des Archives Contemporaines, 2011), 22–32.

15   Lawrence Gostin, 'Meeting Basic Survival Needs of the World's Least Healthy People toward a Framework Convention on Global Health', *Georgetown Law Journal*, 2008, 96: 331–92; Lawrence Gostin and Allyn Lisa Taylor, 'Global Health Law: A Definition and Grand Challenges', *Public Health Ethics*, 2008, 1: 53–63; see also Gostin's chapter in this book.

Adaptive governance: The scope

Adaptive governance institutions are those 'capable of generating long-term, sustainable policy solutions' to complex and dynamic natural resource problems through collaboration among diverse resource users and governmental agencies.[16] This form of governance is adaptable, flexible and responsive and extends from natural systems to human organizations. It reacts to surprises from ecological and human institutions and systems.[17] Adaptive governance recognizes that, because science is constantly evolving, our understanding of natural systems or the effect of human interactions on them is rarely complete.[18] Scientific answers are social constructs and instead of long-term scientific predictions of outcomes and adopting one-time static policies, adaptive management monitors outcomes and maintains flexibility to alter policies, should predictions prove inaccurate or scientific understanding advance. The concept would ensure that institutions, laws and policies are appropriately flexible to address the dynamic global health challenges as the science, learning and other evidence evolve.

Adaptive governance has its origins in complexity theory. Rooted in physical and biological sciences its scope is now broad.[19] At the core of complexity theory is not a cluster of unrelated systems but a complex adaptive system.[20] The relationships between the inter-related parts of this system, the combination of their autonomy and interaction, the capacity of the system for self-adaptation, self-reorganization and the potential for new properties emerge.[21] Over time, several fields of study have developed within the social sciences unified by three common themes: the complexity and uncertainty associated with various aspects of social life; the need for some intensified form of 'social learning' as a response to this uncertainty; and the role of institutions and governance systems in facilitating such learning processes. The increasing complexity and volatility of modern markets has led many to focus on the role of innovation

16 John T. Scholz and Bruce Stiftel (eds), *Adaptive Governance and Water Conflict: New Institutions for Collaborative Planning* (Washington, DC: Resources for the Future Press, 2005), 5.
17 Ibid., 2.
18 J. B. Ruhl, 'Thinking of Environmental Law as a Complex Adaptive System: How to Clean up the Environment by Making a Mess of Environmental law', *Houston Law Review*, 1997, 34: 933; Carl Folke, Thomas Hahn, Per Olsson and Jon Norberg, 'Adaptive Governance of Socio-ecological Systems', *Annual Review of Environment and Resources*, 2005, 30: 441; James Oglethorpe, *Adaptive Management: From Theory to Practice* (Gland, Switzerland: IUCN, 2002).
19 Paul Cilliers, *Complexity and Post Modernism* (London: Routledge, 1998), 112–40.
20 James N. Rosenau, *Distant Proximities: Dynamics beyond Globalization* (Princeton, NJ: Princeton University Press, 2003), 212–13.
21 James N. Rosenau, 'NGOs and Fragmented Authority in Globalizing Space', in Yale Ferguson and Barry R. J. Jones (eds), *Political Space: Frontiers of Change and Governance in a Globalizing World* (New York: State of New York Press, 2002).

and adaptability in economic life. This has necessitated research into learning processes within organizations, as well as the problem of creating reflexive institutional frameworks to facilitate constant learning and innovation across national, regional and global institutions. Secondly, in international relations, scholarship on the behaviour of states in complex interdependence has focused on developing flexible and adaptive international institutions, to respond to rapidly changing global conditions and knowledge of their causes. Others focus on the role of international institutions in counteracting potentially paralysing uncertainty, helping states to develop cognitive models to survive in a complex world, and to identify the interests in it.

Thirdly, work in public law, on learning-centred alternatives to traditional command-and-control regulatory frameworks, has spurred experimentalist and new governance approaches.[22] The integration of the social sciences enriches adaptive governance transcending natural, ecological, human and social processes and institutions. Adaptive governance in social spheres and institutions, including health, requires refinements augmented by social theories. This chapter focuses on five key features of adaptive governance: continuous learning, policy making as experimentation, avoiding irreversible harm, monitoring and feedback and pluralism and process.

Continuous learning

Adaptive governance focuses on facilitating continuous learning as a sine qua non of any response to uncertainty and systemic unpredictability of a social system. A one-time view of the world, scientific or normative, is inadequate to reflect dynamic and evolving realities and to respond to continually changing information and understanding. In global health, policy-making is often based on scientific or other form of evidence. This reflects the importance of continuous learning as a key element of adaptive governance.

Learning in adaptive governance is both simple and complex. Simple learning refers to the acquisition of information, the development of new skills and the building of new competencies.[23] In simple learning, actors participate in the regulatory process, receive new and updated information, learn how to resolve defined problems more effectively and adapt their problem-solving skills to changing conditions. This would require adjustment to health policies to achieve set goals. However, complex learning is not simply a response to inadequate information but to the fundamental limitations of human cognition. It goes beyond learning better solutions to defined problems to redefining

---

22 Peter Hill, 'Understanding Global Health Governance as a Complex Adaptive System', *Global Public Health*, 2011, 6(6): 593–605.
23 Meric S. Gertler and David A. Wolfe, *Innovation and Social Learning: Institutional Adaptation in an Era of Technological Change* (Macmillan/Palgrave: Basingstoke, 2002).

the particular problem and knowledge about it.[24] Complex learning entails expanding awareness of the inherently limited nature of human knowledge and recognizes people's intrinsic ignorance and capacity for mistake. This learning may require reconstitution of actors' preferences, identities and beliefs and the reconstruction of policy-makers' cognitive map which they use to make sense of their world and redefine it.[25]

Policy-making as experimentation

Policy interventions are often viewed as separate from knowledge accumulation and risk-analysis. In adaptive governance, policy-making is a central component of the learning process. Policy interventions are learning by doing and quasi-experiments. Unforeseen consequences are treated as valuable opportunities for learning. This experimental approach implies that policy makers must act despite uncertainties. Adaptive governance is designed to trigger action in conditions of incomplete knowledge without postponing action until 'enough' is known. It acknowledges that time and resources are too short to defer action to tackle urgent problems.[26] Policy interventions in adaptive governance are focused towards generating critical information to enhance certainty, knowledge and experience base. Adaptive governance requires deliberate experimentation to generate the information.[27] However, active policy changes must be reversible without risk-taking in decision making.[28] Such deliberate experimental interventions require resilience, supervisory and accountability mechanisms and the assurance that adaptive management interventions do not risk unacceptable and irreversible outcomes.[29]

24 Joanne Scott and David M. Trubek, 'Mind the Gap: Law and New Approaches to Governance in the European Union', *European Law Journal*, 2002, 8(1): 1–18; Charles F. Sabel, 'Learning by Monitoring: The Institutions of Economic Development', in Neil J. Smelser and Richard Swedberg (eds), *The Handbook of Economic Sociology* (Princeton, NJ: Princeton University Press, 2005).

25 David Schlosberg, 'Reconceiving Environmental Justice: Global Movements and Political Theories', *Environmental Politics*, 2004, 13(2): 517–40; Alexander Wendt, *Social Theory of International Politics* (Cambridge: Cambridge University Press, 1999), 1–6.

26 Ronald D. Brunner, Lindy Coe-juell, Christina Cromley, Christine Edwards, Toddi A. Steelman and Donna Tucker, *Adaptive Governance: Integrating Science, Policy and Decision Making* (New York: Columbia University Press, 2005), 2; Kai N. Lee, 'Appraising Adaptive Management', *Conservation Ecology*, 1999, 3(2): 3.

27 Catherine Allan and George B. Stankey (eds), *Adaptive Environmental Management, a Practitioners Guide* (London: Springer, 2009); Carl Walters, 'Challenges in Adaptive Management of Riparian and Coastal Ecosystems', *Conservation Ecology*, 1997, 1(2).

28 Brunner, Coe-juell, Cromley, Edwards, Steelman and Tucker, *Adaptive Governance*, 2.

29 Derek Armitage, Fikret Berkes and Nancy Doubleday, *Collaboration, Learning and Multi-Level Governance: Adaptive Co-Management* (UBC Press, 2007), 19, 83; Lance Gunderson, 'Resilience, Flexibility and Adaptive Management – Antidotes for Spurious Certitude?', *Conservation Ecology*, 1999, 3(1), 7.

Avoiding irreversible harm

Recognition of the uncertain, dynamic and evolving character of environmental, social and economic systems leads to a strong emphasis on maintaining the resilience of a system.[30] As it is impossible to predict exactly what a complex system will do, or to engineer a static desired policy condition, one pivotal goal of policy becomes the maintenance of system resilience, and its ability to adapt and evolve. This helps avoid irreversible negative environmental or social conditions, but can restrain subsequent policy options, experimentation and learning. Adaptive governance favours impermanent, reversible policy interventions and adoption of strict oversight mechanisms to encourage or ensure reversibility. Policy responses to uncertainties are selected on their robustness. In this way, irreversible and damaging global health policy is minimized or avoided and options for improved health decision making is unfettered.

Monitoring and feedback

Policy-making in adaptive governance is an iterative process of review and revision. Scientific knowledge is not definitive or final, but subject to review as new information and priorities emerge.[31] The smooth functioning of this iterative process depends critically on the progressive development of mechanisms for regular monitoring of specificity of processes and outcomes of policy interventions. Outcomes of monitoring processes routinely feed back into the policy process, to reassess policy goals, assumptions and objectives themselves.[32] Such self-conscious monitoring and feedback mechanisms facilitate learning, fine-tune policy instruments, highlight knowledge gaps, reveal the shortcomings of problem-definition and knowledge and create a culture of openness and experimentation in the conduct of policy.[33]

Pluralism and process

Cooney and Lang emphasize that adaptive governance approaches necessitate pluralist approaches to knowledge as its production and application is a socio-political process.[34] They argue that governance structures are not focused towards identifying a single, correct body of knowledge to guide policy, but to

---

30 Ibid.
31 Carl Bruch, 'Adaptive Water Management: Strengthening Laws and Institutions to Cope with Uncertainty', in Asit K. Biswas, Cecilia Tortajada and Rafael Izquierdo-Avino (eds), *Water Management in 2020 and Beyond* (Heidelberg: Springer, 2009).
32 Rosie Cooney and Andrew T. F. Lang, 'Taking Uncertainty Seriously: Adaptive Governance and International Trade', *The European Journal of International Law*, 2007, 18: 523–51.
33 Ibid.
34 Ibid.

mobilize alternative knowledge, map out uncertainties and enable a disciplined process for decision-making in areas of uncertainty.[35] The aim of policy-making is not solely to accumulate knowledge, but also to discover and highlight the inadequacies of prevailing knowledge frameworks. Policy-making is less about the attainment of a single optimal solution and more about providing a forum for creating consensual knowledge and agreed processes to guide policy.[36] This implies that policy-making processes and underlying knowledge assumptions and judgements should be transparent, explicit and open to scrutiny. Adaptive governance emphasizes open forums for discursive and communicative interaction – information exchange and problem-centred negotiation – in policy formulation. A second implication is the need for broader participation in the production and deployment of knowledge. Adaptive governance prioritizes broader participation in the production and deployment of knowledge due to the diverse values and knowledge of different stakeholders. Approaches integrating multiple perspectives often produce better outcomes and 'efficient' public policy becomes redefined as policy which responds as far as possible to the values, interests and concerns of all stakeholders.[37]

Adaptive governance and WHO law

The WHO constitution

The Constitution of the WHO was adopted in 1946 as the UN Charter that empowered the WHO to spearhead global health protection and promotion within the United Nations system.[38] The Constitution endows WHO with the powers to adopt Conventions, regulations and recommendations that deal with any matters within its competence.[39] The Constitution also empowers WHO's World Health Assembly (WHA) to adopt regulations on sanitation and quarantine, nomenclatures of diseases, causes of death, public health practices and standards for international diagnostic procedures. The Constitution has enabled WHO to spearhead the development and implementation of the WHO Framework Convention on Tobacco Control, the International Health Regulations (2005) and the Nomenclature Regulations. WHO has adopted significant Resolutions in areas such as human rights, health workforce,

---

35   Ibid.
36   Mario Giampietro, 'Complexity and Scales: The Challenge for Integrated Assessment', *Scaling in Integrated Assessment*, 2003, 3(2/3): 247.
37   Oglethorpe, *Adaptive Management*.
38   United Nations, United Nations Charter, Article 57.
39   World Health Organization, *Basic Documents, Constitution of the World Health Organization*, Articles 1–2, 45th edn (WHO, 2005).

neglected diseases, public–private partnerships, climate change and intellectual property, innovation and public health.

The WHO Constitution demonstrates the complexities and need for flexibility in WHO law in the following aspects. First, the WHO constitutional definition of health as a state of complete physical, mental and social well-being, and not merely the absence of disease or infirmity, is evolutionary in its implementation.[40] The definition also reflects health as psychosocial and physical, acknowledging that humans adapt in social environments.[41] At WHO's creation in 1946, it was envisaged that the Constitution would provide a framework for international law to play an expanding role in global health. The WHA has broad standard setting functions and addresses public health issues that are often evolutionary, complex, uncertain and requiring new knowledge to inform policy. Secondly, the WHO Constitution is a functional and purposive instrument. It is general and flexible reflecting changing political environments and processes that have enabled WHO to assume roles unforeseen when it was established and its Constitution adopted. Thirdly, the WHO Constitution envisages its operation through multi-sectoral and collaborative actions.[42] Reflective of this approach, WHO constitutional space is inhabited by stakeholders beyond the organization and its member States and includes other UN system organizations and civil society. It is in this context that, for example, WHO houses over 20 public–private partnerships in global health that include the Global Alliance on Vaccine and Immunization (GAVI) and the Medicines for Malaria Venture (MMV). The Constitution also empowers WHO to promote scientific, technical and legal learning and participation of diverse actors. The challenge for WHO is expanding the diversity of inhabitants in its constitutional and policy space in the public interest.

The WHO Framework Convention on Tobacco Control

With over 170 parties to date, the WHO Framework Convention on Tobacco Control (FCTC) has been hailed as one of the major public health treaties.[43] FCTC requires its parties to implement public health protection measures by regulating tobacco advertising, promotion, sponsorship, packaging and labelling.[44] It also regulates the tobacco industry,[45] illicit trade in tobacco products, tobacco price and tax measures, sales of tobacco, treatment of tobacco dependence, smoke-free environments, research and exchange of information,

---

40 WHO, *Basic Documents*, Preamble.
41 Jennifer Prah Ruger, 'Global Health Justice', *Public Health Ethics*, 2009, 2(3) (2009): 261–75, 267.
42 Gian Luca Burci, 'Institutional Adaptation without Reform: WHO and the Challenges of Globalization', *International Organization Law Review*, 2005, 2: 437–43.
43 WHO, Framework Convention on Tobacco Control, 42 I.L.M. 518 (2003).
44 Ibid., Articles 9–10.
45 Ibid., Article 5(3).

scientific, technical and legal cooperation.[46] The Conference of Parties has adopted guidelines on tobacco labelling and packaging, advertisement and promotion, exposure to tobacco smoke and on monitoring the tobacco industry. The development and implementation of the Convention is a catalyst for an adaptive framework of governance for several reasons. First, the Convention requires multi-sectoral tobacco control measures at the global, regional and national levels. Its state negotiators were a mix of health, foreign affairs, trade and finance officials that also exhibited sectoral tensions.[47] Secondly, the Convention adopts a demand control approach to tobacco regulation through tax and price measures that must be reviewed and changed periodically, to meet evolving tobacco control needs.[48] Thirdly, the treaty provides for its implementation without exclusive reliance on protocol,[49] and recognizes Parties' obligations in other international instruments while prioritizing their right to protect public health.[50] Fourthly, the Convention provides for the scientific and technical cooperation among Parties and other actors on tobacco control,[51] and prohibits reservations to it.[52] It also provides for education, training and exchange of information. The progressive development of the Convention entails capacity-building workshops where learning and exchange of information continues to be implemented around the world.[53] Despite FCTC's adaptive features, the Convention has faced complex implementation challenges such as monitoring the tobacco industry, the dearth of domestic comprehensive tobacco control legislation and multi-sectoral coordinating mechanisms adopted by Parties. Embedding a robust adaptive governance strategy in the FCTC would significantly bolster its effective implementation.

The International Health Regulations

The revised International Health Regulations (IHR) 2005 entered into force after a 10-year negotiation.[54] The IHR's purpose is 'to prevent, protect against, control and provide a public health response to the international spread of disease in ways that are commensurate with and restricted to public health risks and which avoid unnecessary interference with international traffic and trade'.[55] The most radical change in IHR (2005) is its application to

---

46   Ibid., Article 8, 11–22.
47   Ibid., Preamble, Article 5(1).
48   Ibid., Articles, 4–16.
49   Ibid., Articles 3–5.
50   Ibid., Articles 2, 13, 16 and Preamble.
51   Ibid., Part VII of the Convention.
52   Ibid., Article 30.
53   Dr Gro-Harlem Brundtland once referred to the treaty's development as a global public health university.
54   World Health Organization, The International Health Regulations, (2005).
55   Ibid., Article 2.

all 'public health emergencies of international concern', including not only infectious disease outbreaks, but also chemical and radio-nuclear events and perhaps other threats to health as well.[56] Disease is defined quite broadly as 'an illness or medical condition, irrespective of origin or source that presents or could present significant harm to humans'.[57]

It requires States to strengthen core surveillance and response capacities at the primary, intermediate and national level, as well as at designated international ports, airports and ground crossings. Core capacities to be developed include contact points, assessing risks, determining public health events of international concern (PHEIC) and recommending measures for use by States during a PHEIC (both after consultation with external experts); provision of technical assistance to States in response to PHEIC; monitoring and evaluation of IHR(2005) implementation. Mechanisms for public health and additional measures under the IHR include various requirements, including basing such measures on scientific principles, evidence and information.[58] There is provision for adopting standing recommendations by WHO,[59] and requirement of consultation with affected States Parties.[60] While the IHR demonstrates some adaptive elements such as continuous monitoring, learning, use of scientific evidence, pluralism[61] and multisectoralism, its implementation continues to face challenges in achieving effective public health outcomes. Ineffective monitoring of reporting outbreaks has been a challenge in the history of the IHR. For example, China failed to report SARS promptly. The standing recommendations adopted under the Regulations do not have the binding force of WHO's standing and temporary recommendations. Sharing of virus samples, despite a successful conclusion through the 2011 WHA Resolution, continues to be a contentious issue. Countries have been slow in undertaking required assessments and legal and policy frameworks for domestic implementation of the IHR remain underdeveloped especially in many developing countries.

A 2011 IHR review report highlighted a number of shortcomings of the IHR legal regime. The reported stated that:

> Despite the positive features of the IHR, many States Parties lack core capacities to detect, assess and report potential health threats and are not on a path to complete their obligations for plans and infrastructure by the 2012 deadline specified in the IHR. Continuing on the current trajectory will not enable countries to develop these capacities and fully implement the IHR. Of the 194 States Parties, 128, or 66 per cent, responded to a recent WHO questionnaire on

56 Ibid., Articles 12 and 13.
57 Ibid., Article 1.
58 Ibid., Article 43.1–2.
59 Ibid., Article 16.
60 Ibid., Article 43.6.
61 The Global Outbreak Alert Response Network (GOARN) provides scientific expertise with operational capacities comprising 100 agencies and research institutes.

their progress. Only 58 per cent of the respondents reported having developed national plans to meet core capacity requirements, and as few as 10 per cent of reporting countries indicated that they had fully established the capacities envisaged by the IHR. Further, as documented by external studies and a WHO questionnaire, in some countries National Focal Points (NFPs) lack the authority to communicate information related to public-health emergencies to WHO in a timely manner. The most important structural shortcoming of the IHR is the lack of enforceable sanctions. For example, if a country fails to explain why it has adopted more restrictive traffic and trade measures than those recommended by WHO, no legal consequences follow[.][62]

The review further stated that there is no systematic monitoring by WHO of instances where human rights are not respected in implementing the IHR.[63] Furthermore, WHO does not have a mandate to investigate whether particular measures constitute violations of this provision in the IHR. During the pandemic, there were media reports of travellers being quarantined and detained as a consequence. It appears to be a weakness that WHO does not monitor whether human rights are being respected in implementing the IHR.[64] Therefore, the IHR requires optimum governance framework as its actors focus on its domestic implementation and adaptive governance offers a compelling framework of action.

Implications for global health law

Benefits of adaptive governance

Facilitates policy experimentation

Adaptive governance enhances cross-sectoral learning beyond narrow medical approaches to broader legal and normative approaches in global health. It could promote regular use of law as a tool for fulfilling WHO's mandate under Article 19 of its Constitution.[65] New areas for legal and normative instruments could become a routine and institutionalized feature of WHO law, with participation of all stakeholders including end-users of global health identified and mandated. Adaptive governance would ensure that some WHA resolutions can potentially become candidates for legally binding treaties. While the WHA resolutions

62 Implementation of the International Health Regulations (2005): Report of the Review Committee on the Functioning of the International Health Regulations (2005) in Relation to Pandemic (H1N1) 2009: Report by the Director-General: Annex (World Health Organization, Sixty-Fourth World Health Assembly, A64/10, 5 May 2011), paragraphs 23–4.
63 Ibid., para 91.
64 Ibid., paras 92–3.
65 Article 19 of the WHO Constitution authorizes the Organization to promote and adopt Conventions, regulations and recommendations that address any matter within its competence.

have flexibilities in global health policy development and implementation, they are not binding in nature. Policy experimentation would also promote a purposive interpretation of WHO constitutional law. Hence renewed options to promote the monitoring and implementation of WHO law could be developed. One key mechanism would be the need to strengthen the good offices of WHO Director-General and regional Directors-General. Traditionally, good offices consist in a third-party government, international organization or an individual attempting to bring conflicting parties to a negotiating table without interfering in the negotiations themselves.[66] In international organizations, good offices are exercised at various levels often by the Head of the Secretariat or some of its officers.[67]

WHO's mandate increasingly emphasizes the importance of prevention and promotion that focus on communities, groups and populations.[68] WHO has adapted its institutional mechanisms to cope with changes resulting from globalization of public health,[69] but these require a versatile framework. Adaptive governance offers it.

Promotes global health co-regulation

Global health agencies including WHO are international institutions endowed with powers and obligations as international administrative agencies. Adaptive governance would promote co-regulation of global health from below to include end-users of global health such as communities in developing countries. This would broaden WHO's stakeholders beyond the state and other actors.[70] Multisectorality ensures that global health legal regime becomes an administrative practice and shared exercise where multi-stakeholder processes are sites where regulatory problems are defined, innovative solutions devised and institutional relationships enhanced to ensure quality and legitimacy of regulatory actions.[71] This broadening of stakeholders enhances WHO supervision of global health normative frameworks. WHO has routine reporting systems through the WHA and additional stakeholders could help scrutinize such reports to promote normative implementation. Adaptive

---

66 The Hague Conventions of 1899 and 1907 on the Pacific Settlement of Disputes provides for good offices as a mechanism for settling any disputes between the powers.
67 Bertrand G. Ramcharan, *Humanitarian Good Offices in International Law: The Good Offices of the United Nations Secretary-General in the Field of Human Rights* (The Hague: Martinus Nijhoff, 1983).
68 William Onzivu, '(Re)invigorating the World Health Organization's Governance of Health Rights: Repositioning an Evolving Legal Regime, Its Challenges and Prospects', *African Journal of Legal Studies*, 2011, 4(3): 225–56.
69 Burci, *Institutional Adaptation without Reform*, 437–43.
70 Bradley C. Karkkainen, 'Collaborative Ecosystem Governance: Scale, Complexity, and Dynamism', *Virginia Environmental Law Journal*, 2002, 21: 189–243.
71 Jody Freeman, 'Collaborative Governance in the Administrative State', *UCLA Law Review*, 1997, 45(1): 1–98.

governance can reinforce WHO's public health management functions to promote global health law.[72]

Promotes implementation of WHO law and policy

The implementation of Doha Agreement on Trade-Related Aspects of Intellectual Property Rights (TRIPS) and Public Health[73] and the need for utilization of TRIPS flexibilities to provide access to essential medicines especially for developing countries has led to WHO normative action in this area. This has included the adoption of a WHA Resolution.[74] The Resolution requested United Nations and other intergovernmental organizations to critically examine TRIPS including its human rights implications. It echoed a UN Resolution which recognized this conflict and sought to establish 'the primacy of human rights obligations over economic agreements'.[75]

In May 2003, the WHA adopted a resolution recommending the creation of a Committee on Intellectual Property Rights, Innovation and Public Health (CIPIH), to evaluate the impact of IP protections on the development of new drugs.[76] The resolution urged members 'to reaffirm that public health interests are paramount in both pharmaceutical and health policies and to adapt national legislation to use TRIPS flexibilities'.[77] The subsequent plan of action contains concrete action points to promote innovation, research and access to medicine. However, its follow-up remains problematic, with a number of richer countries negotiating adverse bilateral agreements that undermine public health protection.[78]

This scenario reflects the challenges of implementing WHO soft law. Adaptive governance would ensure a strong functional basis to reinforce their implementation and follow-up.

Monitoring and feedback mechanisms would be re-examined to promote participation of all stakeholders. Adaptive governance would promote evaluation that facilitates enforcement of and compliance with international health legal and normative instruments. Evaluation refers to a careful

---

72   Benjamin Mason Meir and Ashley M. Fox, 'International Obligations through Collective Rights: Moving from Foreign Health Assistance to Global Health Governance', *Health and Human Rights*, 2010, 12(1): 61.

73   WT/MIN(01)/DEC/2 14, 14 November 2001, 41 *ILM* 755 (2002).

74   World Health Organization, Intellectual Property Rights, Innovation and Public Health, 2003 WHA 56.27, 28 May 2003.

75   Office of the High Commissioner for Human Rights Sub-Comm. on the Promotion and Protection of Human Rights, Res. 2000/7, U.N. Doc. E/CN.4/Sub/2/2000/L.20 (17 August 2000).

76   World Health Organization, Intellectual Property Rights, Innovation and Public Health, 2003 WHA 56.27, 28 May 2003.

77   Ibid., para 1(1).

78   Equinet, SEATINI, TARSC Policy Brief 21, Policy Series 17: Protecting Health in the Proposed Economic Partnership Agreement between East and Southern African Countries and the European Union, 2007, Harare.

retrospective assessment of the merit, worth and value of administration, output and outcome of government interventions, which is intended to play a role in future, practical action situations.[79] The IHR review committee is an evaluative mechanism for adaptive governance in action and a similar mechanism for the WHO FCTC would promote its monitoring and implementation.

Limits of adaptive governance

Undermines WHO law as binding global health law

The WHO Constitution, the FCTC and the IHR 2005 are binding instruments but adaptive governance would require that they are flexible, regularly modified and reviewed. While the progressive development of global health law is concomitant with reviews, laws must be predictable to facilitate their effectiveness. Rapid changes to WHO laws could undermine their legitimacy. Adaptive governance has been viewed as a political project undertaken by Western Nations to foster an international legal order that perpetuates a neo-colonialist status quo, a so-called gentler civiliser of (developing) nations:[80] It is thus viewed as a potential ploy by the developed world to capture the global health political and normative agenda to the detriment of developing nations.

Regulatory capture

Critics argue that the United Nations, in its quest for resources, faces regulatory capture by powerful vested interests. Global health normative instruments that promote commercial companies' participation have been criticized as a slippery slope towards the commercialization of the UN system and legitimization of illegitimate private self-regulation.[81] For example, some public–private partnerships have been seen to undermine the promotion of equity in health. Critics argue that commercial sector participation at WHO potentially misdirects global health priorities.[82] Profit-seeking corporations' participation in global health could impact on WHO's leadership and adversely affect the promotion of equitable global health. [83]

---

79 Evert Vedung, *Public Policy and Program Evaluation* (New Brunswick, NJ: Transaction Publishers, 1997).

80 Mónica García-Salmones, 'Taking Uncertainty Seriously: Adaptive Governance and International Trade: A Reply to Rosie Cooney and Andrew Lang', *European Journal of International Law*, 2009, 20(1): 167–86.

81 Kent Buse and Amalia Waxman, 'Public–Private Health Partnerships: A Strategy for WHO', *Bulletin of the World Health Organization*, 2001, 8: 79.

82 Gavin Yamey, 'Faltering Steps towards Partnerships', *British Medical Journal*, 2002, 325: 1236–40.

83 Augustine D. Asante and Anthony B. Zwi, 'Public–Private Partnerships and Global Health Equity: Prospects and Challenges', *Indian Journal of Medical Ethics*, 2007, IV(4): 179.

Squeezing out the public character of global health law

Global health governance is subject to the scrutiny of public international law. Yet adaptive governance requires a pluralistic amalgam of public and private actors shaping a (public) legal regime. Corporate private actors in global health inhabit public, not private, space and deal with health, which is a core global public good.[84] The UNDP (United Nations Development Programme) defines a global public good as a public good with benefits that are strongly universal in terms of countries, people and generations.[85] The over 20 Global Public–Private Partnerships housed within WHO contain constituents from both public and private sectors with heterogeneous legal features and inherent conflicting and competing interests. Their governance reflects nodal governance, a social adaptation accomplished in significant part through the creation and operation of 'nodes'.[86] While power is transmitted across networks, the actual point where knowledge and capacity are mobilized for transmission is the node.[87] Adaptive governance contradicts the public character of global health law because it embodies competing private and public nodes with often divergent vested interests in the global health enterprise.[88]

Conclusion

In the face of increasing disease threats, global health law continues to explore appropriate governance frameworks. Adaptive governance provides a concrete model and enables participation, pluralism, continuous learning and experimentation, use of science as well as evaluation and monitoring. These elements can strengthen the effectiveness of WHO law. The WHO Constitution, the FCTC and IHR provide precedents for effective progressive development and implementation of global health law. However, adaptive governance is not a panacea to the malaise that faces the functional effectiveness of WHO law and policy. It has the potential to breed unpredictability in the legal regime due to its over-emphasis on regular amendments to legal and normative instruments.

---

84   David Woodward and Richard Smith, 'Global Public Goods and Health: Concepts and Issues', in Richard Smith, Robert Beaglehole, David Woodward and Nick Drager (eds), *Global Public Goods for Health: Health Economic and Public Health Perspectives* (Oxford: Oxford University Press, 2003), 10–12.

85   United Nations Development Programme, *Providing Global Public Goods: Managing Globalization, 25 Questions and Answers* (New York: UNDP, 2002).

86   Scott Burris, Peter Drahos and Clifford Shearing, 'Nodal Governance', *Australian Journal of Legal Philosophy*, 2005, 30: 30.

87   Scott Burris, 'Symposium: SARS, Public Health, and Global Governance: Governance, Micro Governance and Health', *Temple Law Review*, 2004, 77: 335.

88   Burris, Drahos and Shearing, 'Nodal Governance'.

Its emphasis on multisectorality ignores potential capture by vested interests of the public interest in global health law and policy. Despite its shortcomings, adaptive governance provides a useful framework for reinforcing the effectiveness of global health and the overall improvement of WHO law and policy. However, to reinforce global health legal and normative frameworks, adaptive governance tools must redistribute global health benefits; promote participation of all actors as legitimate inhabitants of global health in a public regulatory space. Finally, institutionalized evaluation of laws and policies, underpinned by public health ethics, must be embedded at the core of global health governance.

15

Meeting Basic Survival Needs of the World's Least Healthy People: Toward a Framework Convention on Global Health

Lawrence O. Gostin[1]

Introduction

This chapter searches for solutions to the most perplexing problems in global health – problems so important that they affect the fate of millions of people, with economic, political and security ramifications for the world's population. No State, acting alone, can insulate itself from major health hazards. The determinants of health (e.g. pathogens, air, food, water, even lifestyle choices) do not originate solely within national borders. Health threats inexorably spread to neighbouring countries, regions and even continents. It is for this reason that safeguarding the world's population requires cooperation and global governance.

If I am correct that ameliorating the most common causes of disease, disability and premature death require global solutions, then the future is demoralizing. The States that bear the disproportionate burden of disease have the least capacity to do anything about it. And the States that have the wherewithal are deeply resistant to expending the political capital and economic resources necessary to truly make a difference to improve health outside their borders. When rich countries do act, it is often more out of narrow self-interest or humanitarian instinct than a full sense of ethical or legal obligation. The result

1 Lawrence O. Gostin is University Professor, the Linda D. and Timothy J. O'Neill Professor of Global Health Law, and Faculty Director of the O'Neill Institute on National and Global Health Law at Georgetown University Law Center. He is also Professor of Public Health, the Johns Hopkins University and Director of the WHO Collaborating Center on Public Health Law and Human Rights. Prof. Gostin was a Distinguished Professorial Fellow at the Institute for Science, Ethics and Innovation, University of Manchester, in June 2011 when he delivered this keynote address. An expanded version of this paper was published in the *Georgetown Law Journal* in 2008. See Lawrence O. Gostin, 'Meeting Basic Survival Needs of the World's Least Healthy People: Toward a Framework Convention on Global Health', *Georgetown Law Journal*, 2008, 96: 331–92, available at http://ssrn.com/abstract=1014082.

is a spiraling deterioration of health in the poorest regions, with manifest global consequences for cross-border disease transmission and systemic effects on trade, international relations and security.

This chapter first inquires why global health is a shared responsibility – for the Global South and North – and then reconceptualizes the global health enterprise. Second, I examine the compelling issue of global health equity, and ask whether it is fair that people in poor countries suffer such a disproportionate burden of illness and death. Here, I briefly explore what I call a 'theory of human functioning' to support a more robust understanding of the transcending value of health. Third, I describe how the international community focuses on a few high profile, heart-rending, issues while largely ignoring deeper, systemic problems in global health. By focusing on what I call 'basic survival needs', the international community could fundamentally improve prospects for the world's population. Finally, I explore the value of international law itself, and propose an innovative mechanism for global health reform – a Framework Convention on Global Health (FCGH).[2]

A global coalition of civil society and academics recently launched the Joint Action and Learning Initiative on National and Global Responsibilities for Health (JALI). Following international stakeholder meetings in Oslo, Berlin, Johannesburg, Delhi and Bellagio, JALI is developing a post–Millennium Development Goal (MDG) framework for global health. JALI's goal is a Framework Convention on Global Health.[3] In March 2011, the UN General Secretary endorsed the FCGH, calling on the United Nations to adopt it.[4] Moreover, the World Health Organization Director-General Margaret Chan proposed a 'framework' for global health as part of the Organization's major reform agenda.[5]

---

2   Lawrence O. Gostin, 'The Unconscionable Health Gap: A Global Plan for Justice', *The Lancet*, 2010, 375: 1504–5; Lawrence O. Gostin, 'Redressing the Unconscionable Health Gap: A Global Plan for Justice', *Harvard Law & Policy Review*, 2010, 4: 271–94. For an explanation of the progression from a Joint Learning Initiative for National and Global Responsibilities for Health, to a Global Plan for Justice, through to a Framework Convention on Global Health, see www.acslaw.org/node/16479.

3   Lawrence O. Gostin, Eric A. Friedman, Gorik Ooms, Thomas Gebauer, Narendra Gupta, Devi Sridhar, Wang Chenguang, John-Arne Røttingen and David Sanders, 'The Joint Action and Learning Initiative: Towards a Global Agreement on National and Global Responsibilities for Health', *PLOS Medicine*, 2011, 8(5): www.plosmedicine.org/article/info%3Adoi%2F10.1371%2Fjournal.pmed.1001031.

4   UN Secretary-General, *Uniting for Universal Access: Towards Zero New HIV Infections, Zero Discrimination and Zero AIDS-Related Deaths: Report of the Secretary-General*, U.N. Doc A/65/979 (New York: United Nations, 2011), para. 73, www.unaids.org/en/media/unaids/contentassets/documents/document/2011/A-65-797_English.pdf.

5   WHO, *Reform for a Healthy Future: An Overview* (Geneva: WHO, 2011) proposing a charter or framework for global health governance as a key output; WHO, *Reforms for a Healthy Future: Report by the Director-General*, Doc. EBSS/2/2 (Geneva: WHO, 2011): http://apps.who.int/gb/ebwha/pdf_files/EBSS/EBSS2_2-en.pdf, proposing a framework, code or charter to guide all global health stakeholders, with agreed targets and indicators or rights and responsibilities.

My proposal for a Framework Convention in a nutshell is to establish fair terms of international cooperation, with agreed-upon mutually binding obligations to create enduring health-system capacities, meet basic survival needs and reduce unconscionable inequalities in global health.

Reconceptualizing 'Health Aid': From 'Aid' to global justice

Global health means different things to different people. Often, it is used as shorthand for the aggregate of health assistance provided by the affluent to the poor in a donor–recipient relationship as a form of charity, together with the volume and the modalities of this assistance – a concept I refer to as 'Health Aid'.

Framing the global health endeavour as Health Aid provided by the affluent to the poor is fundamentally flawed. This suggests that the world is divided between donors and countries in need. This is too simplistic. Collaboration among countries, both as neighbours and across continents, is also about responding to health risks together and building capacity collaboratively – whether it is through South–South partnerships, gaining access to essential vaccines and medicines, or demanding fair distribution of scarce life-saving technologies.

Likewise, the concept of 'aid' both presupposes and imposes an inherently unequal relationship where one side is a benefactor and the other a dependent. This leads affluent states and other donors to believe that they are giving 'charity', which means that financial contributions and programs are largely at their discretion. It also means that donors make decisions about how much to give and for what health-related goods and services. The level of financial assistance, therefore, is not predictable, scalable to needs, or sustainable in the long term. These features of Health Aid could, in turn, mean that host countries might not accept full responsibility for their inhabitants' health, as they can blame the poor state of health on the shortcomings of aid, rather than their own failures.

Conceptualizing international assistance as 'aid' masks the greater truth that human health is a globally shared responsibility reflecting common risks and vulnerabilities – an obligation of health justice that demands a fair contribution from everyone – North and South, rich and poor. Global governance for health must be seen as a partnership, with financial and technical assistance understood as an integral component of the common goal of improving global health and reducing health inequalities.

The framework of mutual responsibilities should prove attractive to both the Global South and North, creating incentives to develop a far-reaching global health agreement. Southern countries would benefit from increased respect for their strategies, greater and more predictable funding from more coordinated and accountable development partners, reform of politics that harm health, such as those in trade and agriculture and, most importantly, better health for their populations. Countries of the North will benefit from increased confidence that development assistance is spent effectively and the prospect of reduced financing needs over time as host countries increase their health spending and build sustainable health systems. All will benefit from lessons on shared health challenges, from economic and educational gains that will come with improved global health, and from increased protection from global public health threats – and from mutual goodwill derived from participating in an historic venture to make unprecedented progress towards global health equity.

Are profound health inequalities fair?

Perhaps it does not, or should not, matter if global health serves the interests of the richest countries. After all, there are powerful humanitarian reasons to help the world's least healthy people. But even ethical arguments have failed to capture the full attention of political leaders and the public.

It is well known that the poor suffer, and suffer more than the rich. Unfortunately, this is also true with respect to global health. What is less often known is the degree to which the poor suffer unnecessarily. The global burden of disease is not just shouldered by the poor, but disproportionately so, such that health disparities across continents render a person's likelihood of survival drastically different based on where she is born. These inequalities have become so extreme and the resultant effects on the poor so dire, that health disparities have become an issue no less important than global warming or the other defining problems of our time.

Over a decade into the twenty-first century, billions of people have yet to benefit from the health advances of the twentieth century. Average life expectancy in Africa is nearly 30 years less than in the Americas or Europe[6] – only two years higher than in the United States a century ago,[7] and 27 years lower than in high-income countries today. Life expectancy in Sierra Leone or Zimbabwe is half that in Japan;[8] a child born in Angola is 65 times more likely to die in the first few years of life than a child born in Norway;[9] and a woman giving birth in sub-Saharan Africa is 100 times more likely to die in labour than a woman in a rich country.[10] The most basic human needs continue to elude

6   WHO, *World Health Statistics* (Geneva: WHO, 2009), www.who.int/whosis/whostat/ EN_WHS09_Table1.pdf reporting that average life expectancy at birth in Africa is 52 years compared with 76 years in the Americas. The gap between rich and poor is still higher when measured by the number of years of healthy life (i.e. life without significant illness or disability).

7   Elizabeth Arias, 'United States Life Tables 2006', *National Vital Statistics Reports*, 2010, 58(21): 1–40, available at www.cdc.gov/nchs/data/nvsr/nvsr58/nvsr58_21.pdf.

8   Ibid.

9   UNICEF, *The State of the World's Children 2007* (New York: UNICEF, 2006): www.unicef. org/sowc07/docs/sowc07.pdf.

10 UNICEF, *Progress for Children: A Report Card on Maternal Mortality* (New York: UNICEF, 2008): www.childinfo.org/files/progress_for_children_maternalmortality.pdf.

the world's poorest people. In 2010, approximately 925 million people were suffering from chronic hunger,[11] 884 million people lacked access to clean water and 2.6 billion people were without access to proper sanitation facilities.[12]

While life expectancy in the developed world has consistently increased throughout the twentieth and early twenty-first centuries, it actually has been decreasing in the least-developed countries and in transitional states such as Russia.[13] Infectious disease epidemics, particularly HIV/AIDS (which kills 4,000 Africans, but only 63 North Americans, each day),[14] and increased chronic disease erased hard-won gains in life expectancy that took decades to achieve.[15]

As little as one concrete example offers a sense of perspective on the global health gap between the rich and the poor. The World Bank reports that in one year alone, 14 million of the poorest people in the world died, while only 4 million would have died if this population had the same death rate as the global rich.[16]

The yawning health gap cannot be fully understood by using the over-simplified division of the world into the global rich (the North) and the global poor (the South). In fact, 20 percent of the largest fortunes in the world are in so-called poor countries. Even within countries, dramatic health differences exist that are closely linked with degrees of social disadvantage. The poorest people in Europe and North America often have life expectancies equal to those in the least-developed countries.

A great deal of the variation in health outcomes within countries and among population subgroups can be explained by where people live (urban/rural), their wealth and their education.[17] The differences can sometimes be striking. For example, in Calton, Glasgow, life expectancy at birth for men is 54 years, while in Lenzie, a few kilometres away, it is 82.[18] And in Baltimore, Maryland, a

11   Food and Agricultural Organization, *925 Million in Chronic Hunger Worldwide* (Rome: FAO, 2010): www.fao.org/news/story/en/item/45210/icode/.

12   United Nations General Assembly, *The Human Right to Water and Sanitation*, U.N. Doc. A/Res/64/292 (New York: UN, 2010): www.un.org/en/ga/64/resolutions.shtml.

13   WHO, *World Health Statistics* (Geneva: WHO, 2009): www.who.int/whosis/whostat/EN_WHS09_Full.pdf.

14   UNAIDS, *Global Facts and Figures: Report on the Global AIDS Epidemic 2008* (Geneva: UNAIDS, 2008) (last modified August 2008): http://data.unaids.org/pub/GlobalReport/2008/20080715_fs_global_En.pdf.

15   UNAIDS, Report on the Global AIDS Epidemic (Geneva: UNAIDS, 2008): www.unaids.org/en/KnowledgeCentre/HIVData/GlobalReport/2008/default.asp; Economic and Social Research Council, *Global Health Disparities Fact Sheet*, available at www.esrcsocietytoday.ac.uk/ESRCInfoCentre/facts/health.aspx.

16   Davidson R. Gawtkin and Michel Guillot, *The Burden of Disease among the Global Poor: Current Situation, Future Trends, and Implications for Strategy* (Washington: World Bank, 2000), 19–20.

17   World Health Organization, *World Health Statistics 2009: Table 8 Health Inequities* (Geneva: WHO, 2009): www.who.int/whosis/whostat/EN_WHS09_Table8.pdf.

18   WHO Commission on Social Determinants of Health, *Closing the Gap in a Generation: Health Equity through Action on the Social Determinants of Health* (Geneva: WHO, 2008): http://whqlibdoc.who.int/publications/2008/9789241563703_Eng.pdf.

black unemployed youth has a lifespan 32 years shorter than a white corporate professional.[19]

The world's 400 million indigenous people have remarkably low standards of health compared with non-indigenous populations. The gap in life expectancy is estimated to be 19–21 years in Australia, 8 years in New Zealand, 5–7 years in Canada and 4–5 years in the United States.[20] This poor health is associated with poverty, malnutrition, poor hygiene, environmental contamination and prevalent infections. Some indigenous groups, as they move from traditional to transitional and modern lifestyles, are rapidly acquiring lifestyle diseases such as cardiovascular disease, diabetes, mental illness and dependency on drugs and alcohol.[21]

As vividly enunciated by Vicente Navarro, 'It is not the North versus the South, it is not globalization, it is not the scarcity of resources – it is the power differentials between and among classes in these countries and their influence over the state that are at the root of the poverty [and health] problem.'[22]

The diseases of poverty are endemic in the world's poorest regions, but barely get noticed among the wealthy. Diseases such as elephantiasis, guinea worm, malaria, river blindness, schistosomiasis and trachoma are common in poor countries, but are largely unheard of in rich countries. Beyond morbidity and premature mortality, the diseases of poverty cause physical and mental anguish, for example, when a two-foot-long guinea worm parasite emerges from the genitals, breasts, extremities and torso with excruciating pain; or filarial worms cause disfiguring enlargement of the arms, legs, breasts and genitals; or river blindness leads to unbearable itching and loss of eyesight.

Human instinct tells us that it is unjust for large populations to have such poor prospects for good health and long life simply by happenstance of where they live. Although almost everyone believes it is unfair that the poor live miserable and short lives, there is little consensus about whether there is an ethical, let alone legal, obligation to help the downtrodden. What do wealthier societies owe as a matter of *justice* to the poor in other parts of the world?

Perhaps the strongest claim that health disparities are unethical is based on what I call a theory of human functioning. Health has special meaning and importance to individuals and the community as a whole. Health is necessary for much of the joy, creativity and productivity that a person

---

19 Vicente Navarro, 'What We Mean by Social Determinants of Health', *International Journal of Health Services*, 2009, 39(3): 423–41.
20 Editorial, 'The Health Status of Indigenous Peoples and Others,' *British Medical Journal*, 2003, 327: 404–5.
21 Michael Gracey and Malcolm King, 'Indigenous Health Part 1: Determinants and Disease Patterns', *The Lancet*, 2009, 374(9683): 65–75; Malcolm King, Alexandra Smith and Michael Gracey, 'Indigenous Health Part 2: The Underlying Causes of The Health Gap', *The Lancet*, 2009, 374(9683): 76–85.
22 Navarro, 'What We Mean by Social Determinants of Health', 430.

derives from life. Individuals with physical and mental health recreate, socialize, work and engage in family and social activities that bring meaning and happiness to their lives. Perhaps not as obvious, health also is essential for the functioning of populations. Without minimum levels of health, people cannot fully engage in social interactions, participate in the political process, exercise rights of citizenship, generate wealth, create art and provide for the common security.

Amartya Sen famously theorized that the capability to avoid starvation, preventable morbidity and early mortality is a substantive freedom that enriches human life.[23] Depriving people of this capability strips them of their freedom to be who they want to be and 'to do things that a person has reason to value'.[24] Other ethicists have expanded on this theory, claiming that health, specifically, is important to the ability to live a life one values – one cannot function who is barely alive.[25] Under a theory of human functioning, health deprivations are unethical because they unnecessarily reduce one's ability to function and the capacity for human agency. Health, among all the other forms of disadvantage, is special and foundational, in that its effects on human capacities impact one's opportunities in the world and, therefore, health must be preserved to ensure equality of opportunity.[26]

But Sen's theory does not answer the harder question about who has the corresponding obligation to do something about global inequalities. Even liberal egalitarians who believe in just distribution, such as Nagel,[27] Rawls[28] and Walzer,[29] frame their claims narrowly and rarely extend them to international obligations of justice. Their theories of justice are 'relational' and apply to a fundamental social structure that people share. States may owe their citizens

---

23 See generally Amartya Sen, *Development as Freedom* (Oxford: Oxford University Press, 1999).

24 Ibid.; *see also* Jennifer Ruger, 'Ethics and Governance of Global Health Inequalities', *Journal of Epidemiology & Community Health*, 2006, 60: 998–9; Amartya Sen, 'Equality of What?', *Tanner Lecture on Human Values at Stanford University*, 1979: www.tannerlectures.utah.edu/lectures/sen80.pdf.

25 See Ruger, 'Ethics and Governance of Global Health Inequalities'. See also Jennifer Ruger, 'Rethinking Equal Access: Agency, Quality, and Norms', *Global Public Health*, 2007, 2(1): 84; Martha C. Nussbaum, 'Human Functioning and Social Justice: In Defense of Aristotelian Essentialism', *Political Threory*,1992, 20(2): 202–46. See also, John Coggon, *What Makes Health Public? A Critical Evaluation of Moral, Legal, and Political Claims in Public Health* (Cambridge: Cambridge University Press, 2012), chapter 8.

26 See Norman Daniels, 'Justice, Health, and Healthcare', *American Journal of Bioethics*, 2001, 1(2): 2–16. See also Sridhar Venkatapuram, *Health Justice* (Malden, MA: Polity Press, 2011).

27 See generally Thomas Nagel, 'The Problem of Global Justice', *Philosophy & Public Affairs*, 2005, 33(2): 113–47.

28 See generally John Rawls, *The Law of Peoples* (Cambridge, MA: Harvard University Press, 1999).

29 See generally Michael Walzer, *Spheres of Justice: A Defense of Pluralism and Equality* (New York: Basic Books, 1983).

basic health protection by reason of a social compact.[30] But positing such a relationship among different countries and regions is much more difficult.

Basic survival needs: Ameliorating suffering and early death

Suppose that States were convinced that amelioration of global health hazards was in their national interests or that they otherwise accepted the claim that they have an ethical responsibility to act. Would the consequent funding and efforts make a difference? If past history is any guide, the answer is no. Most development assistance is driven by high-profile events that evoke public sympathy, such as a natural disaster in the form of a hurricane, tsunami, draught or famine; or an enduring catastrophe such as AIDS; or politicians may lurch from one frightening disease to the next, irrespective of the level of risk ranging from anthrax and smallpox to SARS, novel influenza (H5N1 and H1N1) and bioterrorism.

What is truly needed, and which richer countries instinctively (although not always adequately) do for their own citizens, is to meet what I call 'basic survival needs'. By focusing on the major determinants of health, the international community could dramatically improve prospects for good health. Basic survival needs include sanitation and sewage, pest control, clean air and water, tobacco reduction, diet and nutrition, essential medicines and vaccines and well-functioning health systems. Meeting everyday survival needs may lack the glamour of high-technology medicine or dramatic rescue, but what they lack in excitement they gain in their potential impact on health, precisely because they deal with the major causes of common disease and disabilities across the globe. Mobilizing the public and private sectors to meet basic survival needs, comparable to a Marshall Plan, could radically transform prospects for good health among the world's poorest populations.

Meeting basic survival needs can be disarmingly simple and inexpensive, if only it could rise on the agendas of the world's most powerful countries. It does not take advanced biomedical research, huge financial investments or complex programs. Consider what human benefits would accrue from highly cost-effective interventions such as vaccines, essential medicines, sanitation and pest abatements. Vaccine-preventable diseases are virtually extinct in developed countries, but still kill millions of children and adults annually in poorer regions. A single annual dose of ivermectin (Mectizan®) and albendazole (Albenza®) costing a couple of dollars rids the body of intestinal worms and the itching symptoms of river blindness, prevents blindness and revives sex drive, so it

---

30 See generally Thomas Hobbes, *Leviathan*, (Touchstone, 1997 [1651]). See also Michael O. Hardimon, 'Role Obligations', *The Journal of Philosophy*, 1994, 91(7): 333–63; Robin West, 'Unenumerated Duties', *University of Pennsylvania Journal of Constitutional Law*, 2006, 9: 221–61.

helps regenerate populations in decline.[31] Basic sanitation and water systems would vastly improve global health at minimal cost, such as clean water kits costing as little as $3. An insecticide-treated bednet, which costs roughly $5 and provides protection for up to five years, is highly effective in reducing malaria, river blindness, elephantiasis and other insect-borne diseases among children.[32] But only about one in seven children in Africa sleep under a net, and only 3 per cent of children use a net impregnated with insecticide.[33]

Consequently, what poor countries need is not foreign aid workers parachuting in to rescue them. Nor do they need foreign-run state-of-the-art facilities. Rather, they need to gain the capacity to provide basic health services themselves.

Global governance for health: A proposal for a Framework Convention on Global Health

If meeting basic survival needs can truly make a difference for the world's population, and if this solution is preferable to other paths, then can international law structure legal obligations accordingly? The answer is that extant health governance has been lamentably deficient, and a fresh approach is badly needed.

If law is to play a constructive role, innovative models are essential and here I make the case for a Framework Convention on Global Health. I am proposing a global governance for health scheme incorporating a bottom-up strategy that strives to: build health-system capacity; set priorities to meet basic survival needs; engage stakeholders to bring to bear their resources and expertise; harmonize the activities among the proliferating number of actors operating around the world; and evaluate and monitor progress so that goals are met and promises kept.

The framework convention approach is becoming an essential strategy of powerful transnational social movements to safeguard health and the

---

31 World Health Organization, 'Lymphatic Filariasis', *Weekly Epidemiological Record*, 2001, 76: 149–54; see also Eric A. Ottesen, B.O. Duke, M. Karam and K. Behbehani, 'Strategies and Tools for the Control/Elimination of Lyphatic Filariasis', *Bulletin of WHO*, 1997, 75: 491–503.

32 David Molyneux and Vinad Nantulya, 'Linking Disease Control Programmes in Rural Africa: A Pro-Poor Strategy to Reach Abuja Targets and Millenium Development Goals', *British Medical Journal*, 2004, 75: 1129–32; see also C. Lengeler, 'Insecticide-Treated Bed Nets and Curtains for Preventing Malaria', *Cochrane Database of Systematic Reviews*, 2004, 2: CD000363; Donald G. McNeil, Jr, 'Beyond Swollen Limbs, a Disease's Hidden Agony', *New York Times*, 9 April 2006.

33 World Health Organization, *Africa Malaria Report 2003* (Geneva: WHO, 2003): www.rbm. who.int/amd2003/amr2003/amr_toc.htm; John M. Miller, Eline L. Korenromp, Bernard L. Nahlen and Richard W. Steketee, 'Estimating the Number of Insecticide-Treated Nets Required by African Households to Reach Continent-Wide Malaria Coverage Targets', *Journal of the American Medical Association*, 2007, 297: 2241.

environment.[34] A series of international environmental treaties serve as models for global health governance, including the Barcelona Convention for Protection of the Mediterranean Sea Against Pollution (1976),[35] the Convention on Long-Range Transboundary Air Pollution (1979),[36] and the Vienna Convention for the Protection of the Ozone Layer (1985)[37] (leading to the Montreal Protocol on Substances that Deplete the Ozone Layer in 1987).[38]

The UN Framework Convention on Climate Change (UNFCCC) (1992), the most prominent international environmental treaty, is designed to stabilize greenhouse gas concentrations in the atmosphere.[39] The 1997 Kyoto protocol required ratifying States to reduce their total greenhouse gas emissions, with specific quantitative levels assigned to each country.[40] Although the United States failed to ratify,[41] and highly polluting transitional States such as China and India are largely exempt, the Kyoto Protocol represents a nascent attempt at global cooperative governance to reduce global climate change.[42] But even this approach can be painstakingly difficult, as the stalled climate change negotiations make clear.

These framework conventions recognize that the world's atmosphere and bodies of water are shared resources, and that a collective effort is necessary to mitigate the threat that humans pose to the global environment. Although far from perfect, international environmental treaties offer innovative approaches to global governance. The Montreal protocol, for example, adopted a 'common but differentiated responsibility', with disparate legal obligations on developing and developed countries; created a multilateral implementation fund administered by the World Bank to provide technical and financial assistance to developing countries;[43] and utilized trade sanctions for enforcement.[44]

34   Ibid.
35   Convention for Protection of the Mediterranean Sea against Pollution 1976 and Protocols 1980 and 1982 (12 February 1978): http://eelink.net/~asilwildlife/barcelona.html.
36   Convention on Long-Range Transboundary Air Pollution 1979 (establishing a broad agreement between European and North American countries to address the problem of emissions that cross borders, causing regional environmental and health effects).
37   Vienna Convention for the Protection of the Ozone Layer 1985.
38   Montreal Protocol on Substances that Deplete the Ozone Layer 1987.
39   United Nations Framework Convention on Climate Change 1992.
40   Kyoto Protocol to the United Nations Framework Convention on Climate Change 1998 [hereinafter Kyoto Protocol]; see David Dreisen, 'Free Lunch or Cheap Fix: The Emissions Trading Idea and the Climate Change Convention', *Boston College Environmental Affairs Law Review*, 1998, 26: 5.
41   Kyoto Protocol: Status of Ratification: http://unfccc.int/files/kyoto_protocol/background/status_of_ratification/application/pdf/kp_rat_131206.pdf.
42   United Nations, *United Nations Framework Convention on Climate Change: The First Ten Years* (New York: United Nations, 2004): http://unfccc.int/resource/docs/publications/first_ten_years_En.pdf.
43   World Bank, *The Multilateral Fund for Implementation of the Montreal Protocol* (Washington: World Bank, 2004).
44   World Bank, *The World Bank and the Montreal Protocol: Reducing Health Risks by Restoring the Ozone Layer* (Washington: World Bank, 2003): http://web.worldbank.org/servlets/ECR?contentMDK=20489383&sitePK=407352.

The Framework Convention on Tobacco Control, one of only two treaties negotiated under the WHO's constitutional authority, was modelled on environmental framework conventions, notably the UNFCCC.[45] It too has inventive governance approaches to tobacco control that include: *demand reduction* – price and tax measures, as well as non-price measures; *supply reduction* – control of illicit trade and sales to minors, as well as creation of economically viable alternatives to tobacco production; and, most controversially, *tort litigation* – international cooperation on tort actions and criminal prosecutions, such as information exchange and legal assistance.

The key modalities of an FCGH

An FCGH would represent an historical shift in global health, with a broadly imagined global governance regime. The initial framework would establish the key modalities, with a strategy for subsequent protocols on each of the most important governance parameters. It is not necessary, or perhaps even wise, to specify in detail the substance of an initial FCGH, but it may be helpful to state the broad principles:

- *FCGH mission* – Convention Parties seek innovative solutions for the most pressing health problems facing the world in partnership with non-state actors and civil society, with particular emphasis on the most disadvantaged populations.

- *FCGH objectives* – establish fair terms of international cooperation, with agreed-upon mutually binding obligations to create enduring health-system capacities, meet basic survival needs and reduce global health disparities.

- *Engagement and coordination* – finding common purposes and process among a wide variety of State and non-state actors, setting priorities and coordinating activities to achieve the mission of the FCGH.

- *State Party and other stakeholder obligations* – incentives, forms of assistance (e.g. financial aid, debt relief, technical support, subsidies, tradable credits) and levels of assistance, with differentiated responsibility for developed, developing and least-developed countries.

- *Institutional structures* – conference of Parties, secretariat, technical advisory body and financing mechanism, with integral involvement of non-state actors and civil society.

---

45   Ruth Roemer, Allyn Taylor and Jean Lariviere, 'Origins of the WHO Framework Convention on Tobacco Control', *American Journal of Public Health*, 2005, 95: 936–8; Allyn Taylor and Douglas Bettcher, 'WHO Framework Convention on Tobacco Control: A Global "Good" for Public Health', *Bulletin of WHO*, 2000, 78: 920–9.

- *Empirical monitoring* – data gathering, benchmarks and leading health indicators, such as maternal, infant and child survival.

- *Enforcement mechanisms* – inducements, sanctions, mediation and dispute resolution.

- *Ongoing scientific analysis* – processes for ongoing scientific research and evaluation on cost-effective health interventions, such as the creation of an Intergovernmental Panel on Global Health, comprised of prominent medical and public health experts.

- *Guidance for subsequent law-making process* – content, methods and timetables to meet framework convention goals.

Strengths of the framework convention-protocol approach

Facilitating global consensus

The framework convention-protocol approach has a number of advantages resulting from the incremental nature of the process, and its ability to evolve over a longer time horizon. The framework agreement allows for the initial codification of normative parameters, with the expectation of building detailed standards in the future. The incremental nature of the governance strategy allows the international community to focus on a problem in a stepwise manner, avoiding potential political bottlenecks over contentious elements. A comprehensive international governance regime can emerge from a long-term negotiation process as political will develops.[46] Although the graduated nature of framework conventions can frustrate those desiring rapid results, it can offer the only realistic strategy for finding global consensus.

Facilitating a shared humanitarian instinct

The creation of international norms and institutions provides an ongoing and structured forum for States and stakeholders to develop a shared humanitarian instinct on global health. A high-profile forum for normative discussion can help educate and persuade Parties, and influence public opinion, in favour of decisive action. And it can create internal pressure for governments and others to actively participate in the framework dialogue. The creation of such a normative community, therefore, may be an essential element of building an international consensus.[47] The imperatives of global health have to be framed

46 Allyn Taylor, 'An International Regulatory Strategy for Global Tobacco Control', *Yale Journal of International Law*, 1996, 12: 257–304.
47 Marc Levy, 'Improving the Effectiveness of International Environmental Institutions', in Peter Haas, Rober O. Keohane and Marc A. Levy (eds), *Institutions for the Earth* (Cambridge, MA and London, England: MIT, 1993).

not just as a series of isolated problems in far-off places, but as a common concern of humankind.

Building factual and scientific consensus

The framework convention-protocol approach can be used to build international consensus about the essential facts of global health, such as the causes of extremely poor health and stark disparities, as well as the most cost-effective solutions. Just as the normative process can shape values, it can also serve as a forum for experts and policy-makers to collect and analyse health data and scientific evidence. The FCTC process, for example, facilitated discussion about the harms of tobacco and role of the industry, which was vital to the adoption of the treaty. At the same time, the incremental approach of a Framework Convention allows for normative development to accommodate evolving scientific evidence.

Transcending shifts in political will

An ongoing diplomatic forum can also help to transcend the inevitable ebbs and flows of interest in international cooperation around global health. As political environments change, governments can become more or less interested in creating new international obligations, or complying with existing obligations. One of the strengths of an FCGH is that it can serve as a lasting entity that is resistant to temporary shifts in political will.

Engaging multiple actors and stakeholders

The really interesting and vital aspect of a FCGH is not merely how it governs inter-State responsibilities. The critical challenge is how to make it do the really hard work of mobilizing the diverse drivers of health, including NGOs, private industry, foundations, public/private hybrids, researchers and the media. It is essential to harness the ingenuity and resources of these non-state actors. The FCGH, therefore, should actively engage major stakeholders in the process of negotiation, debate and information exchange, as well as reducing barriers for them to actively engage in capacity-building.

Political difficulties of a Framework Convention on Global Health

An FCGH offers an intriguing approach, potentially creating a process and structure for an innovative international mechanism for ameliorating complex problems in global health. It will not, however, be a panacea, and there are multiple social, political and economic barriers to the creation of such a framework convention. The framework convention-protocol approach cannot easily circumvent many of the seemingly intractable problems of global health governance: the domination of the most economically and politically powerful countries; the deep resistance to creating obligations to expend, or transfer, wealth; the lack of confidence in international legal regimes and trust in international organizations; and the vocal concerns about the integrity and competency of governments in many of the poorest countries.

Although the framework convention-protocol approach can help create the political, scientific and normative space for agreement to be reached, it does not ensure consensus on contentious issues. In fact, this approach has a number of structural problems that could hinder the creation of a universal, cooperative solution to global health problems. Loss of momentum is one potential barrier. The extended, incremental process can be seen as detrimentally long and drawn out.[48] After an initial framework convention, if years pass without an agreement on subsequent protocols, there is a risk that political momentum will wane. Furthermore, the long timeframe can be used to derail the imposition of binding obligations. Parties that were initially reluctant to engage in negotiations about an issue, can take advantage of the political capital achieved by signing a framework convention, then subtly disengage from, or even subvert, the subsequent protocol creation process.

But given the dismal nature of extant global health governance, an FCGH is a risk worth taking. It will, at a minimum, identify the truly important problems in global health. Solutions will not be found solely in increased resources, although that is important. Rather, an FCGH can demonstrate the imperative of targeting the major determinants of health, prioritizing and coordinating currently fragmented activities, and engaging a broad range of stakeholders. It also will provide a needed forum to raise visibility of one of the most pressing problems facing humankind. An FCGH would represent an historical shift in global health, with a broadly imagined global governance regime.

A tipping point

I have sought to demonstrate why politically and economically powerful countries should care about the world's least healthy people. It may be a matter of national interest for the Global South and North so that helping the poor makes everyone safer and more secure. Or global health assistance simply may be ethically the right thing to do to avert an unfolding humanitarian catastrophe. Or there may be a growing sense of legal obligation, whether through WHO treaties and regulations or the international right to health. Although no single argument may be definitive in itself, the cumulative weight of the evidence is now overwhelmingly persuasive. Whatever the reasons, perhaps we are coming to a tipping point where the status quo is no longer acceptable and it is time to take bold action. Global health, like global climate change, may soon become

---

48 Lawrence Susskind, 'The Weaknesses of the Existing Environmental Treaty-Making System', in Lawrence Susskind (ed.), *Environmental Diplomacy: Negotiating More Effective Global Agreements* (New York: Oxford University Press, 1993), 11–39.

a matter so important to the world's future that it demands international attention, and no State can escape the responsibility to act.

If that were the case, States would need an innovative international mechanism to bind themselves, and others, to take an effective course of action. Amelioration of the enduring and complex problems of global health is virtually impossible without a collective response. No State or stakeholder, acting alone, can avert the ubiquitous threats of pathogens as they rapidly migrate and change forms. If all States and stakeholders voluntarily accepted fair terms of cooperation through an FCGH, then it could dramatically improve life prospects for millions of people. But it would do more than that. Cooperative action for global health, like global warming, benefits everyone by diminishing our collective vulnerabilities.

The alternative to fair terms of cooperation through a Framework Convention is that everyone would be worse off, particularly those who suffer compounding disadvantages. Absent a binding commitment to help, rich States might find it politically or economically easier to withhold their fair share of global health assistance, hoping that others will take up the slack. Major outbreaks of infectious disease, including extensively drug-resistant forms, would become increasingly more likely. Even if the economically and politically powerful escaped major health hazards, they would still have to avert their eyes from the mounting suffering among the poor. And they would have to live with their consciences knowing that much of this physical and mental anguish is preventable.

What is most important is that if the global community does not accept fair terms of cooperation on global health soon, there is every reason to believe that affluent States, philanthropists and celebrities simply will move on to another cause. And when they do, the vicious cycle of poverty and endemic disease among the world's least healthy people will continue unabated. That is a consequence that none of us should be willing to tolerate.

Bibliography

Abbott, F., 'The Enduring Enigma of TRIPS: A Challenge for the World Economic System', *Journal of International Economic Law* (1998) 1, 497–521.

Adema, W. and Ladaique, M., *How Expensive is the Welfare State? Gross and Net Indicators in the OECD Social Expenditure Database (SOCX)*, Paris: OECD, 2009.

Aginam, O., 'Health or Trade? A Critique of Contemporary Approaches to Global Health Diplomacy', *Asian Journal of WTO and International Health Law and Policy* (2010) 5:2, 355–80.

Allan, C. and Stankey, G. B., (eds), *Adaptive Environmental Management, A Practitioners Guide*, London: Springer, 2009.

Ambassador Laura Kennedy, *Statement of the US Special Representative for the Biological and Toxin Weapons Convention Issues at the Preparatory Committee for the BWC Review Conference*, Geneva: United Nations, 14 April 2011.

Anand, S., Peter, F. and Sen, A. (eds), *Public Health, Ethics, and Equity*, Oxford: Oxford University Press, 2004.

Anomaly, J., 'Combating Resistance: The Case for a Global Antibiotics Treaty', *Public Health Ethics* (2010) 3:1, 13–22.

Arias E., *United States Life Tables 2006*, National Vital Statistics Reports 58, 2010, www.cdc.gov/nchs/data/nvsr/nvsr58/nvsr58_21.pdf.

Armitage, D., Berkes, F. and Doubleday, N., Collaboration, Learning and Multi-Level Governance: Adaptive Co-Management, Vancouver: UBC Press, 2007.

Arras, J., 'Theory and Bioethics', in E. N. Zalta (ed.), *Stanford Encyclopedia of Bioethics*, http://plato.stanford.edu/archives/sum2010/entries/theory-bioethics/.

Asante, A. D. and Zwi, A. B., 'Public-Private Partnerships and Global Health Equity: Prospects and Challenges', *Indian Journal of Medical Ethics* (2007) IV:4, 179.

Ashcroft. R., 'Fair Process & the Redundancy of Bioethics: A Polemic', *Public Health Ethics* (2008) 1:1, 3–9.

Asslaber, M. and Zatloukal, K., 'Biobanks: Transnational, European and Global Networks', *Briefings in Functional Genomics & Proteomics* (2007) 6, 193–201.

Attfield, R., 'Ecological Issues of Justice', in H. Widdows and N. J. Smith (eds), *Global Social Justice: Rethinking Globalizations*, London and New York: Routledge, 2011, 82–9.

Australia, Japan and Switzerland on behalf of 'JACKSNNZ', and Sweden, *Possible Approaches to Education and Awareness-Raising among Life Scientists*, BWC/CONF. VII/PC/INF.4, Geneva: United Nations, 2011.

Australia, *Raising Awareness: Approaches and Opportunities for Outreach*. BWC/MSP/2005/MX/WP.29, 21 June 2005, available at www.opbw.org

Avert, *Aids, Drug Prices and Generic Drugs*, www.avert.org/generic.htm

Bakker, I. C. and Gill, S., 'Towards a New Common Sense: The Need for New Paradigms of Global Health', in S. R. Benatar and G. Brock (eds), *Global Health and Global Health Ethics*, Cambridge: Cambridge University Press, 2011.

—, *Power, Production and Social Reproduction*, London: Zed Books, 2003.

Banerjee, A., Hollis, A. and Pogge, T., 'The Health Impact Fund: Incentives for Improving Access to Medicines', *The Lancet* (2010) 375, 166–9.

Barlow, P., 'Health Care Is Not a Human Right', *British Medical Journal* (1999) 319, 321.

Barnett, A. and Smith, H., 'Cruel Cost of the Human Egg Trade', *Observer*, 29 April 2006, 6.

Barnett, J. and Adger W. N., 'Climate Dangers and Atoll Countries', *Climatic Change* (2003) 61, 321–37.

Baron, M. W., *Kantian Ethics Almost Without Apology*, Ithaca: Cornell University Press, 1995.

Baron, M. W., Pettit, P. and Slote, M., *Three Methods of Ethics: A Debate*, Malden, MA: Blackwell Publishers Ltd, 1997.

Barr, M. D., *Cultural Politics and Asian Values: The Tepid War*, London and New York: Routledge, 2002.

Barrett, C. B., 'Measuring Food Insecurity', *Science* (2010) 327, 825.

Barry, B., *Theories of Justice*, Berkeley, CA: University of California Press, 1989.

Barton, J. H., 'TRIPS and the Global Pharmaceutical Market', *Health Affairs* (2004) 23, 146–54.

Battin, M. P., Francis, L. P., Jacobson, J. A. and Smith, C. B., *The Patient as Victim and Vector: Ethics and Infectious Disease,* Oxford: Oxford University Press, 2008.

Bauer, J. R. and Bell, D. A. (eds), *The East Asian Challenge for Human Rights*, Cambridge, UK: Cambridge University Press, 1999.

BBC News Online, 'Dignitas: Swiss Suicide Helpers', *BBC News: Health*, 2009, http://news.bbc.co.uk/2/hi/4643196.stm.

Beaglehole, R. and Bonita, R. (eds), *Global Public Health – A New Era*, 2nd edn, Oxford: Oxford University Press, 2009.

Beauchamp, T. L. and Childress, J. F., *Principles of Biomedical Ethics*, 6th edn, Oxford: Oxford University Press, 2009.

Belanger, M., *Global Health Law, an Introduction*, Cambridge: Cambridge Scientific Publishers, 2011.

Benatar, D., 'Animals, the Environment and Global Health', in S. R. Benatar and G. Brock (eds), *Global Health and Global Health Ethics*, Cambridge: Cambridge University Press, 2011.

Benatar, S. R., 'Global Disparities in Health and Human Rights: A Critical Commentary', *American Journal of Public Health* (1998) 88, 295–300.

—, 'Global Health and Human Rights: Working with the 20th Century Legacy', *Annual Human Rights Lecture*, University of Alberta, 2011.

—, 'Global Leadership, Ethics and Global Health: The Search for New Paradigms', in S. Gill (ed.), *The Global Crisis & the Crisis of Global Leadership*, Cambridge: Cambridge University Press, 2011.

—, 'Justice and Priority Setting in International Health Research', in R. Ashcroft, A. Dawson, H. Draper and J. R. McMillan (eds), *Principles of Health Care Ethics*, 2nd edn, Chichester: John Wiley and Sons, 2007.

—, 'Millennial Challenges for Medicine & Modernity', *J Roy Coll Phys Lond* (1998) 32, 160–5.

—, 'Moral Imagination: The Missing Component in Global Health', *PLoS Medicine* (2005) 2:12, e400.

—, 'Reflections and Recommendations on Research Ethics in Developing Countries', *Social Science & Medicine* (2002) 54, 1131–41.

—, 'South Africa's Transition in a Globalizing World. HIV/AIDS as a Window and a Mirror', *International Affairs* (2001) 77:2, 347–75.

—, 'The Coming Catastrophe in International Health', *Canadian Journal of International Affairs* (2001) 4, 611–31.

—, 'War, or Peace & Development: S. Africa's Message for Global Peace & Security', *Medicine, Conflict and Survival* (1997) 13, 125–34.

Benatar, S. R. and Brock, G. (eds), *Global Health and Global Health Ethics,* Cambridge: Cambridge University Press, 2011.

Benatar, S. R. and Doyal, L., 'Human Rights Abuses: Balancing Two Perspectives', *International Journal of Health Services* (2009) 39:1, 139–59.

Benatar, S. R., Daar, A. and Singer, P. A., 'Global Health Ethics: The Rationale for Mutual Caring', in S. R. Benatar and G. Brock (eds), *Global Health and Global Health Ethics*, Cambridge: Cambridge University Press, 2011.

Benatar, S. R., Gill, S., and Bakker, I. C., 'Global Health and the Global Economic Crisis', *American Journal of Public Health* (2011) 101:4, 646–53.

Benatar, S. R. and Upshur, R., 'What is Global Health?', in S. R. Benatar and G. Brock (eds), *Global Health and Global Health Ethics,* Cambridge, Cambridge University Press, 2011.

Bennett, B. and Tomossy, G. F. (eds), *Globalization and Health: Challenges for Health Law and Bioethics,* New York: Springer, 2006.

Bhatia, G. S., O'Neill, J. S., Gall, G. L. and Bendin, P. D. (eds), *Peace, Justice and Freedom: Human Rights Challenges for the New Millennium*, Alberta: University of Alberta Press 2000.

Biobank UK, *UK Biobank: Protocol for a Large-Scale Prospective Epidemiological Resource,* Stockport: Biobank UK, 2007.

Birn, A.-E., 'Addressing the Societal Determinants of Health: The Key Global Health Ethics Imperative', in S. R. Benatar and G. Brock (eds), *Global Health and Global Health Ethics*, Cambridge: Cambridge University Press, 2011.

—, 'Gates' Grandest Challenge: Transcending Technology as Public Health Ideology', *The Lancet,* (2005) 366:9484, 514–19.

Board of Science and Education, *Biotechnology, Weapons and Humanity II*, London: British Medical Association, 2004.

Boylan, M., *Morality and Global Justice: Justifications and Applications*, Westview Press, 2011.

Boylan, M. (ed.), *The Morality and Global Justice Reader*, Boulder: Westview Press, 2011.

Boyle, A., 'Human Rights or Environmental Rights: A Reassessment', *Fordham Environmental Law Review* (2007) 18, 471.

Boyle, J., *The Public Domain: Enclosing the Commons of the Mind*, New Haven: Yale University Press, 2008.

Brand Frank, Z., *Google Baby*, Brandcom Productions and HBO Documentary Films, 2009.

Brecher, J., Costello, T. and Smith, B., *Globalisation from Below: The E Power of Solidarity,* Cambridge, MA: South End Press, 2000.

Brian G. Spratt, *Independent Review of the Safety of UK Facilities Handling Foot-and-Mouth Disease Virus*, Defra: UK, 2007.

Brock, G., *Global Justice: A Cosmopolitan Account*, Oxford: Oxford University Press, 2009.

Brock, G., 'Taxation and Global Justice: Closing the Gap between Theory and Practice', *Journal of Social Philosophy* (2008) 39:2, 161–84.

Brown, E. M. and Nathanwi, D., 'Antibiotic Cycling or Rotation: A Systematic Review of the Evidence of Efficacy', *Journal of Antimicrobial Chemotherapy* (2005) 55, 6–9.

Bruch, C., 'Adaptive Water Management: Strengthening Laws and Institutions to Cope with Uncertainty', in A. K. Biswas, C. Tortajada and R. Izquierdo-Avino (eds), *Water Management in 2020 and Beyond*, Heidelberg: Springer, 2009.

Brunner, R. D., Steelman, T. A., Coe-Juell, L., Cromley, C. M., Edwards, C. M. and Tucker, D. W., *Adaptive Governance: Integrating Science, Policy and Decision Making*, New York: Columbia University Press, 2005.

Building a Global Community. Globalization and the Common Good, Copenhagen: Royal Danish Foreign Ministry for Foreign Affairs, 2000.

Bunting, M., 'Profits that Kill', *The Guardian* 12 February 2001, www.guardian.co.uk/world/2001/feb/12/wto.aids.

Burci, G. L., 'Institutional Adaptation without Reform: Who and the Challenges of Globalization', *International Organization Law Review* (2005) 2, 437–43.

Burris, S., 'Symposium: SARS, Public Health, and Global Governance: Governance, Micro governance and Health', *Temple Law Review* (2004) 77, 335.

Burris, S., Drahos, P. and Shearing, C., 'Nodal Governance', *Australian Journal of Legal Philosophy* (2005) 30, 30.

Buse, K. and Walt, G., 'An Unruly Melange? Coordinating External Resources To The Health Sector: A Review', *Social Science & Medicine* (1997) 45, 449–63.

Buse, K. and Waxman, A., 'Public–Private Health Partnerships: A Strategy for WHO', *Bulletin of the World Health Organization* (2001) 8, 79.

Campbell-Lendrum, D., Corvalán, C. and Prüss-Ustün, A., 'How Much Disease Could Climate Change Cause?', in A. McMichael, D. Campbell-Lendrum, C. Corvalán, C. Ebi, A. Githeko, J. Scheraga and A. Woodward (eds), *Climate Change and Human Health: Risks and Responses*, Geneva: World Health Organization, 2003.

Caney, S., 'Climate Change and the Future: Discounting for Time, Wealth, and Risk', *Journal of Social Philosophy* (2009) 40, 163–86.

—, 'Cosmopolitan Justice and Equalizing Opportunities', *Metaphilosophy* (2001) 32, 113–34.

—, 'Justice and the Distribution of Greenhouse Gas Emissions' in H. Widdows and N. J. Smith (eds), *Global Social Justice*, London and New York: Routledge, 2011.

—, *Justice beyond Borders, a Global Political Theory*, Oxford, UK: Oxford University Press, 2005.

Chan, M., 'Strengthening Multilateral Cooperation on Intellectual Property and Public Health', in *World Intellectual Property Organisation Conference on Intellectual Property and Public Policy Issues*, Geneva: WIPO, 2009.

Chandra, R., *Knowledge as Property: Issues in the Moral Grounding of Intellectual Property Rights*, New Delhi: Oxford University Press, 2010.

Chaudhuri, S., Goldberg, P. K. and Jia, P., 'Estimating the Effects of Global Patent Protection in Pharmaceuticals: A Case Study of Quinolones in India', *The American Economic Review* (2006) 96, 1477–514.

Chien, C., 'Cheap Drugs at What Price to Innovation: Does the Compulsory Licensing of Pharmaceuticals Hurt Innovation?', *Berkeley Technology Law Journal* (2003) www.law.berkeley.edu/journals/btlj/articles/vol18/Chien.web.pdf.

Cilliers, P., *Complexity and Post Modernism*, London: Routledge, 1998.

Clarke, S. G. and Simpson, E., 'Introduction: The Primacy of Moral Practice', in S. G. Clarke and E. Simpson (eds), *Anti-Theory in Ethics and Moral Conservatism*, Albany: State University of New York, 1989.

Codex Alimentarius Commission, *Codex Principles for the Risk Analysis of Foods Derived from Modern Biotechnology 2003*, Rome: FAO, 2011.

—, *Guideline for the Conduct of Food Safety Assessment of Foods Derived from Recombinant-DNA Plants 2003*, Rome: FAO, 2008.

—, *Guideline for the Conduct of Food Safety Assessment of Foods Produced Using Recombinant-DNA Microorganisms, 2003*, Rome: FAO, 2003.

—, *Guideline for the Conduct of Food Safety Assessment of Foods Derived from Recombinant-DNA Animals, 2008*, Rome: FAO, 2008.

Coggon, J., *What Makes Health Public? A Critical Evaluation of Moral, Legal, and Political Claims in Public Health*, Cambridge: Cambridge University Press, 2012.

Cohen, L. R. and Noll, R. G., 'Intellectual Property, Antitrust and the New Economy', *University of Pittsburgh Law Review* (2000) 62, 453–73.

Cohen-Kohler, J. C., 'The Morally Uncomfortable Global Drug Gap', *Clinical Pharmacology & Therapeutics* (2007) 82:5, 610–4.

Collier, P., *The Bottom Billion Why the Poorest Countries are Failing and What Can Be Done About It*, Oxford: Oxford University Press, 2008.

Commission on Intellectual Property Rights, Innovation and Public Health, *Intellectual Property Rights, Innovation and Public Health*, Geneva: WHO, 2006.

Committee on Science, Engineering and Public Policy, *On Being a Scientist: A Guide to Responsible Conduct in Research*, 3rd edn, Washington DC: National Academies Press, 2009.

Committee on the Conduct of Science, *On Being a Scientist*, US National Academy of Sciences, Washington DC: National Academies Press, 1989.

Conference Statement, *Strengthen Local Campaigns for National and International Accountability for Health and Health Services*, Johannesburg Conference Statement and Resolutions, 2011, www.section27.org.za/wp-content/uploads/2011/04/Johann esburg-Conference-Consensus-and-Resolutions-final.pdf.

Connell, J., 'Medical Tourism: Sea, Sun, Sand and . . . Surgery', *Tourism Management* (2006) 27, 1093–100.

Convention on Biodiversity Secretariat, *Nagoya Protocol on Access to Genetic Resources and the Fair and Equitable Sharing of the Benefits Arising Out of their Utilisation*, Montreal: CBD Secretariat, 2010.

Cooney, R. and Lang, A. T. F., 'Taking Uncertainty Seriously: Adaptive Governance and International Trade', *The European Journal of International Law* (2007) 18, 523–51.

Cooper, A. F., Kirton, J. J. and Schrecker, T. (eds), *Governing Global Health: Challenge, Response, Innovation*, London: Ashgate, 2007.

Correa, C. M., 'Implications of Bilateral Free Trade Agreements on Access to Medicines', *Bulletin of the World Health Organisation* (2006) 84, 399–404.

Costello, A., Abbas, M., Allen, A., Ball, S., Bell, S., Bellamy, R., et al. 'Managing the Health Effects of Climate Change', *The Lancet* (2009) 373, 1693.

D'Costa, V., King, C., Kalan, L., Morar, M., Sung, W., Schwartz, C., Froese, D., Zazula, G., et al., 'Antibiotic Resistance Is Ancient', *Nature* (2011) 477:7365, 457–61.

Daar, A. S., Singer, P. A., Persad, D. L., Pramming, S. K., Matthews, D. R., Beaglehole, R., et al., 'Grand Challenges In Chronic Non-Communicable Diseases', *Nature* (2007) 450, 494–6.

Dalrymple, T., 'Is There a "Right" to Health Care?', *Wall Street Journal*, 28 July 2009.

Dando, M. R. and Rappert, B., 'In-depth Implementation of the BTWC: Education and Outreach', *Review Conference Paper No. 18*, Bradford: University of Bradford, 2006.

Daniels, N., 'Is There a Right to Health Care and, if so, What Does It Encompass?' in H. Kuhse and P. Singer (eds) *A Companion to Bioethics*, Oxford, UK: Wiley-Blackwell, 2009, 362–72.

—, 'Justice, Health, and Healthcare', *Am. J. Bioethics* (2001) 1:2, 2–16.

—, *Just Health Care*, Cambridge, UK: Cambridge University Press, 1985.

—, *Just Health: Meeting Health Needs Fairly*, Cambridge, UK: Cambridge University Press, 2008.

—, 'Social Responsibility and Global Pharmaceutical Companies', *Developing World Bioethics* (2001) 1, 38–41.

Daniels, N. and Sabin, J. E., *Setting Limits Fairly: Can We Learn to Share Medical Resources?* Oxford: Oxford University Press, 2002.

—, *Setting Limits Fairly: Learning to Share Resources for Health Second Edition,* New York, USA: Oxford University Press, 2008.

Danzon, P. M. and Towse, A., 'Differential Pricing for Pharmaceuticals: Reconciling Access, R&D and Patents', *International Journal of Health Care Finance and Economics* (2003) 3, 183–205.

David DeGraw, 'The Economic Elite Have Engineered an Extraordinary Coup, Threatening the Very Existence of the Middle Class,' Alternet.org, 2010.

Dentico, N. and Ford, N., 'The Courage to Change the Rules: A Proposal for an Essential Health R&D Treaty', *PLoS Medicine* (2005) 2, 96–9.

Devos, Y., Reheul, D., Waele, D. D. and Spreybroeck, L. V., 'The Interplay between Societal Concerns and the Regulatory Frame on GM Crops in the European Union', *Environmental Biosafety Research* (2006) 5:3, 127–49.

DiMasi, J. A. and Grabowski, H. G., 'Patents and R&D Incentives: Comments on the Hubbard and Love Trade Framework for Financing Pharmaceutical R&D', in Submission for WHO Commission on Intellectual Property Rights, Innovation and Public Health, Geneva: WHO, 2004.

Donchin, A. and Purdy, L., *Embodying Bioethics. Recent Feminist Advances,* Oxford: Rowman & Littlefield Publishers, 1999.

Donnelly, J., *Universal Human Rights in Theory and Practice,* London: Cornell University Press, 1989.

Doyal, L. and Gough, I., *A Theory of Human Need,* London: McMillan, 1991.

Drahos, P., 'The Universality of Human Rights: Origins and Development', in *World Intellectual Property Organisation Panel Discussion to Commemorate the 50th Anniversary of the Universal Declaration of Human Rights,* Geneva, 1999.

Drain, P. K., Huffman, A., Pyrtle, S. E. and Chan, K., *Caring for the World: A Guidebook to Global Health Opportunities,* Toronto: University of Toronto Press, 2009.

Dreisen, D., 'Free Lunch or Cheap Fix: The Emissions Trading Idea and the Climate Change Convention', *Boston College Environmental Affairs Law Review* (1998) 26, 5.

Dresner, S., *The Principles of Sustainability,* London: Earthscan, 2002.

Drlica, K. and Perlin, D. S., *Antibiotic Resistance: Understanding and Responding to an Emerging Crisis,* New Jersey: FT Press, 2011.

Dutfield, G., 'Delivering Drugs to the Poor: Will the TRIPS Amendment Help?', *American Journal of Law & Medicine* (2008) 34, 107–24.

Dworkin, R., 'Rights as Trumps', in J. Waldron (ed.), *Theories of Rights,* Oxford: Oxford University Press, 2004.

Dyzenhaus, D., 'The Politics of Deference: Judicial Review and Democracy', in M. Taggart (ed.), *The Province of Administrative Law,* Oxford: Hart, 1997.

Editorial, *India's Choice,* The New York Times, January 18, 2005.

—, 'Right-to-Health Responsibilities of Pharmaceutical Companies', *The Lancet* (2009) 373, 1998.

—, 'The Health Status of Indigenous Peoples and Others', *BMJ* (2003) 327, 404–5.

Engelhardt, T. H., 'Critical Care: Why There Is No Global Bioethics', *Journal of Medicine and Philosophy* (1998) 23, 643–51.

European Food Safety Authority, 'Scientific Opinion, Guidance on the Environmental Risk Assessment of Genetically Modified Plants, EFSA Panel on Genetically Modified Organisms (GMO), Summary', *EFSA Journal* (2010) 8:11, 1879.

European Medicines Agency and European Centre for Disease Prevention and Control, *Joint Technical Report: The Bacterial Challenge – time to React*, 2009, http://ecdc.europa.eu/en/publications/Publications/0909_TER_The_Bacterial_Challenge_Time_to_React.pdf.

Fanu, J. L., *The Rise and Fall of Modern Medicine*, London: Little, Brown and Company, 1999.

FAO/WHO, *Understanding the Codex Alimentarius*, Rome: FAO, 2006, ftp://ftp.fao.org/codex/Publications/understanding/Understanding_EN.pdf.

Farmer, P., *Infections and Inequalities: The Modern Plagues*, Berkeley, CA: University of California Press, 1999.

—, *Pathologies of Power: Health, Human Rights and the New War on the Poor*, 2nd edn, Berkeley, CA: University of California Press, 2004.

Fedoroff, N. V., Battisti, D. S. Beachy, R. N., Cooper, P. J. M., Fischhoff, D. A., Hodges, C. N., et al., 'Radically Rethinking Agriculture for the 21st Century', *Science* (2010) 327, 833–34.

Fidler, D., 'International Law and Global Public Health', *Kansas Law Review* (1999) 48, 1–26.

—, *International Law and Public Health*, Ardsley, NY: Transnational Publishers, 2000.

Fink, C. and Reichenmiller, P., *Tightening TRIPS: The Intellectual Property Provisions of Recent US Free Trade Agreements*, Geneva: International Centre for Trade and Sustainable Development, 2005.

Finkelstein, L. S., 'What Is Global Governance?', *Global Governance* (1995) 1:3, 363–72.

Folke, C., Hahn, T., Olsson, P. and Norberg, J., 'Adaptive Governance of Socio-Ecological Systems', *Annual Review of Environment and Resources* (2005) 30, 441.

Food and Agricultural Organisation, *925 Million in Chronic Hunger Worldwide*, Rome: FAO, 2010, www.fao.org/news/story/en/item/45210/icode/.

—, 'World Hunger Report 2011: High, Volatile Prices Set to Continue', *Press Release 10 October 2011*, Rome: FAO, www.fao.org/news/story/en/item/92495/icode/.

—, *Current FAO Mechanisms for Dealing with the Deliberate Release of Detrimental Biological Agents – Biological Weapons Convention (BWC) Meeting of States*, Geneva: BWC Implementation Support Unit, 2007.

—, *International Plant Protection Convention*, Rome: FAO, 1997, www.ippc.int/file_uploaded//publications/13742.New_Revised_Text_of_the_International_Plant_Protectio.pdf.

—, *International Treaty on Plant Genetic Resources for Food and Agriculture*, Rome: FAO, 2001, ftp://ftp.fao.org/docrep/fao/011/i0510e/i0510e.pdf.

—, *The Scourge of 'Hidden Hunger': Global Dimensions of Micronutrient Deficiencies*, Rome: FAO, 2003, ftp://ftp.fao.org/docrep/fao/005/y8346my8346m01.pdf.

Foot, P., 'Utilitarianism and the Virtues', *Mind* (1985) 94, 196–209.

—, *Virtues and Vices and Other Essays in Moral Philosophy*, Berkeley, CA: University of California Press, 1978.

Forsythe, D. P., *Human Rights in International Relations*, Cambridge: Cambridge University Press, 2006.

Foster K. R. and Grundmann, H., 'Do We Need To Put Society First? The Potential for Tragedy in Antimicrobial Resistance', PLoS Med (2006) 3, e29.

Fox, J., The Myth of the Rational Market: A History of Risk, Reward, and Delusion on Wall Street, New York: Harper Business/Harper Collins, 2009.

Fox, W., A Theory of General Ethics: Human Relationships, Nature, and the Built Environment, Cambridge, MA: MIT Press, 2007.

Franklin, U., The Real World of Technology, Massey Lectures 1989, Revised Edition, Toronto: House of Anansi Press, 1999.

Fredman, S., Human Rights Transformed, Oxford: Oxford University Press, 2008.

Freeman, J., 'Collaborative Governance in the Administrative State', UCLA Law Review (1997) 45:1, 1–98.

Freidson, E., Professionalism the Third Logic, Chicago: University of Chicago Press, 2003.

Friel, S., Butler, C. and McMichael, A., 'Climate Change and Health Risks and Inequities', in S. R. Benatar and G. Brock (eds), Global Health and Global Health Ethics, Cambridge: Cambridge University Press, 2011, 198–219.

Friel, S., Marmot, M., McMichael, A., Kjellstrom, T. and Vågerö D., 'Global Health Equity and Climate Stabilisation: A Common Agenda', The Lancet (2008) 372, 1677.

Galbraith, J. K., The Affluent Society, Boston: Houghton Mifflin, 1958.

—, The Culture of Contentment, New York: Houghton-Mifflin Company, 1992, 156–57.

—, The Economics of Innocent Fraud; Truth for Our Times, Boston: Houghton Mifflin, 2004.

—, The Good Society, Boston: Houghton Mifflin, 1996.

—, The New Industrial State, Boston: Houghton Mifflin, 1976.

—, The Socially Concerned Today, Toronto: University of Toronto Press, 1998.

Galtung, J., True Worlds, New York: Free Press, 1980.

García-Salmones, M., 'Taking Uncertainty Seriously: Adaptive Governance and International Trade: A Reply to Rosie Cooney and Andrew Lang', European Journal of International Law (2009) 20:1, 167–86.

Gardiner, S. M., 'Ethics and Global Climate Change', Ethics (2004) 114, 555–600.

Gargarella, R., 'Dialogic Justice in the Enforcement of Social Rights: Some Initial Arguments', in A. Yamin and S. Gloppen (eds), Litigating Health Rights, Cambridge, MA: Harvard University Press, 2011.

Gaskell, G., Allansdottir, A., Allum, N., Corchero, C., Fischler, C., Hampel, J., et al., 'Europeans and Biotechnology in 2005: Patterns and Trends, Eurobarometer 64.3', Report to the European Commission's Directorate-General for Research, 2006.

Gauri, V. and Brinks, D. (eds), Courting Social Justice, Cambridge: Cambridge University Press, 2008.

Gawtkin, D. R. and Guillot, M., The Burden of Disease among the Global Poor: Current Situation, Future Trends, and Implications for Strategy, Washington: World Bank, 2000.

Gebauer, T., 'Universal Coverage – A Shift in the International Debate in Global Health', Equinet Newsletter (2011) 119, 1.

George, A., A Fate Worse than Debt, London: Penguin Books, 1988.

Gertler, M. S. and Wolfe, D. A., Innovation and Social Learning: Institutional Adaptation in an Era of Technological Change, Basingstoke: Palgrave, 2002.

Giampietro, M., 'Complexity and Scales: The Challenge for Integrated Assessment', Scaling in Integrated Assessment (2003) 3:2/3, 247.

Gilbert, D., Walley, T. and New, B., 'Lifestyle Medicines', *British Medical Journal* (2000) 321, 1341–4.

Gill, S., *Power and Resistance in the New World Order*, 2nd edn, New York: Palgrave MacMillan, 2008.

Gill, S. (ed.), *Global Crises and the Crisis of Global Leadership*, Cambridge: Cambridge University Press, 2011.

Gill, S. and Bakker, I. C., 'The Global Crisis and Global Health', in S. R. Benatar and G. Brock (eds), *Global Health and Global Health Ethics*, Cambridge: Cambridge University Press, 2011, 221–38.

Global Fund to Fight AIDS, Tuberculosis and Malaria, *By-laws, as amended 21 November 2011*, Geneva: Global Fund to fight AIDS, Tuberculosis and Malaria, 2011, www.theglobalfund.org/documents/core/bylaws/Core_GlobalFund_Bylaws_En/.

Global Health Watch, *Global Health Watch 1: 2005–2006*, London: Zed Books, 2007.

Glover, J., 'Poverty, Distance and Two Dimensions of Ethics', in S. R. Benatar and G. Brock (eds), *Global Health and Global Health Ethics*, Cambridge: Cambridge University Press, 2011, 311–18.

Gostin, L. O., *Global Health Law: International Law, Global Institutions, and World Health*, Cambridge, MA: Harvard University Press, forthcoming.

—, 'Meeting Basic Survival Needs of the World's Least Healthy People toward a Framework Convention on Global Health', *Georgetown Law Journal (2008) 96*, 331–92.

—, 'Redressing the Unconscionable Health Gap: A Global Plan for Justice', *Harvard Law & Policy Rev* (2010) 4, 271–94, http://ssrn.com/abstract=1635895.

—, 'The Unconscionable Health Gap: A Global Plan for Justice', *The Lancet* (2010) 375, 1504–05, http://ssrn.com/abstract=1635902.

Gostin, L. O. and Taylor, A. L., 'Global Health Law: A Definition and Grand Challenges', *Journal of Public Health Ethics* (2008) 1, 53–63.

Gostin L. O., Friedman E. A., Ooms G., Gebauer T., Gupta N., Sridhar D., Chenguang W., Røttingen J.-A. and Sanders D., 'The Joint Action and Learning Initiative: Towards a Global Agreement on National and Global Responsibilities for Health', *PLoS Medicine* (2011) 8:5.

Gottret, P. E., and Schieber, G., *Health Financing Revisited – A Practitioner's Guide*, Washington DC: The World Bank Publication, 2006.

Gracey, M. and King, M., 'Indigenous Health Part 1: Determinants and Disease Patterns', *The Lancet* (2009) 374:9683, 65–75.

Graham, H., *Unequal Lives: Health and Socioeconomic Inequalities*, Berkshire: McGraw-Hill Open University Press, 2007.

Grover, A., *Promotion and Protection of all Human Rights, Civil, Political, Economic, Social and Cultural Rights, including the Right to Development: A Report of the Special Rapporteur on the Right of Everyone to the Enjoyment of the Highest Attainable Standard of Physical and Mental Health*, A/HRC/11/12, New York: United Nations, 2009.

Gunderson, L., 'Resilience, Flexibility and Adaptive Management – Antidotes for Spurious Certitude?', *Conservation Ecology* (1999) 3:1, 7.

Haimowitz, R. and Sinha, V., *Made In India*, Women Make Movies, 2010.

Halliburton, M., 'Drug Resistance, Patent Resistance: Indian Pharmaceuticals and the Impact of a New Patent Regime', *Global Public Health* (2009) 4, 515–27.

Hampton, J., *Political Philosophy*, Boulder, CO: Westview Press, 1997.

Hardimon, M. O., 'Role Obligations', *The Journal of Philosophy* (1994) 91:7, 333–63.

Hawks, N. and Cohen, D., 'What Makes an Orphan Drug?', *British Medical Journal* (2010) 341, 1076–8.

Heald, P. J., 'A Skeptical Look at Mansfield''s Famous 1994 Survey', *Information Economics and Policy* (2004) 16, 57–65.

Heilbroner, R., *An Inquiry into the Human Prospect*, New York: W.W. Norton, 1974.

Hein, W. and Kohlmorgen, L. (eds), *Globalisation, Global Health Governance and National Health Politics in Developing Countries – An Exploration Into the Dynamics of Interfaces*, Hamburg: DÜI, 2003.

Held, V., 'Care and Justice in the Global Context', *Ratio Juris* (2004) 17, 141–55.

—, *The Ethics of Care: Personal, Political, and Global*, Oxford, UK: Oxford University Press, 2006.

Helfer, L. R., *Intellectual Property Rights In Plant Varieties – International Legal Regimes And Policy Options For National Governments*, FAO Legislative Study 85, Rome: United Nations, 2004.

Henry, D. and Lexchin, J., 'The Pharmaceutical Industry as a Medicines Power', *The Lancet,* (2002) 360, 1590–5.

Hill, P., 'Understanding Global Health Governance as a Complex Adaptive System', *Global Public Health* (2011) 6:6, 593–605.

Hobbes, T., *Leviathan*, Touchstone, 1997.

Hollis, A. and Pogge, T., *The Health Impact Fund: Making New Medicines Accessible for All*, New Haven, Connecticut: Incentives for Global Health, 2008.

Hooker, B., *Ideal Code, Real World*, Oxford: Clarendon Press, 2000.

Howells, J., 'The Internationalization of R & D and the Development of Global Research Networks', *Regional Studies: The Journal of the Regional Studies Association* (1990) 24, 495–512.

Hubbard, T. and Love, J., 'A New Trade Framework for Global Healthcare R&D', *PLoS Biology* (2004) 2, 147–150.

Hunt, P., *Report of the Special Rapporteur on the Right of Everyone to the Enjoyment of the Highest Attainable Standard of Health: Annex – Mission to Glaxosmithkline*, New York: United Nations, 2009.

Hunt, P. and Backman, G., 'Health Systems and the Right to the Highest Attainable Standard of Health', *Health and Human Rights* (2008) 10, 81.

Hurst, S. A., Mezger, N., Mauron, A., 'Allocating Resources in Humanitarian Medicine', in S. R. Benatar and G. Brock (eds), *Global Health and Global Health Ethics*, Cambridge: Cambridge University Press, 2011, 173–83.

Hursthouse, R., *On Virtue Ethics*, Oxford, UK: Oxford University Press, 2001.

—, 'Virtue Theory and Abortion', *Philosophy & Public Affairs* (1991) 20, 223–46.

Ignatieff, M., *The Needs of Strangers,* New York: Viking Press, 1984.

Ikeme, J., 'Equity, Environmental Justice and Sustainability: Incomplete Approaches in Climate Change Politics', *Global Environmental Change* (2003) 13, 95–206.

Intergovernmental Panel on Climate Change, *Climate Change 2007, Synthesis Report – A Report of the Intergovernmental Panel on Climate Change*, Cambridge: Cambridge University Press, 2007.

Intergovernmental Panel on Climate Change, 'Food, Fibre and Forest Production', in M. Parry, O. Canziani, J. Palutikof, P. Linden and C. Hanson (eds), *Climate Change 2007: Impacts, Adaptation and Vulnerability*, Cambridge: Cambridge University Press, 2007.

Jefferson, T., *Letter to Isaac McPherson*, 13 August 1813, in Writings 13, 333–5, http://press-pubs.uchicago.edu/founders/documents/a1_8_8s12.html.

Johnson, J., 'Teaching Ethics to Science Students: Challenges and a Strategy', in B. Rappert (ed.), *Education and Ethics in the Life Sciences*, Canberra: ANUE Press, 2010.

Johnston, J. and Wasunna, A. A., 'Patents Biomedical Research and Treatments – Examining Concerns, Canvassing Solutions', *A Hastings Centre Special Report* (2007) 37:1, S1–S36.

Jonsen, A. R., Seigler, M. and Winslade, W. J., *Clinical Ethics: A Practical Approach to Ethical Decisions in Clinical Medicine*, 7th edn, New York: McGraw Hill Medical, 2010.

Jørgensen, R. B., 'GMO: En løsning på ændrede klimaforhold', in M. Gjerris, C. Gamborg, J. E. Olesen and J. Wolf (eds), *Jorden Braender – Klimaforandringerne i videnskabsteoretisk og etisk perspektiv*, Forlaget: Alfa Frederiksberg, 2009.

Judt, T., *Ill Fares the Land*, New York: Penguin Books, 2010.

Kades, E., 'Preserving a Precious Resource: Rationalising the Use of Antibiotics', *Northwestern Law Review* (2005) 99:2, 611–675.

Kaebnick, G., 'It's Against Nature', *The Hastings Centre Report* (2009) 39:1, 24–6.

Kant, I., *Grundlegung zur Metaphysik der Sitten*, Hamburg: Felix Meiner Verlag, 1965, [1785]

—, *Metaphysische Anfangsgründe der Tugendlehre*, Hamburg: Felix Meiner Verlag,1990, [1797].

Karkkainen, B. C., 'Collaborative Ecosystem Governance: Scale, Complexity and Dynamism', *Virginia Environmental Law Journal* (2002) 21, 189–243.

Kemp, P. and Nielsen, L. W., *The Barriers To Climate Awareness – A Report On The Ethics Of Sustainability*, Copenhagen: Ministry of Climate and Energy, 2009.

Kerry, V. B. and Lee, K., 'TRIPS, the Doha Declaration and Paragraph 6 Decision: What Are the Remaining Steps for Protecting Access to Medicines?', *Globalisation and Health*, (2007) 3, 3.

King, M., Smith, A. and Gracey, M., 'Indigenous Health Part 2: The Underlying Causes of the Health Gap', *The Lancet* (2009) 374:9683, 76–85.

Knoppers, B. M., Chadwick, R., Takebe, H., Kirby, M., Berg, K., Qiu, R.-Z., Macer, D., Cantu, J.-M., Wertz, D. C., Murray, T. H., Daar, A. S., Verma I. and Engels, E. M., *HUGO Ethics Committee, Statement on Benefit Sharing*, Vancouver: Human Genome Organisation, 2000, www.hugo-international.org/img/benefit_sharing_2000.pdf.

Knoppers, B. M., Chadwick, R. F., Verma, I. C., Berg, K., Cantu, J. M., Daar, A., Engels, E. M., Kato, K., Kirby, M., Macer, D. R. J., Murray, T. H., Qiu, R.-Z., Wertz, D. C., Bovenberg, J. and Cotton, R., *HUGO Ethics Committee: Statement on Human Genomic Databases*, Singapore: Human Genome Organisation, 2002, www.hugo-international.org/img/genomic_2002.pdf.

Knox, J., 'Linking Human Rights and Climate Change at the United Nations', *Harvard Environmental Law Review* (2009) 33, 477.

Koivusalo, M., 'Trade and Health: The Ethics of Global Rights, Regulation and Redistribution', in S. R. Benatar and G. Brock (eds), *Global Health and Global Health Ethics*, Cambridge: Cambridge University Press, 2011.

Krikorian, G., 'New Trends in IP Protection and Health Issues', in B. Coriat (ed.), *The Political Economy of HIV/AIDS in Developing Countries*, Cheltenham: Edward Elgar Publishing Ltd., 2008.

Kronman, A., *The Lost Lawyer: Failing Ideals of the Legal Profession*, Cambridge: Harvard University Press, 1993.

Kydd, J., Haddock, J., Mansfield, J., Ainsworth, C. and Buckwell, A., 'Genetically Modified Organisms: Major Issues and Policy Responses for Developing Countries', *Journal of International Development* (2000) 12:8, 1133–45.

Ladikas, M. and Schroeder, D., 'Too Early for Global Ethics?', *Cambridge Quarterly of Healthcare Ethics* (2005) 14, 404–15.

Lee, K., 'Appraising Adaptive Management', *Conservation Ecology* (1999) 3:2, 3.

—, 'Understanding of Global Health Governance: The Contested Landscape', in A. Kay and O. Williams (eds), *Global Health Governance: Crisis, Institutions and Political Economy*, London: Palgrave, 2009.

Lee, K. and Goodman, H., 'Global Policy Networks: The Propagation of Healthcare Financing Reform since the 1980s', in K. Lee, K. Buse and S. Fustukian (eds), *Health Policy In A Globalising World*, Cambridge: Cambridge University Press, 2002.

Lee, K., Fustukian, S. and Buse, K., 'An Introduction to Global Health Policy', in K. Lee, K. Buse and S. Fustukian (eds), *Health Policy In a Globalising World*, Cambridge: Cambridge University Press, 2002.

Lengeler, C., 'Insecticide-Treated Bed Nets and Curtains for Preventing Malaria', *Cochrance Database Sys. Rev.* (2004) 2, CD000363.

Levinson R., Dewar S., Shepherd S., *Understanding Doctors: Harnessing Professionalism*, London: The King's Fund, 2008.

Levy, M., 'Improving the Effectiveness of International Environmental Institutions', in P. Haas, R. O. Keohane and M. A. Levy (eds), *Institutions for the Earth*, MIT, 1993.

Lewontin, R., *Biology as Ideology*, New York: Harper Collins, 1991.

Lipsitch M., Singer R. S. and Levin B. R., 'Antibiotics in Agriculture: When Is It Time to Close The Barn Door?', *Proc Natl Acad Sci USA* (2002) 99, 5752–4.

Lister, G., 'Interdependence' in Marinker, M., (ed.), *Constructive Conversations about Health: Policy and Values*, Abingdon: Radcliffe Publishing, 2006.

Loefter, I., '"Health Care Is a Human Right" Is a Meaningless and Devastating Manifesto', *British Medical Journal* (1999) 318, 1766.

Longley, D., *Public Law and Health Service Accountability*, Buckingham: Open University Press, 1993.

Madeley, J., *Yours for Food: Plant Genetic Resources and Food Security*, London: Christian Aid, 1996.

Maibach, E., Nisbet, M., Baldwin, P., Akerlof, K. and Diao, G., 'Reframing Climate Change as a Public Health Issue: An Exploratory Study of Public Reactions', *BMC Public Health* (2010) 10, 299.

Mancini, G. and Revill, J., *Fostering the Biosecurity Norm: Biosecurity Education for the Next Generation of Life Scientists*, Como/Bradford: Landau Network and University of Bradford, 2008.

Marmot, M. and Wilkinson, R., *Social Determinants of Health*, Oxford: Oxford University Press, 2005.

Marris, C., 'Public Views on GMOs: Deconstructing the Myths', *EMBO Reports* (2001) 2:7, 545–8.

Martin, D. K., Benatar, S. R., 'Resource allocation: International Perspectives on Resource Allocation', in K. Heggenhougen and S. Quah (eds) *International Encyclopaedia of Public Health, Vol 5.*, San Diego: Academic Press 2008, 538–43.

Martin, D. K., Singer, P. A. and Bernstein, M., 'Access to ICU Needs for Neurosurgery Patients: A Qualitative Case Study', *J Neurology, Neurosurgery and Psychiatry* (2003) 74, 1299–303.

McIntyre, A., 'Doctrine of Double Effect', in Zalta, E. N. (ed.), *The Stanford Encyclopedia of Philosophy*, 2011, http://plato.stanford.edu/archives/fall2011/entries/double-effect/.

McIntyre, L. and Rondeau, K., 'Food Security and Global Health', in S. R. Benatar and G. Brock (eds), *Global Health and Global Health Ethics*, Cambridge: Cambridge University Press, 2011, 261–73.

McLeish, C., 'Reflecting on the Problem of Dual-Use', in B. Rappert and C. McLeish (eds), *A Web of Prevention*, London: Earthscan, 2007, 189–208.

McMichael, A., 'Global Climate Change and Health: An Old Story Writ Large', in A. McMichael, D. Campbell-Lendrum, K. Corvalán, C. Ebi, A. Githeko, J. Scheraga and A. Woodward (eds) *Climate Change and Human Health: Risks and Responses*, Geneva: World Health Organization, 2003.

McMichael, A., Friel, S., Nyong, A. and Corvalán, C., 'Global Environmental Change and Health: Impacts, Inequalities and the Health Sector', *British Medical Journal* (2008) 336, 191.

McMichael, A., Woodruff, R. and Hales, S., 'Climate Change and Human Health: Present and Future Risks', *The Lancet* (2006) 367, 859.

McMichael, A. J., *Planetary Overload: Global Environmental Change and the Health of the Human Species*, Cambridge, UK: Cambridge University Press, 1993.

McMichael, T. and Beaglehole, R., 'The Global Context of Public Health', in R. Begalehole (ed.), *Global Public Health, a New Era*, Oxford: Oxford University Press, 2003.

McNeil, D. G., 'Beyond Swollen Limbs, a Disease's Hidden Agony', *N.Y. Times*, April 9, 2006.

Medecins Sans Frontieres , 'Europe! Hands off Our Medicine', 2010.

Meeting of G8 Foreign Ministers, *Statement on the 7th Review Conference for the Biological and Toxin Weapons Convention*, 14–15 March 2011.

Meir, B. M. and Fox, A. M., 'International Obligations through Collective Rights: Moving from Foreign Health Assistance to Global Health Governance', *Health and Human Rights* (2010) 12:1, 61.

Michael Boylan (ed.), *International Public Health Policy and Ethics*, New York: Springer, 2008.

Mielke, J., Martin, D. K. and Singer P. A., 'Priority Setting in Critical Care: A Qualitative Case Study', *Critical Care Medicine* (2003) 31, 2764–8.

Milanovic, B., *Global Income Inequality: What It Is and Why It Matters*, Washington, DC: World Bank, 2006.

—, *The Haves and the Have-Nots*, New York: Basic Books, 2011.

—, *Worlds Apart: Measuring International and Global Inequality*, Princeton and Oxford: Princeton University Press, 2005.

Millar, M. R., 'Can Antibiotic Use be Both Just and Sustainable . . . or Only More or Less So?', *Journal of Medical Ethics* (2011) 37,153–7.

Miller, D., *National Responsibility and Global Justice*, Oxford: Oxford University Press, 2007.

Miller, J. M., Korenromp, E. L., Nahlen, B. L. and Steketee, R. W., 'Estimating the Number of Insecticide-Treated Nets Required by African Households to Reach Continent-Wide Malaria Coverage Targets', *JAMA* (2007) 297, 2241.

Minehata, M. and Shinomiya, M., *Biosecurity Education: Enhancing Ethics, Securing Life and Promoting Science*, Japan: National Defence Medical College and University of Bradford, 2009, www.dual-use bioethics.net.

Minow, M., *Between Vengeance and Forgiveness: Facing History after Genocide and Mass Violence,* Boston: Beacon Press, 1998.

Moellendorf, D., *Cosmopolitan Justice*, Boulder, CO: Westview Press, 2002.
—, *Global Inequality Matters*, Houndmills, Basingstoke, UK: Palgrave Macmillan, 2009.
Molyneux, D., and Nantulya,V., 'Linking Disease Control Programmes in Rural Africa: A Pro-Poor Strategy to Reach Abuja Targets and Millennium Development Goals', *BMJ* (2004) 75, 1129–32.
Moore, W., 'Keeping Mum', *BMJ* (2007) 334: 7595, 698.
Morales, M. C. P., *The Declaration of Human Duties and Responsibilities: From Human Rights to Responsibilities of the Global Community*, www.onlineunesco.org/conferencias/tele6/human%20duties%20and%20responsibilities.ppt#256,1.
Morel C. M. and Mossialos, E., 'Stoking the Antibiotic Pipeline', *BMJ* (2010) 340, bmj.c2115.
Mrazek, M. F. and Mossialos, E., 'Stimulating Pharmaceutical Research and Development for Neglected Diseases', *Health Policy* (2003) 64, 75–88.
Murdoch, I., *Metaphysics as a Guide to Morals*, New York, USA: Allen Lane, Penguin Press, 1993.
—, 'Vision and Choice in Morality', in *Existentialists and Mystics: Writings on Philosophy and Literature*, New York, USA: Allen Lane, Penguin Press, 1998, 76–98.
Mureinik, E., 'A Bridge to Where? Introducing the Interim Bill of Rights', *South African Journal of Human Rights* (1994) 10, 31.
Murphy, S. D., 'Biotechnology and International Law', *Harvard International Law Journal* (2001) 42:1, 47–139.
Murray, C. J. L. and Lopez, A. D. (eds), *Global Health Statistics*, Cambridge, MA: Harvard University Press, 1996.
Muzaffar, C., *Rights, Religion, and Reform: Enhancing Human Dignity through Spiritual and Moral Transformation*, London, UK: Routledge, 2002.
Myrdal, G., *Rich Lands and Poor: The Road to World Prosperity*, New York: Harper and Row, 1957.
Nagel, T., 'The Problem of Global Justice', *Philosophy & Public Affairs* (2005) 33:2, 113–47.
Nathan, C., 'Aligning Pharmaceutical Innovation with Medical Need', *Nature Medicine* (2007) 13:3, 304–8.
National Academies, *Ethics Education and Scientific and Engineering Research: What's Been Learned? What Should Be Done?* Washington, DC: National Academies Press, 2009.
National Research Council of the National Academies, 'Impact of Genetically Engineered Crops on Farm Sustainability in the United States', *Report by the Committee on the Impact of Biotechnology on Farm-Level Economics and Sustainability*, Board on Agricultural and Natural Resources (BANR) and Earth and Life Studies (DELS), 2010.
National Science Advisory Board for Biosecurity, *Strategic Plan for Outreach and Education on Dual-use Research Issues*, Washington DC: NSABB, 2008.
Navarro, V., 'What We Mean by Social Determinants of Health', *Int'l J. of Health Services* (2009) 39:3, 423–41.
NHS Choices, 'SARS (Severe Acute Respiratory Syndrome)', *NHS Choices*, 2010, www.nhs.uk/conditions/SARS/Pages/Introduction.aspx.
—, 'What Is Swine Flu (H1N1)?', *NHS Choices*, 2011, www.nhs.uk/chq/Pages/2886.aspx?CategoryID=5&SubCategoryID=5.

Nixon, S. and Forman, L., 'Exploring the Synergies between Human Rights and Public Health Ethics: A Whole Greater than the Sum of Its Parts', *BMC International Health and Human Rights* (2008) 8, 2.

Noble, C. N., 'Normative Ethical Theories', in S. G. Clarke and E. Simpson (eds), *Anti-Theory in Ethics and Moral Conservatism*, Albany: State University of New York, 1989.

Nozick, R., *Anarchy, State and Utopia*, New York: Basic Books, 1974.

Nussbaum, M., 'Capabilities as Fundamental Entitlements: Sen and Social Justice', *Feminist Economics,* (2003) 9, 35–59.

Nussbaum, M., 'Creating Capabilities: The Human Development Approach and Its Implementation', *Hyparia* (2009) 24, 211–15.

—, *Creating Capabilities: The Human Development Approach*, Cambridge, MA: Harvard University Press, 2011.

—, *Frontiers of Justice: Disability, Nationality, Species Membership*, Cambridge, MA: Harvard University Press, 2007.

—, 'Human Functioning and Social Justice: In Defense of Aristotelian Essentialism', *Political Theory* (1992) 20:2, 202–46.

—, *Women and Human Development: The Capabilities Approach*, Cambridge, UK: Cambridge University Press, 2000.

O'Brien, K., St Clair A. L. and Kristoffersen, B., 'The Framing of Climate Change: Why It Matters', in K. O'Brien, A. L. St Clair and B. Kristoffersen (eds), *Climate Change, Ethics and Human Security*, Cambridge: Cambridge University Press, 2010.

O'Neill, O., *Civic and Cosmopolitan Justice,* Kansas, USA: Department of Philosophy, University of Kansas, 2000.

—, *Faces of Hunger: An Essay on Poverty, Justice, and Development*, London, UK: G. Allen & Unwin, 1986.

—, 'Justice, Capabilities and Vulnerabilities', in M. Nussbaum and J. Glover (eds) *Women, Culture, and Development: A Study of Human Capabilities*, Oxford, UK: Clarendon Press, 1995, 140–52.

—, *The Bounds of Justice*, Cambridge, UK: Cambridge University Press, 2000.

Office International des Epizooties, *Statement for the Biological and Toxin Weapons Convention Meeting of States Parties,* Geneva: BWC Implementation Support Unit, 2010.

—, *Terrestrial Animal Health Code*, 20th edn, Paris: OIE, May 2011, www.oie.int/international-standard-setting/terrestrial-code/access-online/.

Oglethorpe, J., *Adaptive Management: From Theory to Practice*, Gland, Switzerland: IUCN, 2002.

Okin, S. M., 'Mistresses of their Own Destiny: Group Rights, Gender and Realistic Rights of Exit', *Ethics* (2002) 112, 205–30.

Olesen, J. E., 'Fødevarernes Andel Af Klimabelastningen', in Danish Council of Ethics, *Vores mad og det globale klima – etik til en varmere klode*, Copenhagen: Det Etiske Raad, 2010.

Onzivu, W., 'Globalism, Regionalism or Both: Health Policy and Regional Economic Integration in Developing Countries, an Evolution of a Legal Regime?', *Minnesota Journal of International Law* (2006)15:1, 117.

—, '(Re) Invigorating the World Health Organization's Governance of Health Rights: Repositing an Evolving Legal Regime, Its Challenges and Prospects', *African Journal of Legal Studies* (2011) 4:3, 225–56.

Ooms, G., 'Fiscal Space and the Importance of Long Term Reliability of International Co-financing', *JALI*-Working paper No. 1, 2011.

—, 'Why the West Is Perceived as Being Unworthy of Cooperation', *Journal of Law, Medicine & Ethics* (2010) 38:3, 594–613.

Ooms, G., and Hammonds, R., 'Correcting Globalisation in Health: Transnational Entitlements versus the Ethical Imperative of Reducing Aid-Dependency', *Public Health Ethics* (2008) 1:2, 154–70.

—, 'Taking up Daniels' Challenge: The Case for Global Health Justice', *Health & Human Rights* (2010) 12:1, 29–46.

Osofsky, H., 'The Continuing Importance of Climate Change Litigation', *Climate Law* (2010) 1:3, 29.

—, 'The Inuit Petition as a Bridge? Beyond Dialectics of Climate Change and Indigenous Peoples', Rights' *American Indian Law Review* (2007) 31, 675.

Ottesen, E. A., Duke, B. O., Karam, M. and Behbehani, K., 'Strategies and Tools for the Control/Elimination of Lyphatic Filariasis', *Bulletin of WHO* (1997) 75, 491–503.

Oxfam, *Investing for Life – Meeting poor people's needs for access to medicines through responsible business practices*, Oxfam Briefing Paper 109, 2007, www.oxfam.org/sites/www.oxfam.org/files/bp109-investing-for-life-0711.pdf.

Palmer, A., Tomkinson, J., Phung, C., Ford, N., Res, M. J., Fernandes, K. A., Zeng, L., Lima, V., Montaner, J. S. G., Guyatt, G. H. and Mills, E. J., 'Does Ratification Of Human-Rights Treaties Have Effects On Population Health?', *The Lancet* (2009) 373:9679, 1987–92.

Parker, R. and Sommer, M. (eds), *Routledge Handbook in Global Public Health*, New York: Routledge, 2011.

Patz, J., Gibbs, H., Foley, J., Rogers, J. and Smith, K., 'Climate Change and Global Health: Quantifying A Growing Ethical Crisis', *EcoHealth* (2007) 4, 397.

Pearson, G. S., 'Preparing for the BTWC Seventh Review Conference in 2011', *Review Conference Paper No. 21*, Bradford: University of Bradford, 2010.

Pennings, G., 'Reproductive Tourism as Moral Pluralism in Motion', *Journal of Medical Ethics* (2002) 28, 337–41.

Pogge, T., *Politics as Usual*, Cambridge: Polity, 2010.

—, *Poverty and Human Rights,* Geneva: UN-OHCHR, 2008, www2.ohchr.org/english/issues/poverty/expert/docs/Thomas_Pogge_Summary.pdf.

—, 'Priorities of Global Justice', in Pogge, T., (ed.), *Global Justice*, Oxford: Blackwell Publishers, 2001.

—, 'The Health Impact Fund: How to Make New Medicines Accessible to All', in S. R. Benatar and G. Brock (eds), *Global Health and Global Health Ethics*, Cambridge: Cambridge University Press, 2011, 241–50.

—, *World Poverty and Human Rights*, 2nd edn, Cambridge: Polity, 2008.

—, *World Poverty and Human Rights: Cosmopolitan Responsibilities and Reforms: Second Edition*, Cambridge: Polity Press, 2008.

Potts, H., *Accountability and the Right to the Highest Attainable Standard of Health*, Colchester: University of Essex Human Rights Centre, 2008.

Powers, M. and Faden, R., *Social Justice: The Moral Foundations of Public Health and Health Policy*, Oxford and New York: Oxford University Press, 2006.

Presidential Commission for the Study of Bioethical Issues, *New Directions: The Ethics of Synthetic Biology and Emerging Technologies,* Washington DC: Presidential Commission, 2010.

Price-Smith, A. T., *The Health of Nations: Infectious Disease, Climate Change, and Their Effects on National Security and Development*, Cambridge, MA: The MIT Press, 2002.

Ramcharan, B. G., *Humanitarian Good Offices in International Law: The Good Offices of the United Nations Secretary-General in the Field of Human Rights*, The Hague: Martinus Nijhoff, 1983.

Rapoport, A., *General System Theory*, Tunbridge Wells: Abacus Press, 1986.

Rawls, J., *A Theory of Justice. Revised Edition*, Cambridge, MA: The Belknap Press of the Harvard University Press, 1999.

—, *Justice as Fairness: A Restatement*, Cambridge, MA: The Belknap Press of the Harvard University Press, 2001.

—, *Political Liberalism. Expanded Edition*, New York: Columbia University Press, 2005.

—, *The Law of Peoples*, Cambridge, MA: Harvard University Press, 2001.

Read, A. F., Day, T. and Huijben, S., 'The Evolution of Drug Resistance and the Curious Orthodoxy of Aggressive Chemotherapy', *Proceedings of the National Academy of Sciences*, 2011, forthcoming, doi:10.1073/pnas.110029910.

Report of the Special Rapporteur on the Right to Adequate Food of the UN Sub-Commission on Prevention of Discrimination and Protection of Minorities, *The Right to Adequate Food as a Human Right*, (E/CN.4/Sub.2/1987/23) (7 July 1987).

Revill, J., *Developing Metrics and Measures for Dual-Use Education*, Bradford: University of Bradford, 2010.

Rhodes, C., *International Governance of Biotechnology: Needs, Problems and Potential*, London: Bloomsbury Academic, 2010.

Rice, L. B., 'The Maxwell Finland Lecture: For the Duration – Rational Antibiotic Administration in an Era of Antimicrobial Resistance and Clostridium Difficile', *Clinical Infectious Diseases* (2008) 46:4, 491–6.

Rigney, D., *The Matthew Effect: How Advantage Begets Further Advantage*, New York: Columbia University Press, 2010.

Risse, M., 'Common Ownership of the Earth as a Non-Parochial Standpoint: A Contingent Derivation of Human Rights', *European Journal of Philosophy* (2009) 17:2, 277–304.

Robertson, A., 'Critical Reflections on the Politics of Need: Implications for Public Health', *Social Science and Medicine* (1998) 4:7, 1419–30.

Roderick, P. E., 'Foreword', in W. C. G. Burns and H. M. Osofsky (eds), *Adjudicating Climate Change*, Cambridge, UK: Cambridge University Press, 2009.

Roemer, R., Taylor, A., and Lariviere, J., 'Origins of the WHO Framework Convention on Tobacco Control', *Am. J. Pub. Health* (2005) 95, 936–38.

Rosenau, J. N., *Distant Proximities: Dynamics beyond Globalization*, Princeton, NJ: Princeton University Press, 2003.

—, 'NGOs and Fragmented Authority in Globalizing Space', in Y. Ferguson and B. R. J. Jones (eds), *Political Space: Frontiers of Change and Governance in a Globalizing World*, New York: State of New York Press, 2002.

Rowden, N., *The Deadly Ideas of Neoliberalism: How the IMF Undermined Public Health & the Fight Against AIDS*, London, New York: Zed Books, 2009.

Ruger, J. P., 'Ethics and Governance of Global Health Inequalities', *J. Epidemiology & Community Health* (2006) 60, 998–9.

—, 'Global Health Justice', *Public Health Ethics* (2009) 2:3, 261–75.

—, *Health and Social Justice*, Oxford: Oxford University Press, 2010.

—, 'Rethinking Equal Access: Agency, Quality, and Norms', *Global Pub. Health* (2007) 2:1, 78–96.

Ruhl, J. B., 'Thinking of Environmental Law as a Complex Adaptive System: How to Clean up the Environment by Making a Mess of Environmental Law', *Houston Law Review* (1997) 34, 933.

Ryan, W., *Blaming the Victim: Revised, Updated Edition*, New York, USA: Pantheon Books, 1971.

Rydin, Y., Bleahu, A., Davies, M., Davila, J. D., Friel, S., Grandis, G. D., Groce, N., Hallal, P., Hamilton, I., Howden-Chapman, P., Lai, K. M., Lim, C. J., Martins, J., Osrin, D., Ridley, I., Scott, I., Taylor, M., Wilkinson, P. and Wilson, J., 'Shaping Cities for Health: The Complexity of Planning Urban Environments in the 21st Century', *The Lancet* (2012) 6736:12, 60435–8.

Sabel, C. F., 'Learning by Monitoring: The Institutions of Economic Development', in N. Smelser and R. Swedberg (eds), *The Handbook of Economic Sociology*, Princeton, NJ: Princeton University Press, 2005.

Sachs, J., *The Price of Civilization*, New York: Random House, 2011.

Sakakibara, M. and Branstetter, L., 'Do Stronger Patents Induce More Innovation? Evidence from the 1988 Japanese Patent Law Reforms', *RAND Journal of Economics* (2001) 32, 77–100.

Schedler, A., 'Conceptualising Accountability' in A. Schedler, L. Diamond and M. Plattner (eds), *The Self-Restraining State*, Boulder: Lynne Rienner, 1999.

Scheper-Hughes, N., 'A Beastly Trade in "Parts"; The Organ Market Is Dehumanizing the World's Poor', *Los Angeles Times*, 29 July 2003.

—, 'Keeping an Eye on the Global Traffic in Human Organs', *The Lancet* (2003b) 361, 1645–8.

Schlosberg, D., 'Reconceiving Environmental Justice: Global Movements and Political Theories', *Environmental Politics* (2004) 13:2, 517–40.

Scholz, J. T. and Stiftel B., (eds), *Adaptive Governance and Water Conflict: New Institutions for Collaborative Planning*, Washington, DC: Resources for the Future Press, 2005.

Schroeder, D., 'Does the Pharmaceutical Sector have a Co-Responsibility to Secure the Human Right to Health?', *Cambridge Quarterly of Healthcare Ethics* (2011) 20:2, 298–308.

Schroeder, D., and Singer, P., 'Access to Life-Saving Medicines and Intellectual Property Rights – An Ethical Assessment', *Cambridge Quarterly of Healthcare Ethic* (2011) 20:2, 279–89.

Science and Development Network, *Drug Licences All for the Poor, Says Thai Minister*, SciDevNet, 2007, www.scidev.net/en/news/drug-licences-all-for-the-poor-s ays-thai-minister.html.

Scotcher, S., *Innovation and Incentives*, Cambridge, MA: MIT Press, 2004.

Scott, J. and Trubek, D. M., 'Mind the Gap: Law and New Approaches to Governance in the European Union', *European Law Journal* (2002) 8:1, 1–18.

Segall, S., *Health, Luck and Justice*, Princeton, NJ: Princeton University Press, 2010.

Selgelid, M. J., 'A Full-Pull Program for the Provision of Pharmaceuticals: Practical Issues', *Public Health Ethics* (2008) 1, 134–45.

—, 'Ethics and Drug Resistance', *Bioethics* (2007) 21:4, 218–29.

—, 'Ethics Engagement of the Dual-Use Dilemma: Progress and Potential', in B. Rappert (ed.), *Education and Ethics in the Life Sciences*, Canberra: ANUE Press, 2010.

—, 'Justice, Infectious Diseases and Globalization', in S. R. Benatar and G. Brock (eds), *Global Health and Global Health Ethics*, Cambridge: Cambridge University Press, 2011.

Selgelid, M. J. and Pogge, T., *Health Rights*, London: Ashgate, 2010.

Selgelid M. J. and Sepers, E. M., 'Patents, Profits, and the Price of Pills: Implications for Access and Availability', in P. Illingworth, U. Schuklenk and J. C. Cohen (eds), *The Power of Pills: Social, Ethical and Legal Issues in Drug Development, Marketing and Pricing Policies,* London: Pluto Press, 2006.

Sen, A., 'Development as Capabilities Expansion', *The Journal of Development Planning* (1989) 19, 41–58.

—, *Development as Freedom,* Oxford: Oxford University Press, 1999.

—, 'Equality of What?', *Tanner Lecture on Human Values,* Stanford: Stanford University, 1979, www.tannerlectures.utah.edu/lectures/sen80.pdf.

—, *The Idea of Justice,* London: Penguin, 2010.

Sepúldeva, M., *The Nature of the Obligations under the International Covenant on Economic, Social and Cultural Rights,* Antwerp: Intersentia, 2003.

Shachar, A., 'Group Identity and Women's Rights in Family Law: The Perils of Multicultural Accommodation', *Journal of Political Philosophy* (1998) 6, 285–305.

Shue, H., *Basic Rights: Subsistence, Affluence and U.S. Foreign Policy,* Princeton, NJ: Princeton University Press, 1980.

—, 'Ethics, the Environment and the Changing International Order', *International Affairs* (1995) 71, 453–61.

—, 'Global Environment and International Inequality', *International Affairs* (1999) 75, 531–45.

Sims, N., 'An Annual Meeting for the BTWC', *Review Conference Paper No. 22,* Bradford: University of Bradford, 2010.

Singer, P., 'Famine, Affluence and Morality', *Philosophy and Public Affairs* (1972) 1, 229–43.

—, *One World: The Ethics of Globalization,* New Haven: Yale University Press, 2001.

—, *The Life You Can Save: Acting Now to End World Poverty,* London: Picador, 2009.

Smart, J. J. C. and Williams, B., *Utilitarianism: For and Against,* Cambridge: Cambridge University Press, 1973.

Smith, G. L. and Davison, N., 'Assessing the Spectrum of Biological Risks', *Bulletin of the Atomic Scientists,* (2010) 66:1, 1–11.

Smith, K. E., 'Introduction: Mitigating, Adapting and Suffering: How Much of Each?', *Annual Review of Public Health* (2008) 29, xxxii.

Smith, K. E., Besser, J. M., Hedberg, C. W., Leano, F. T., Bender, J. B., Wicklund, J. H., Johnson, B. P., Moore, K. A. and Osterholm, M. T., 'Q'uinolone-Resistant Campylobacter Jejuni Infections in Minnesota, 1992–1998', *The New England Journal of Medicine* (1999) 340: 20, 1525.

Songkhla, M. N., 'Health before Profits? Learning from Thailand's Experience', *The Lancet* (2009) 373, 441–2.

Sparks, A., *Tomorrow Is Another Country,* New York: Hill and Wang, 1995.

Stiglitz, J., *Making Globalisation Work,* London: W. W. Norton & Company, 2006.

—, 'Scrooge and Intellectual Property Rights', *British Medical Journal* (2006) 333, 1279–80.

Stuckler, D. and McKee, M., 'Five Metaphors about Global-Health Policy', *The Lancet* (2008) 372: 9633, 95–7.

Susskind, L., 'The Weaknesses of the Existing Environmental Treaty-Making System', in Susskind, L. (ed.), *Environmental Diplomacy: Negotiating More Effective Global Agreements,* Oxford: Oxford University Press, 1993.

Swick, H. M., 'Academic Medicine Must Deal with the Clash of Business and Professionalism', *Academic Medicine* (1998) 73, 741–55.

Syrett, K., *Law, Legitimacy and the Rationing of Health Care,* Cambridge: Cambridge University Press, 2007.

Taylor, A., 'An International Regulatory Strategy for Global Tobacco Control', *Yale J. Int'l L.* (1996) 12, 257–304.

—, 'Global Governance, in International Health Law and WHO: Looking Towards the Future', *Bulletin of the World Health Organization* (2002) 80:12, 975–80.

Taylor, A. and Bettcher, D., 'WHO Framework Convention on Tobacco Control: A Global "Good" for Public Health', *Bulletin of WHO* (2000) 78, 920–9.

Taylor, C., *The Malaise of Modernity*, Massey Lectures, Toronto: House of Anansi Press, 1991.

Teik, K. B., *Beyond Mahathir: Malaysian Politics And Its Discontents*, London, UK: Zed Books, 2003.

The Royal Society, *Reaping the Benefits – Science and the Sustainable Intensification of Global Agriculture*, London: The Royal Society, 2009.

Toebes, B., 'Towards an Improved Understanding of the International Human Right to Health', *Human Rights Quarterly* (1999) 21, 661.

Tong, R., 'Towards a Feminist Global Bioethics: Addressing Women's Health Concerns Worldwide', *Health Care Analysis* (2001) 9, 229–46.

Trades Union Congress, *The Missing Billions – The UK Tax Gap*, www.tuc.org.uk/touchstone/missingbillions/1missingbillions.pdf.

Trouiller, P., Olliaro, P., Torreele, E., Orbinski, J., Laing, R. and Ford, N., 'Drug Development for Neglected Diseases: A Deficient Market and a Public-Health Policy Failure', *The Lancet* (2002) 359, 2188–94.

Türmen, T. and Clift, C., 'Public Health, Innovation and Intellectual Property Rights: Unfinished Business', *Bulletin of the World Health Organisation* (2006) 84, 338.

UNAIDS, *Global Facts and Figures: Report on the Global AIDS Epidemic 2008*, Geneva: UNAIDS, 2008.

—, *Report on the Global AIDS Epidemic*, Geneva: UNAIDS, 2008.

UNICEF, *Progress for Children: A Report Card on Maternal Mortality*, New York: UNICEF, 2008.

—, *The State of the World's Children 2007*, New York: UNICEF, 2006.

United Nations, *Cartagena Protocol on Biosafety to the Convention on Biological Diversity, Text and Annexes*, New York: United Nations, 2000.

—, *Final Declaration*, Second Review Conference of the Parties to the *Convention on the Prohibition of the Development, Production, and Stockpiling of Bacteriological (Biological) and Toxin Weapons and on Their Destruction*, BWC/CONF.II/4, Geneva: United Nations, 1986.

—, *Report of the Meeting of States Parties*, BWC/MSP/2008/5, Geneva: United Nations, 2008.

—, *United Nations Framework Convention on Climate Change 1992*, New York: United Nations, 1992.

—, *United Nations Framework Convention on Climate Change: The First Ten Years*, New York: United Nations, 2004.

United Nations Committee on Economic, Social and Cultural Rights, *General Comment No.14: The Right to the Highest Attainable Standard of Health*, E/C.12/2000/4, Geneva: UNCESCR, 2000.

United Nations Development Programme, *Providing Global Public Goods: Managing Globalization, 25 Questions and Answers*, New York: UNDP, 2002.

United Nations Economic Commission for Europe, *Convention on Long-Range Transboundary Air Pollution 1979*, Geneva: UNECE, 1979.

United Nations Environment Program, *Barcelona Convention for Protection of the Mediterranean Sea against Pollution 1976 and Protocols 1980 & 1982*, Nairobi: UNEP, 1976.

—, *Montreal Protocol on Substances that Deplete the Ozone Layer 1987*, Nairobi: UNEP, 1987.

—, *Vienna Convention for the Protection of the Ozone Layer 1985*, New York: UN Treaty Collection, 1988.

United Nations Framework Convention on Climate Change, *Kyoto Protocol to the United Nations Framework Convention on Climate Change 1997*, Bonn: UNFCCC, 1997.

—, *Kyoto Protocol: Status of Ratification,* Bonn: UNFCCC, 1999.

United Nations General Assembly, *Report of the United Nations Special Rapporteur on the Right of Everyone to the Enjoyment of the Highest Attainable Standard of Physical and Mental Health*, A/62/214, Geneva: OHCHR, 2007.

—, *The Human Right to Water and Sanitation*, New York: United Nations, 2010.

—, *United Nations Millennium Declaration*, New York: The United Nations, 2000.

—, *Universal Declaration of Human Rights,* New York: United Nations, 1948.

United Nations Human Rights Council Resolution 7/23, *Human Rights and Climate Change*, Geneva: OHCHR, 2008.

—, *Report of the Office of the United Nations High Commissioner for Human Rights on the Relationship between Climate Change and Human Rights,* A/HRC/10/61, Geneva: OHCHR, 2009.

United Nations MDG Gap Task Force, *Delivering on the Global Partnership for Achieving the Millennium Development Goals*, New York: United Nations, 2008.

United Nations Secretary-General, *Uniting for Universal Access: Towards Zero New HIV Infections, Zero Discrimination and Zero AIDS-Related Deaths: Report of the Secretary-General*, New York: United Nations, 2011.

van der Heijden, H-A *Social Movements, Public Spheres and the European Politics of the Environment – Green Power Europe?* New York: Palgrave Macmillan, 2010.

Van der Walt, J. and Botha, H., 'Democracy and Rights in South Africa: Beyond a Constitutional Culture of Justification', *Constellations* (2000) 7:341, 343–4.

Vedung, E., *Public Policy and Program Evaluation*, New Brunswick, NJ: Transaction Publishers, 1997.

Venkatapuram, S., *Health Justice*, Malden, MA: Polity Press, 2011.

Verhoog, H., *The Reasons for Rejecting Genetic Engineering by the Organic Movement, FORUM TTN*, 2003, www.ecopb.org/fileadmin/ecopb/documents/reasons_reject_gmo.pdf.

Wagner, W., Kronberger, N., Gaskell, G., Allansdottir, A., Allum, N., de Cheveigné, S., et al., 'Nature in Disorder: The Troubled Public of Biotechnology', in G. Gaskell and M. W. Bauer (eds), *Biotechnology 1996–2000 – The Years of Controversy*, London: Science Museum, 2001.

Walters, C., 'Challenges in Adaptive Management of Riparian and Coastal Ecosystems', *Conservation Ecology* (1997) 1, 2.

Walzer, M., *Spheres of Justice: A Defense of Pluralism and Equality*, New York: Basic Books, 1983.

Watt-Cloutier, S., *Presentation to Eleventh Conference of Parties to the UN Framework Convention on Climate Change,* Inuit Circumpolar Council 7 December 2005, www.inuitcircumpolar.com/index.php?ID=318&Lang=En.

Wendt, A., *Social Theory of International Politics,* Cambridge: Cambridge University Press, 1999.

West, R., 'Unenumerated Duties', *U. Pa. J. Const. L.* (2006) 9, 221–61.

Wheelis, M., Rosza, L. and Dando, M. R., *Deadly Cultures: Biological Weapons since 1945,* Cambridge, MA: Harvard University Press, 2006.

Whitby, S. and Dando, M. R., 'Effective Implementation of the BTWC: The Key Role of Awareness Raising and Education', *Review Conference Paper No. 26,* Bradford: University of Bradford, 2010.

Whitehead, M., Townsend, P. and Davidson, N., *Inequalities in Health: The Black Report and the Health Divide,* 2nd edn, London: Penguin, 1992.

WHO, 'Indonesia to Resume Sharing H5N1 Avian Influenza Virus Samples Following a WHO Meeting in Jakarta', *Press Release 27 March 2007,* Geneva: WHO, 2007.

WHO, 'Lymphatic Filariasis', *Wkly. Epidemiolgy Rec.* (2001) 76, 149–54.

WHO, *Africa Malaria Report 2003,* Geneva: WHO, 2003.

WHO, *Biorisk Management: Laboratory Biosecurity Guidance,* Geneva: WHO, 2006.

WHO, *Fact Sheet 194: Antimicrobial Resistance,* Geneva: WHO, 2011.

WHO, *Genomics and World Health,* Geneva: WHO, 2002.

WHO, *Global Burden of Disease Report Update,* Geneva: WHO, 2008.

WHO, *Global Report: UNAIDS Report on the Global AIDS Epidemic 2010,* Geneva: WHO, 2010.

WHO, *Health Internetwork Access to Research Initiative,* Geneva: WHO, www.who. int/hinari/en.

WHO, *Interim Statement of the Intergovernmental Meeting on Pandemic Influenza Preparedness: Sharing of Influenza Viruses and Access to Vaccines and Other Benefits,* Geneva: WHO, 2011.

WHO, *Laboratory Biosafety Manual,* Geneva: WHO, 2004.

WHO, *Micronutrient Deficiencies: Vitamin A Deficiency,* Geneva: WHO, no date.

WHO, *Patent Applications for SARS Virus and Genes,* Geneva: WHO, 2003.

WHO, *Preamble to the Constitution of the World Health Organization as Adopted by the International Health Conference,* Geneva: WHO, 1946.

WHO, *Preparedness for Deliberate Epidemics,* Geneva: WHO, no date.

WHO, *Reform for a Healthy Future: An Overview,* Geneva: WHO, 2011.

WHO, *Reforms for a Healthy Future: Report by the Director-General,* Geneva: WHO, 2011.

WHO, *Spending on Health: A Global Overview: Fact sheet No. 319,* Geneva: WHO, 2007.

WHO, *The Ethical, Legal and Social Implications of Pharmacogenomics in Developing Countries: Report of an International Group of Experts,* Geneva: WHO, 2007.

WHO, *The International Health Regulations,* Geneva: World Health Organisation, 2005.

WHO, *The World Health Report: Health Systems Financing: The Path to Universal Coverage,* Geneva: World Health Organisation, 2010.

WHO, *WHO's Response in the Case of an Alleged Use of a Biological Agent,* Geneva: BWC Implementation Support Unit, 2010.

WHO, *World Health Report 1999: Making a Difference,* Geneva: WHO, 1999.

WHO, *World Health Report 2008: Primary Health Care – Now More Than Ever,* Geneva: WHO, 2009.

WHO, *World Health Report: Health Systems Financing – The Path to Universal Coverage,* Geneva: WHO, 2010.

WHO, *World Health Statistics 2009*, Geneva: WHO, 2009.

WHO, *World Health Statistics 2009: Table 8 Health Inequities*, Geneva: WHO, 2009.

WHO, *World Health Statistics 2011*, Geneva: WHO, 2011.

WHO, *Worldwide Prevalence of Anaemia Report 1993–2005*, Geneva: WHO, 2008.

WHO Commission on Social Determinants of Health, *Closing the Gap in a Generation: Health Equity Through Action on the Social Determinants of Health*, Geneva: WHO, 2008.

WHO Regional Office for Africa, *The Work of WHO in the African Region 2008: Annual Report of the Regional Director*, AFR/RC59/2, Geneva: WHO, 2009.

Widdows, H., 'Border Disputes across Bodies: Exploitation in Trafficking for Prostitution and Egg Sale for Stem Cell Research', *International Journal of Feminist Approaches to Bioethics* (2009) 2, 5–24.

—, 'Conceptualising the Self in the Genetic Era', *Health Care Analysis* (2007) 15, 5–12.

—, 'Is Global Ethics Moral Neo-Colonialism? An Investigation of the Issue in the Context of Bioethics', *Bioethics* (2007) 21, 305–15.

—, 'Localized Past, Globalized Future: Towards an Effective Bioethical Framework Using Examples from Population Genetics and Medical Tourism', *Bioethics* (2011) 25, 83–91.

—, 'Western and Eastern Principles and Globalised Bioethics', *Asian Bioethics Review* (2011) 3, 14–22.

—, *Global Ethics: An Introduction*, Durham: Acumen Publishing, 2011.

Widdows, H. and Cordell, S., 'The Ethics of Biobanking: Key Issues and Controversies', *Health Care Analysis* (2011) 19, 207–19.

—, 'Why Communities and Their Goods Matter: Illustrated with the Example of Biobanks', *Public Health Ethics* (2011) 4, 14–25.

Wiist, W. H., 'Public Health and the Anticorporate Movement', *American Journal of Public Health* (2006) 96:8, 1370–5.

Wilkinson, R. and Pickett, K., *The Spirit Level: Why Equality is Better for Everyone*, London: Penguin, 2010.

Willetts, P., *What is a Non-Governmental Organization?* UNESCO Encyclopaedia of Life Support Systems, City University London, 2002, www.staff.city.ac.uk/p.willetts/CS-NTWKS/NGO-ART.HTM#Part1.

Williams, B., *Morality: An Introduction to Ethics*, Cambridge: Cambridge University Press, 1972.

—, *Moral Luck*, Cambridge, MA: Harvard University Press, 1981.

Wilson, J., 'Could There Be a Right to Own Intellectual Property?', *Law and Philosophy* (2009) 28:4, 393–427.

—, 'Ontology and the Regulation of Intellectual Property', *The Monist* (2010) 93:3, 453–66.

—, 'Why Paying for Patented Drugs is Difficult to Justify', (ms., 2011).

—, *Why Paying for Patented Drugs Is Hard to Justify: An Argument about Time Discounting and Medical Need*, Manuscript, 2011.

Winslow, C.-E. A., 'The Untilled Fields of Public Health', *Science* (1920) 51:1306, 23–33.

Wolff, J., 'The Human Right to Health', in S. R. Benatar and G. Brock (eds), *Global Health and Global Health Ethics*, Cambridge: Cambridge University Press, 2011.

—, *The Human Right to Health*, New York, NY: W. W. Norton & Company, 2012.

Wolff, J. and de-Shalit, A., *Disadvantage*, Oxford: Oxford University Press, 2007.

Wolff, S. M. (ed.), *Feminism and Bioethics: Beyond Reproduction*, New York, USA: Oxford University Press, 1996.

Woodward, D. and Smith, R., 'Global Public Goods and Health: Concepts and Issues', in R. Smith, R. Beaglehole, D. Woodward and N. Drager (eds), *Global Public Goods for Health: Health Economic and Public Health Perspectives*, Oxford: Oxford University Press, 2003.

World Bank, *The Multilateral Fund for Implementation of the Montreal Protocol*, Washington: World Bank, 2004.

—, *The World Bank and the Montreal Protocol: Reducing Health Risks by Restoring the Ozone Layer*, Washington: World Bank, 2003.

World Commission on Environment and Development, *Our Common Future*, Oxford: Oxford University Press, 1987.

World Health Assembly, *Pandemic Influenza Preparedness Framework: Sharing of Influenza Viruses and Access to Vaccines and Other Benefits*, Geneva: WHO, 2011.

World Intellectual Property Organisation, 'Leading Pharmaceutical Companies and Research Institutions Offer IP and Expertise for use in Treating Neglected Tropical Diseases as Part of WIPO Re:Search', *Press Release PR/2011/699*, Geneva: WIPO, 2011.

—, *Access to Research for Development and Innovation*, Geneva: WIPO, www.wipo.int/ardi/.

—, *Patent Issues Related to Influenza Viruses and their Genes*, Geneva: WIPO, 2007.

—, *Patent Landscape for the H5 Virus: Interim Report*, Geneva: WIPO, 2007.

World Medical Association General Assembly, *WMA Declaration of Helsinki – Ethical Principles for Medical Research Involving Human Subjects*, Adopted by the 18th WMA General Assembly, Helsinki, Finland, June 1964, http://wma.net/en/30publications/10policies/b3/.

World Trade Organisation, *Agreement on the Application of Sanitary and Phytosanitary Measures*, Geneva: WTO, 1995.

—, *Agreement on Trade Related Aspects of Intellectual Property Rights*, Geneva: WTO, 1995.

—, *Amendment of the TRIPS Agreement*, Geneva: WTO, 2005.

—, *Decision on Implementation of Paragraph 6 of the Doha Declaration on the TRIPS Agreement and Public Health*, Geneva: WTO, 2003.

—, *Declaration on the TRIPS Agreement and Public Health*, Geneva: WTO, 2001.

—, *Doha Ministerial Declaration*, WT/MIN(01)/DEC/1, Geneva: WTO, 2001.

Wynia, M. K., 'The Short History and Tenuous Future of Medical Professionalism: The Erosion of Medicine's Social Contract', *Perspectives in Biology & Medicine* (2008) 51:4, 565–78.

Xu, K., Evans, D. B., Carrin, G., Aguilar-Rivera, A. M., Musgrove, P. and Evans, T., 'Protecting Households from Catastrophic Health Spending – Moving Away from Out-of-Pocket Health Care Payments to Prepayment Mechanisms Is the Key to Reducing Financial Catastrophe', *Health Affairs* (2007) 26:4, 972–83.

Yamey, G., 'Faltering Steps towards Partnerships', *British Medical Journal* (2002) 325, 1236–40.

Ziegler, J., *La Haine de l'Occident*, Paris: Editions Albin Michel, 2008.

Zilberman, D., Ameden, H. and Qaim, M., 'The Impact of Agricultural Biotechnology on Yields, Risks and Biodiversity in Low Income Countries', *Journal of Development Studies Special Issue – Transgenics and the Poor: Biotechnology in Development Studies* (2007) 43:1, 63–78.

Zumla, A., 'Drugs for Neglected Diseases', *The Lancet: Infectious Diseases* (2002) 2, 393.

Index